Cardiovascular Diseases and Disorders Sourcebook

Cardiovascular Diseases and Disorders Sourcebook

Basic Information about Cardiovascular Diseases and Disorders Featuring Facts about the Cardiovascular System, Demographic and Statistical Data, Descriptions of Pharmacologic and Surgical Interventions, Lifestyle Modifications, and a Special Section Focusing on Heart Disorders in Children.

Health Reference Series
Volume Five

Edited by
**Karen Bellenir and
Peter D. Dresser**

Omnigraphics, Inc. • Penobscot Building • Detroit, MI 48226

1995

BIBLIOGRAPHIC NOTE

This volume contains individual publications issued by the National Institutes of Health (NIH), its sister agencies, and subagencies. Numbered publications are: NIH 78-1058; 86-2700; 90-747; 90-2696; 91-3029; 92-737 92-2264; 92-2720; 92-2920; 92-3028; 92-3099; 92-3291; 93-0119; 93-1088; 93-1677; 93-2256; 93-2263; 93-2922; 94-0604; 94-0614; 94-923; 94-3182; and FDA 95-3212. Unnumbered publications from the National Heart, Lung, and Blood Institute and the Department of Health and Human Services' Health Resources and Services Administration are also included along with selected articles from the National Center for Research Resources *Reporter*, CDC's *Morbidity and Mortality Weekly Report*, and FDA's *FDA Consumer*.

In addition, this volume contains excerpts from 15 copyrighted documents produced by the American Heart Association: 50-047; 50-058; 50-074; 50-078; 50-1002; 50-1003; 50-1006; 50-1014; 50-1020; 50-1030; 50-1037; 50-1061; 50-1064; 50-1109; and 51-1005. These are used by permission.

RC
667
.C392
1995

Karen Bellenir
Peter D. Dresser
Editors

Omnigraphics, Inc.

Matthew P. Barbour, *Production Coordinator*
Laurie Lanzen Harris, *Vice President, Editorial*
Peter E. Ruffner, *Vice President, Administration*
James A. Sellgren, *Vice President, Operations and Finance*
Jane J. Steele, *Vice President, Research*

Frederick G. Ruffner, Jr., *Publisher*
Copyright © 1995 Omnigraphics, Inc.

Library of Congress Cataloging-in-Publication Data

Cardiovascular diseases and disorders sourcebook : basic information about cardiovascular diseases and disorders . . . / edited by Karen Bellenir and Peter D. Dresser.
    p. cm. — (Health reference series ; v. 5)
"This volume contains individual publications issued by the National Institutes of Health, its sister agencies, and subagencies"—T.p. verso.
    ISBN 0-7808-0032-X (library binding : alk. paper)
    1. Cardiovascular system—Diseases. 2. Cardiovascular system—Diseases—Epidemiology.
    I. Bellenir, Karen. II. Dresser, Peter D. III. National Institutes of Health (U.S.)
IV. Series.
    [DNLM: 1. Heart Diseases—collected works. 2. Vascular Diseases—popular works. 3. Vascular Diseases—collected works. 4. Vascular Diseases—popular works. W1 HE506R
v.5 1995 / WG 113 C267 1995]
RC667.C392 1995
616.1—dc20
DNLM/DLC   95-10583
for Library of Congress   CIP

∞

This book is printed on acid-free paper meeting the ANSI Z39.48 Standard. The infinity symbol that appears above indicates that the paper in this book meets that standard.

Printed in the United States of America

32278251

Contents

Part II: Statistical and Demographic Data

PART III: Heart Disorders in Children

PART IV: Cardiovascular Pharmacological Interventions

PART VII: Lifestyle Choices for a Healthier Cardiovascular System

Preface

About This Book

This book contains publications produced by several government agencies (including the National Heart, Lung, and Blood Institute, other agencies of the National Institutes of Health, and the Food and Drug Administration) and excerpts from several publications produced by the American Heart Association (AHA). The documents selected for inclusion were chosen to present basic medical information for the interested layperson and for the patient with cardiovascular disease and his or her family.

How to Use This Book

The *Introduction* offers information on how to recognize and respond to cardiac emergencies.

Part I: Facts about Cardiovascular Diseases and Disorders provides a description of many common heart and vascular problems. It includes information about how the heart works and the conditions that lead to compromised health. Vascular disorders, such as high blood pressure, aneurysms, and Raynaud's Phenomenon are also covered.

Part II: Statistical and Demographic Data reports on cardiovascular risk factors and the prevalence, morbidity, and mortality from cardiovascular diseases in the United States. It also looks at special heart-health issues of concern to minority populations.

Part III: Heart Disorders in Children offers parents background information that will be helpful in understanding cardiac illness in children. It covers congenital defects as well as disease-related conditions such as Kawasaki Syndrome and rheumatic heart disease. The chapter on cholesterol in children focuses on helping children develop heart-healthy habits.

Part IV: Cardiovascular Pharmacological Interventions gives cardiovascular patients and family members information about various drug-related interventions including thrombolytic agents, anti-arrhythmic drugs, estrogen therapy, and aspirin. A chapter describing the AHA's official position regarding chelation therapy is also included.

Part V: Surgical Interventions describes the types of surgical procedures that may be used to help restore health to the cardiovascular patient. It offers background information on defibrillators, pacemakers, coronary bypass graft surgery, balloon angioplasty, heart valve surgery, and organ transplantation.

Part VI: Living with Cardiovascular Disease provides information related to day-to-day living for cardiovascular patients and their families.

Part VII: Lifestyle Choices for a Healthier Cardiovascular System offers suggestions for avoiding cardiovascular disease. Prevention issues include dietary modification, exercise, and smoking cessation. A chapter on finding resources for healthy heart programs provides sources of further information for employers, community groups, and private citizens.

Acknowledgements

The editors wish to thank the American Heart Association for their permission to include exerpts from 15 AHA publications. Thanks also go to Margaret Mary Missar who searched diligently to find all the information included in this volume. Bruce the Scanman, and his special assistant Mike, made its production possible.

Introduction

How to Recognize and Respond to a Heart Attack

The symptoms of a heart attack vary, but the usual warning signs are:

1. Uncomfortable pressure, fullness, squeezing or pain in the center of the chest lasting more than a few minutes.

2. Pain spreading to the shoulders, neck or arms.

3. Chest discomfort with lightheadedness, fainting, sweating, nausea or shortness of breath.

These signs aren't always present. Many times a heart attack victim will experience some—but not all—of these symptoms. And in some cases, the symptoms subside and then return.

It's very common for heart attack victims to deny they're having a heart attack. In fact, if you're with someone showing the signs of a heart attack, **expect** a denial. The thought of having a heart attack is scary—many people don't want to face that possibility. Also, they may be afraid to risk the embarrassment of a "false alarm." As a result, they delay getting help by ignoring their symptoms or rationalizing that "it's just indigestion."

Execrpts from American Heart Association Pub. No. 50-078-A (CP). Used by Permission.

Don't let this happen. Don't Wait! Get help or get to a hospital immediately!

1. Call the emergency medical service system. Depending on your community, this could be the fire department or ambulance service.

2. If you can get the victim to the hospital quicker by driving yourself, do so. If you think you're having a heart attack, don't drive—ask someone to drive you. Go to the nearest medical facility with 24-hour emergency cardiac care.

3. If necessary and if you're properly trained, give CPR (mouth-to-mouth breathing and chest compression) while you're waiting for an emergency vehicle to arrive.

Part One

Facts about Cardiovascular Diseases and Disorders

Chapter 1

The Human Heart: A Living Pump

Clench your fist, relax it, clench your fist, relax it. You have just imitated the beating of your heart, a muscular, fist-sized organ that lies near the center of your chest, between your lungs and just behind your breastbone. The heart's constant beating pumps your blood to keep it circulating throughout your body. Your heart is truly a living pump.

The heart is a hollow, muscular organ with four chambers. The upper two are blood-receiving chambers called atria. The lower two are blood-pumping chambers called ventricles. Openings permit the flow of blood from each atrium to the ventricle below. but a thick wall divides the right side of the heart from the left side.

Although the two sides are separated, they beat at the same time. Both ventricles relax and refill (diastole) with blood flowing in, through valves, from the atria above. Then both ventricles contract and pump (systole) the blood out through another set of valves into the arteries which supply blood to the lungs and rest of the body.

One complete heartbeat consists of one diastolic phase and one systolic phase.

The heart beats between 70 and 80 times per minute, or about 100,000 times per day. While you rest or sleep, your heart pumps about 2 1/2 ounces (70 milliliters) of blood with each beat. It may not sound like much, but it adds up to nearly 5 quarts (approximately 5

NIH Pub. No. 78-1058.

liters) of blood pumped by the heart in one minute, or about 75 gallons (300 liters) per hour.

The output of the heart can vary according to the body's needs. For example, during periods of vigorous exercise, when the body demands more oxygen and nutrient-rich blood, the heart can increase its output by nearly five times.

A vast web of blood vessels supplies all areas of the body with blood. Some blood vessels carry fresh, oxygen-rich blood; some carry used, oxygen-poor blood. The pumping heart keeps the blood moving through the vessels—so that blood in the heart can travel to the big toe and back in less than 60 seconds.

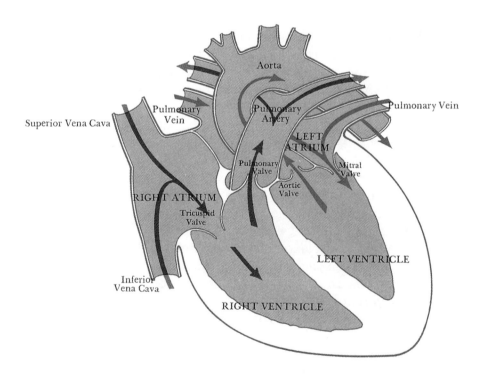

Figure 1.1. The Human Heart

Oxygen-poor blood from the body flows down through the right atrium to fill the right ventricle which pumps the blood out through the pulmonary artery to the lungs.

As blood flows through the lungs it gives up the waste carbon dioxide and gains more oxygen from the inhaled air. The freshly oxygenated blood returns to the left atrium of the heart by way of the pulmonary veins.

Oxygen-rich blood from the lungs flows down through the left atrium to fill the left ventricle which pumps it into the aorta, the main artery to the body.

The blood passes from the aorta into smaller arteries which carry it to all body organs and tissues. There it flows into the smallest arterial branches, the arterioles.

From the arterioles, blood flows into dense networks of tiny, thin-walled blood vessels called capillaries. Oxygen and nutrients in the blood easily pass through the thin capillary walls to the cells, and carbon dioxide and other cellular waste products can pass back through the walls into the blood to be carried away.

From the capillaries, the blood flows into the smallest veins, the venules, and then into larger and larger veins. Eventually all blood from the body enters either the superior vena cava or the inferior vena cava, which empty into the right atrium.

Basic Heart Terms

Artery: A blood vessel which carries blood away from the heart. All arteries carry oxygen-rich blood except the pulmonary artery and its branches, through which oxygen-poor blood is pumped from the right ventricle to the lungs.

The aorta is the largest artery. It originates in the left ventricle, arches up over the heart, and passes down behind it through the chest and abdomen. It gives off many smaller arteries which conduct blood to all body organs and tissues. The smallest arteries are called arterioles.

Atrium: One of the two upper chambers of the heart. Each receives blood through veins from the body or lungs.

Capillaries: The tiniest blood vessels. Capillary networks connect the arterioles and venules. Their thin walls permit the exchange of gases and of nutrients or waste materials between the blood and the body tissues.

Carbon Dioxide: A gaseous waste product of chemical reactions in the cells. It passes from the cells to the blood which eventually releases it in the lungs to be breathed out.

Heartbeat: Each beat of the heart lasts less than one second and has two phases:

- **Diastole:** The time during which the ventricular muscles relax and the ventricles refill with blood flowing in from the atria above.
- **Systole:** The time during which the blood-filled ventricles contract and pump blood out of the heart into the pulmonary artery (to the lungs) and the aorta (to the rest of the body).

Oxygen: A gas which is the most important component of the air we breathe. It is vital to energy-producing chemical reactions in the living cells of the body. Breathed into the lungs, it enters the bloodstream and is carried by the blood to the body tissues.

Valve: A flap of tissue which prevents backflow of blood to keep it moving in one direction. For example, in the heart there are large valves at the entrances of the ventricles (the tricuspid valve of the right ventricle and the mitral valve of the left) and at the exits of the ventricles (the pulmonary valve of the right ventricle and the aortic valve of the left). There are also small valves along the inside of the veins which promote flow of blood toward the heart.

Vein: A blood vessel that carries blood to the heart. All veins carry oxygen poor blood except the pulmonary vein and its branches, which carry oxygen-rich blood to the heart from the lungs. The veins of the body carry blood to the superior and inferior venae cavae which return it to the right atrium of the heart. The smallest veins are called venules.

Ventricle: One of the two lower chambers of the heart. Each pumps blood out through arteries to the lungs or body.

Chapter 2

Heart Attacks

The Magnitude of the Problem

Cardiovascular disease is a major health problem, with 60 million Americans having high blood pressure or one or more forms of heart or blood vessel disease. Heart disease has been the number one cause of death since 1910. Since 1949 it has caused about one-half the deaths in the United States, accounting for 987,000 deaths in 1983. Two forms of cardiovascular disease, heart disease and stroke, rank as the first and third causes of death respectively.

In economic terms data available for 1982 give an idea of the huge cost of cardiovascular diseases to the Nation. That year, the cost to the U.S. for cardiovascular diseases was an estimated $94 billion. Of this total, $41 billion was for direct health care costs; and an additional $53 billion was the estimated loss of productivity resulting from illness and premature deaths from cardiovascular diseases.

How the Heart Works

To understand what happens in a heart attack, think of the heart as a four-chambered pump. Blood from the body enters the upper chamber, atrium, on the right side of the heart and flows from there into the lower chamber, the ventricle. The blood is then pumped under

Taken from NIH Pub. No. 86-2700.

relatively low pressure into the lungs where it releases excess carbon dioxide and picks up oxygen. The oxygenated blood flows from the lungs to the atrium on the left side of the heart and then into the lower chamber, left ventricle. The left ventricle, the main pumping chamber, then pumps the blood under relatively higher pressure to the rest of the body to supply oxygen and nutrients to the tissues.

So, the heart is like a pump, squeezing and forcing blood throughout the body. The most important part of the heart is the heart muscle, or myocardium. Like all muscles in the body, the myocardium must have oxygen and nutrients in order to do its work. The myocardium cannot use oxygen and nutrients directly from the blood within the chambers of the heart. Instead, nutrients and oxygen are furnished by three main blood vessels outside the heart. These are the left anterior descending and circumflex coronary arteries (which start out together as the left coronary artery) and the right coronary artery. They in turn have further branches.

What Causes Heart Attacks?

Arteriosclerosis, which involves both hardening and blocking of the blood vessels, is the major cause of cardiovascular disease. Arteriosclerosis of the coronary arteries, also known as coronary artery disease, continues to be the most important medical problem, in spite of a number of advances in medical and surgical treatment. It causes the most death, severely limits activity, and is the leading cause of social security disability. It also ranks first in number of hospital bed days utilized.

Arteriosclerosis is a general medical term for a number of diseases of the arteries. Atherosclerosis is the most common form of arteriosclerosis and it affects primarily the larger arteries of the body. In this condition the lining of the artery becomes thickened and irregular with deposits of fatty substances.

Atherosclerosis develops by a process that is totally silent. At birth the vessels are perfectly smooth and open, but all through one's life fatty deposits, or atheromata, develop in the blood vessels. Fortunately, in most people they develop at a very slow rate and only in certain areas.

Moreover, medical evidence shows that more than two-thirds of a coronary artery may be filled with fatty deposits without causing symptoms. Symptoms may show themselves as chest pain, called angina pectoris; heart attack, or sudden death. Arteriosclerosis is responsible for 77 percent of all cardiovascular disease, or using 1981 statistics, for more than 760,000 deaths a year. Twenty percent of deaths due to arteriosclerosis, about 150,000 a year, occur in people younger than 65.

Heart attacks account for nearly 56 percent of all cardiovascular deaths. In 1983 more than 550,000 deaths were due to arteriosclerosis of the coronary arteries resulting in heart attack. Another 160,000 deaths were due to strokes caused by arteriosclerosis of the vessels of the brain.

When a Heart Attack Occurs

A heart attack happens when any of the coronary vessels become blocked and blood reaches the more distant heart muscle. Recent studies have shown that most heart attacks are caused by the formation of a clot, thrombus, in a coronary vessel at the site of narrowing and hardening. If an area of the myocardium is supplied by more than one vessel, the heart muscle may live for a period of time even if one vessel becomes blocked. However, the extent of heart muscle damage occurring with a heart attack depends on which vessel is blocked, on whether it is a big or small one, and on the remaining blood supply to that area of the myocardium. When heart muscle does not get adequate oxygen and nutrients, it dies. This process is called a myocardial infarction. A further area of heart muscle may be deprived of blood flow and oxygen to a lesser degree causing a temporary injury called myocardial ischemia. This dead and injured heart muscle causes the heart to lose some of its effectiveness as a pump, since reduced muscle contraction means reduced blood flow.

Symptoms

Many different symptoms may indicate a heart attack. Certainly the one most people have is chest pain, but this pain differs among individuals. Most often the pain is under the breastbone, or sternum. Sometimes it radiates to the neck, jaw or left shoulder or goes down the left arm. Some describe the pain as viselike, or constricting, as if a rope were being pulled tightly around the chest. Heart attack patients often experience weakness, shortness of breath and nausea. A patient acutely ill with a heart attack often appears pale, cold and sweaty.

Unfortunately, the first sign of disease in the heart and its vessels in about one-quarter of the patients who suffer heart attacks is sudden death. Also, approximately 60 percent of the deaths due to heart attacks occur outside of the hospital.

Risk of death is greatest within the first 2 hours of the heart attack. What does this mean? It means that anyone who has a new onset of chest pain or anyone with coronary disease who has continuing chest pain should seek medical help as quickly as possible.

What To Do, Where To Go for Help

If you have any sign of a heart attack, have someone get you to a hospital and obtain medical help as quickly as possible. But what if you or someone in a crowd suddenly collapses? A lifesaving technique has been developed to help someone who suffers heart arrest before an ambulance comes. This procedure is called cardiopulmonary resuscitation.

Cardiopulmonary Resuscitation (CPR)

If someone has had a heart attack so severe that the heart and breathing have stopped, CPR can keep the person alive until an ambulance and medical treatment is available. CPR is an emergency procedure that can be started immediately when the heart stops. CPR involves using a combination of mouth-to-mouth resuscitation to maintain the patient's breathing and compression of the chest to maintain circulation. It has been used successfully for some time by doctors and nurses and an increasing fraction of the general public. It is recommended that the public be trained to use CPR. If you are interested in learning CPR, consult the white pages of your telephone book and call your local chapter of the American Heart Association or the American Red Cross.

Medical Aid

What happens when an ambulance does come, when a paramedic or doctor arrives on the scene? The first effort is to relax the patient and relieve pain. Doctors handle this primarily by giving an injection of pain-relieving drugs which will relieve chest pain and relax the patient. In addition, oxygen often may be given to try to make up for a deficient blood supply and to keep the heart muscle working.

Electrocardiograms are used to find out whether a heart attack really is happening. By placing electrodes on the chest and arms, the area of heart damage can be located. An electrocardiogram can also characterize rhythm disturbances.

Defibrillators

Should the heart develop ventricular fibrillation, a quivering of the heart with no effective beat, what happens then? Most ambulances now carry special equipment called defibrillators. Using a defibrillator, a paramedic or physician shocks the heart with an electrical impulse that can correct a chaotic, ineffective rhythm or start the heart beating again. Defibrillation is very effective and has saved many lives that otherwise would have been lost.

Coronary Care Units

When the ambulance reaches the hospital, the patient is admitted immediately to a coronary care unit where vital signs—blood pressure, heart rate, temperature, respiration—can be monitored.

Blood pressure is measured in order to determine the adequacy of blood circulation and blood is drawn for tests that can help diagnose a heart attack.

In the coronary care unit, medicines will be given that can relax the patient, relieve pain, or control the blood pressure. Also there are medicines that can help the heart to beat regularly.

Electrical Heart Problems

The heart is normally paced by electrical impulses from specific areas of the heart. If part of the heart's electrical system is injured by disease or heart attack, it may slow dramatically or it may stop beating. A much more common electrical problem is early or extra beats, which may progress to the chaotic, fatal ventricular fibrillation if not treated with drugs.

Twenty-five years ago, over half the heart attack deaths were from electrical problems in the heart. Today, in-hospital deaths due to electrical rhythm disturbances of the heart have become relatively uncommon because of the ability to monitor electrical impulses, to control heart rhythm with drugs or pacemakers, and to restart the heart with defibrillators. As a result, the death rate in hospitalized heart at-

11

tack patients has been reduced from 30-40 percent to 15 percent or even less. Most of these remaining deaths result from weakening of the heart. The heart muscle may have been so extensively damaged that the heart cannot beat effectively. The result is not enough blood pumped out to serve the rest of the body.

Problems of Heart Function

Doctors are also making inroads in problems of maintaining adequate heart function. Techniques are now available that allow estimating the amount of heart muscle that has been damaged when a patient has a heart attack. Blood tests measure the amount of specific enzymes released by dying and dead heart muscle and help diagnose how severe the heart attack is. Using a still experimental procedure, doctors can find and measure specific areas of heart damage and follow the extent of a heart attack by mapping the heart. This is done by placing a special vest with many small electrodes on the patient's chest.

In addition, new tests allow visualization of the area of heart damage. When certain radioisotopes are injected into a patient's vein, they accumulate in heart tissue. Some radioisotopes have an affinity for dead tissue, which allows the doctor to determine the extent of the damaged area. Others collect in healthy heart muscle, and thus indicate areas of inadequate perfusion or injury. Still others remain in the blood, allowing measurement of the dimensions and movements of the heart chambers. The amount of muscle damaged during a heart attack is not fixed when a patient enters a coronary care unit. There are now treatments that may decrease the amount of heart muscle damage. These include giving oxygen or altering the blood pressure in some circumstances. Clinical studies are being conducted to identify other treatments to decrease the amount of heart muscle damage. Some studies are testing thrombolytic agents which are infused by catheter into the coronary circulation or injected into a vein to enter the general circulation. A thrombolytic agent is one that dissolves (lyses) a blood clot (thrombus) that may be obstructing a vein or coronary artery. Also being tested are special catheters that may dilate partially obstructed vessels. These agents and techniques may reduce heart muscle damage and mechanical failure, which are the major causes of death in patients hospitalized with heart disease.

After a Heart Attack

Rehabilitation for the patient with a heart attack begins at the time of hospitalization, as the patient enters the coronary care unit. Doctors now know that many symptoms experienced by patients after heart attacks are not due to heart muscle damage but to physical inactivity. Today, patients begin to exercise arm and leg muscles while in the coronary care unit. Shortly after hospital discharge, they can go on to full activity under medical supervision. Often, an exercise test is done before leaving the hospital to test endurance and to look for abnormal heart rhythm associated with exercise.

Chapter 3

Facts about Coronary Heart Disease

Some 7 million Americans suffer from coronary heart disease (CHD), the most common form of heart disease. This type of heart disease is caused by a narrowing of the coronary arteries that feed the heart.

CHD is the number one killer of both men and women in the U.S. Each year, more than 500,000 Americans die of heart attacks caused by CHD.

Many of these deaths could be prevented because CHD is related to certain aspects of lifestyle. Risk factors for CHD include high blood pressure, high blood cholesterol, smoking, obesity, and physical inactivity—all of which can be controlled. Although medical treatments for heart disease have come a long way, controlling risk factors remains the key to preventing illness and death from CHD.

Who Is At Risk for CHD?

Risk factors are conditions that increase your risk of developing heart disease. Some can be changed [Controllable], and some cannot [Uncontrollable]. Although these factors each increase the risk of CHD they do not describe all the causes of the disease; even with none of these risk factors, you might still develop CHD.

NIH Pub. No. 93-2265.

Controllable

- High blood pressure
- High blood cholesterol
- Smoking
- Obesity
- Physical inactivity
- Diabetes
- Stress (Although stress **may** be a risk factor for CHD, scientists still do not know exactly how stress might be involved in heart disease.)

Uncontrollable

- Gender
- Heredity (family history of CHD)
- Age

What Is CHD?

Like any muscle, the heart needs a constant supply of oxygen and nutrients that are carried to it by the blood in the coronary arteries. When the coronary arteries become narrowed or clogged and cannot supply enough blood to the heart, the result is CHD. If not enough oxygen-carrying blood reaches the heart, the heart may respond with a pain called angina. The pain is usually felt in the chest or sometimes in the left arm and shoulder. (However, the same inadequate blood supply may cause no symptoms, a condition called silent angina.)

When the blood supply is cut off completely, the result is a heart attack. The part of the heart that does not receive oxygen begins to die, and some of the heart muscle may be permanently damaged.

What Causes CHD?

CHD is caused by a thickening of the inside walls of the coronary arteries. This thickening, called atherosclerosis, narrows the space through which blood can flow, decreasing and sometimes completely cutting off the supply of oxygen and nutrients to the heart.

Atherosclerosis usually occurs when a person has high levels of cholesterol, a fat-like substance, in the blood. Cholesterol and fat, circulating in the blood, build up on the walls of the arteries. This buildup narrows the arteries and can slow or block the flow of blood. When the level of cholesterol in the blood is high, there is a greater chance that it will be deposited onto the artery walls. This process begins in most people during childhood and the teenage years, and worsens as they get older.

In addition to high blood cholesterol, high blood pressure and smoking also contribute to CHD. On the average, each of these doubles your chance of developing heart disease. Therefore, a person who has all three risk factors is eight times more likely to develop heart disease than someone who has none. Obesity and physical inactivity are other factors that can lead to CHD. Overweight increases the likelihood of developing high blood cholesterol and high blood pressure, and physical inactivity increases the risk of heart attack. Regular exercise, good nutrition, and smoking cessation are key to controlling the risk factors for CHD.

What Are the Symptoms of CHD?

Chest pain (angina) or shortness of breath may be the earliest signs of CHD. A person may feel heaviness, tightness, pain, burning, pressure or squeezing, usually behind the breastbone but sometimes also in the arms, neck, or jaws. These signs usually bring the patient to a doctor for the first time. Nevertheless, some people have heart attacks without ever having any of these symptoms.

It is important to know that there is a wide range of severity for CHD. Some people have no symptoms at all, some have mild intermittent chest pain, and some have more pronounced and steady pain. Still others have CHD that is severe enough to make normal everyday activities difficult.

Because CHD varies so much from one person to another, the way a doctor diagnoses and treats CHD will also vary a lot. The following descriptions are general guidelines to some tests and treatments that may or may not be used, depending on the individual case.

Are There Tests for CHD?

There is no one simple test—some or all of the following procedures may be needed. These diagnostic procedures are used to establish CHD, to determine its extent and severity, and to rule out other possible causes of the symptoms.

After taking a careful medical history and doing a physical examination, the doctor may use some tests to see how advanced the CHD is. The only certain way to diagnose and assess the extent of CHD is coronary angiography (see below); other tests can indicate a problem but do not show exactly where it is.

An examination for CHD may include the following tests:

- An **electrocardiogram** (ECG or EKG) is a graphic record of the electrical activity of the heart as it contracts and rests. Abnormal heartbeats and some areas of damage, inadequate blood flow, and heart enlargement can be detected on the records.

- A **stress test** (also called a treadmill test or exercise ECG) is used to record the heartbeat during exercise. This is done because some heart problems only show up when the heart is working hard. In the test, an ECG is done before, during, and after exercising on a treadmill; breathing rate and blood pressure may be measured as well. Exercise tests are useful but are not completely reliable; false positives (showing a problem where none exists) and false negatives (showing no problem when something is wrong) are fairly common.

- **Nuclear scanning** is sometimes used to show damaged areas of the heart and expose problems with the heart's pumping action. A small amount of radioactive material is injected into a vein, usually in the arm. A scanning camera records the nuclear material that is taken up by heart muscle (healthy areas) or not taken up (damaged areas).

- **Coronary angiography** (or arteriography) is a test used to explore the coronary arteries. A fine tube (catheter) is put into an artery of an arm or leg and passed through this blood vessel to the heart. A fluid that shows up on x rays is injected through the tube into the arteries of the heart. The heart and blood vessels are then filmed while the heart pumps. The picture that is seen, called an **angiogram** or **arteriogram**, will show problems such as a blockage caused by atherosclerosis.

How Is CHD Treated?

CHD is treated in a number of ways, depending on the seriousness of the disease. For many people, CHD is managed with lifestyle changes and medications. Others with severe CHD may need surgery. In any case, once CHD develops, it requires lifelong management.

What Kind of Lifestyle Changes Can Help a Person with CHD?

Although great advances have been made in treating CHD, changing one's habits remains the single most effective way to stop the disease from progressing.

If you know that you have CHD, changing your diet to one low in fat, especially saturated fat, and cholesterol will help reduce high blood cholesterol, a primary cause of atherosclerosis. In fact, it is even more important to keep your cholesterol low after a heart attack to help lower your risk of having another one. Eating less fat should also help you lose weight. If you are overweight, losing weight can help lower blood cholesterol and is the most effective lifestyle way to reduce high blood pressure, another risk factor for atherosclerosis and heart disease.

People with CHD can also benefit from exercise. Recent research has shown that even moderate amounts of physical activity are associated with lower death rates from CHD. However, people with severe CHD may have to restrict their exercise somewhat. If you have CHD, check with your doctor to find out what kinds of exercise are best for you.

Smoking is one of the three major risk factors for CHD. Quitting smoking dramatically lowers the risk of a heart attack and also reduces the risk of a second heart attack in people who have already had one.

What Medications Are Used to Treat CHD?

Medications are prescribed according to the nature of the patient's CHD and other problems. The symptoms of angina can generally be controlled by "beta-blocker" drugs that decrease the workload on the heart, by nitroglycerine and other "nitrates" and by "calcium-channel blockers" that relax the arteries, and by other classes of drugs. The tendency to form clots is reduced by aspirin or by other platelet inhibitory and anticoagulant drugs. Beta-blockers are given to decrease the recurrence of heart attack. For those with elevated blood cholesterol that is unresponsive to dietary and weight loss measures, cholesterol-lowering drugs may be prescribed, such as lovastatin, colestipol, cholestyramine, gemfibrozil, and niacin. Impaired pumping function of the heart may be treated with digitalis drugs or ACE inhibitors. If there is high blood pressure or fluid retention, these conditions are also treated.

Ask your doctor which medication you are taking, what it does, and whether there are any side effects. Knowing more about this will help you stick to the schedule that has been prescribed for you.

What Types of Surgery Are Used to Treat CHD?

Many patients can control CHD with lifestyle changes and medication. Surgery may be recommended for patients who continue to have frequent or disabling angina despite the use of medications, or people who are found to have severe blockages in their coronary arteries.

Coronary angioplasty or **balloon** angioplasty begins with a procedure similar to that described under angiography. However, the catheter positioned in the narrowed coronary artery has a tiny balloon at its tip. The balloon is inflated and deflated to stretch or break open the narrowing and improve the passage for blood flow. The balloon-tipped catheter is then removed.

Strictly speaking, angioplasty is not surgery. It is done while the patient is awake and may last 1 to 2 hours. If angioplasty does not widen the artery or if complications occur, bypass surgery may be needed.

In a **coronary artery bypass operation**, a blood vessel, usually taken from the leg or chest, is grafted onto the blocked artery, bypassing the blocked area. If more than one artery is blocked, a bypass can be done on each. The blood can then go around the obstruction to supply the heart with enough blood to relieve chest pain.

Bypass surgery relieves symptoms of heart disease but does not cure it. Usually you will need to make a number of changes in your lifestyle after the operation. If your normal lifestyle includes smoking, a high-fat diet, or no exercise, changes are advised.

Several experimental catheter-surgical procedures for unblocking coronary arteries are under study; their safety and effectiveness have not yet been established. They include:

- Atherectomy, a procedure in which surgeons shave off thin strips of the plaque blocking the artery and remove these strips.
- Laser angioplasty; instead of using a balloon to open up the blocked artery, doctors insert a catheter with a laser tip that burns or breaks down the plaque.
- Insertion of a stent, a metal coil that can be permanently implanted in a narrowed part of an artery to keep it propped open.

Chapter 4

Cardiomyopathy

Defining Cardiomyopathy

Cardiomyopathy refers to a number of diseases that weaken the heart muscle. Doctors classify cardiomyopathies by the way they affect the anatomy and function of the heart.

In dilated cardiomyopathy, the chambers of the heart are large and the heart can't pump blood effectively. In hypertrophic cardiomyopathy, the heart muscle thickens, reducing the size of the left heart ventricle. Usually, the septum (dividing wall) between the ventricles enlarges more than the outside walls of the heart. The ventricles can't expand well and fill with enough blood. In restrictive cardiomyopathy, the inside of the ventricle walls becomes stiff and unable to expand. Again, enough blood cannot fill the ventricles.

Tests used to detect cardiomyopathy are described below. The causes, symptoms, treatments, and prognosis for the three types of cardiomyopathy are then given.

Diagnostic Tests

Chest X-ray. A picture of the chest, including the heart.

An unnumbered fact sheet produced by the National Heart, Lung, and Blood Institute dated 11/89.

Electrocardiogram (EKG). A record of the heart's electrical activity. It shows when the heart contracts and rests. Disks are placed on the chest and connected by wires to a recording machine. As the heart beats, its electrical signals cause a pen to draw lines across a strip of graph paper in the EKG machine. Abnormal heartbeats, areas of damage, and heart enlargement can be detected from these graphs.

Echocardiogram. A picture of the heart produced by sound waves, which are sent out over the patient's heart from an "transducer" (measuring device) placed on the chest. The sound waves bounce off the heart muscle and change into electrical signals that are recorded onto graph paper. Problems in the heart muscle and valves can be detected this way.

Nuclear Scan. A picture of blood movement through the heart. A small amount of radioactive material is injected into a vein, usually in the arm. As the material moves through the heart, a scanning camera records its images. Sometimes the scan is done while the patient is resting; it may also be done while the patient is exercising.

Cardiac Catheterization. A procedure in which a fine tube (catheter) is put into an artery or vein of an arm or leg and forwarded to the hart. Some catheters measure the heart's electrical activity; others measure the blood pressure inside the chambers of the heart. **Angiography** is a special type of catheterization in which a colorless dye is injected through the catheter into the heart or arteries of the heart. The heart and blood vessels are then filmed while the heart pumps. The picture that results is called an **angiogram**.

Dilated Cardiomyopathy

Cause

This type of cardiomyopathy may be caused by alcohol or infections. Other conditions associated with it include high blood pressure, pregnancy, and cigarette smoking. If the cause cannot be found, doctors call it "idiopathic." Dilated cardiomyopathy is generally found in middle-aged people, more commonly men.

Symptoms

Symptoms often develop gradually, and many patients with this disease may not have symptoms for awhile. Patients may feel tired and weak. In later stages, they may experience chest or abdominal pains. Dilated cardiomyopathy that progresses may lead to congestive heart failure, in which the heart fails to pump blood well.

Treatment

Doctors try to treat what causes dilated cardiomyopathy. For instance, alcoholics with this disease must stop drinking. If the cause is unknown, doctors treat the symptoms of congestive heart failure. They give medicines to reduce the workload of the heart. These may include hydralazine and nitrates, vasodilator drugs that relax the blood vessel walls. Patients' activities may need to be restricted. Sometimes, a heart transplant is necessary.

Prognosis

Dilated cardiomyopathy is a serious disease that may be difficult to control if doctors do not know the underlying cause. Because each patient's outlook depends on many factors, you should discuss any questions about prognosis with the doctor.

Hypertrophic Cardiomyopathy (also called Idiopathic Hypertrophic Subaortic Stenosis)

Cause

The cause of hypertrophic cardiomyopathy is unknown. However, the tendency to develop this disease is inherited in over half the cases. Oftentimes, family members of a patient with hypertrophic cardiomyopathy are also examined by a cardiologist to determine whether they have signs of the disease. Most patients with this disease who experience symptoms are young adults, but hypertrophic cardiomyopathy is found in all ages and equally in men and women.

Symptoms

Many times, patients with this problem do not have symptoms. The most common symptom is difficulty breathing. Angina pectoris (chest discomfort), fatigue, and fainting are also common in those who have symptoms. Exercise may bring on symptoms.

Treatment

Doctors give medicines to help the ventricles fill better and to decrease the contraction of the ventricles. These may include drugs called beta-adrenoreceptor blockers or calcium antagonists. Medications are also prescribed to control arrhythmias that may develop as a result of hypertrophic cardiomyopathy.

If a patient does not respond to drug therapy and has severe symptoms, surgery may be considered. In a procedure called septal myotemy-myectomy, doctors remove a piece of the septal well to improve blood flow out of the left ventricle. Sometimes, the surgeon may replace the mitral valve at the same time. (The mitral valve connects the left ventricle and the left atrium, where oxygenated blood is received from the lungs).

Patients with hypertrophic cardiomyopathy must also avoid strenuous exercise. This lifestyle change, in addition to medical treatment, is important in reducing the risk of sudden cardiac death, or sudden death due to heart failure. (Unfortunately, sudden cardiac death is sometimes the only sign of hypertrophic cardiomyopathy in a person who has no symptoms.)

Prognosis

The prognosis for patients with hypertrophic cardiomyopathy varies. In most patients, symptoms remain the same, although improvement may occur over five to ten years. Women with this disease can have children.

Restrictive Cardiomyopathies

Cause

Restrictive cardiomyopathies are the least common of the cardiomyopathies in the western world. Several diseases may cause the ventricle walls to become rigid, although many times the cause is unknown. Diseases include fibrosis (the formation of tough, fibrous tissue in the heart), collagen-vascular diseases (connective tissue disorders of the heart), and amyloidosis (the accumulation of protein fibers in the heart).

Some diseases that cause restrictive cardiomyopathy are inherited. These include Fabry's disease (accumulation of a metabolic product in the heart), hemochromatosis (accumulation of iron in the heart), and sarcoidosis (appearance of tumor-like growths in the heart).

Symptoms

Symptoms vary, but often include weakness and difficulty breathing, particularly during exercise.

Treatment and Prognosis

Treatments differ according to what is causing the disease. Generally, restrictive cardiomyopathies are difficult to treat and prognosis for this disease remains poor. For this reason, doctors may try different investigational therapies to improve a patient's outcome.

Chapter 5

Understanding Angina

Angina

Angina, or angina pectoris, is a recurring discomfort. It's usually located near the center of the chest. The pain or discomfort occurs when the blood supply to part of the heart muscle doesn't meet the heart's needs. As a result, the heart doesn't get enough oxygen and nutrients.

The discomfort occurs most often during exercise or emotional stress. That's when the heart rate and blood pressure increase, and the heart muscle needs more oxygen.

Anginal pain or discomfort is usually brief, lasting just a few minutes. People describe it as a heaviness, tightness, oppressive pain, burning, pressure or squeezing. Usually it's located behind the breastbone. Sometimes it spreads to the arms, neck or jaws. It may also cause a numbness in the shoulders, arms or wrists.

Angina and Heart Attack

Angina is different from a heart attack. Both relate to the blood flow through the coronary arteries (which bring blood to the heart muscle), but there's a key difference. With angina, the blood flow is re-

---

Excerpts from American Heart Association Pub. No. 50-1064. Used by Permission. Editor's comments are bracketed.

duced, especially when the heart must do more work. This reduced blood flow to the heart muscle is temporary and leads to discomfort in the chest. [For information about what happens during a heart attack, see Chapter 2.]

Diagnosing Your Condition

Usually your doctor can accurately diagnose angina from your description of symptoms. If you're suffering from it, it's possible for your physical examination and resting electrocardiogram to be entirely normal. That's why your doctor may recommend an exercise test to increase your heart's demand for blood and oxygen. An electrocardiogram recorded during an exercise test can show if your heart isn't getting enough oxygen.

Sometimes it's hard to diagnose angina even after a medical history, a physical examination and an exercise test. If that's the case, your doctor may order a thallium stress test. This is a special exercise test in which a radioisotope (thallium) is injected into a vein during exercise. It uses radioactivity detectors and computers to measure the blood flow to the heart muscle during exercise.

Your doctor may decide that a coronary arteriogram is necessary. This is an x-ray movie of your coronary arteries. It shows blood flow patterns as a radiopaque substance (a liquid that blocks x-rays) is injected into your arteries. If you have angina, an arteriogram will show if your coronary arteries are blocked or constricted, where the blockage is and how severe it is.

Medical Treatment

Nitroglycerin [is one of the most frequently prescribed medications to treat angina. Typically, nitroglycerin comes in small tablets that dissolve in the mouth under the tongue. Nitroglycerin] may also be prescribed as an oral spray.

[The American Heart Association offers this caution to angina patients:]

> If you have angina that does not go away after 15 minutes of taking 1 nitroglycerin tablet every 5 minutes, you should call the emergency medical service or have someone drive you to the nearest hospital emergency room.

[Other medications that can sometimes help angina patients include beta blockers and calcium blockers. For more information about beta blockers see Chapter 47. Calcium blockers] work by reducing the blood pressure—and sometimes the heart rate—during exercise. They also relax and widen the arteries to the heart muscle like nitroglycerin does.

Surgery

[Sometimes medication alone does not give appropriate relief to the angina patient. Your doctor may find it necessary to recommend surgical procedures. Coronary artery bypass surgery and angioplasty are two possible options. For more information about coronary artery bypass surgery, see Chapter 35. For more information about angioplasty, see Chapter 36.]

Chapter 6

Facts about Arrhythmias/ Rhythm Disorders

What Is an Arrhythmia?

An arrhythmia is a change in the regular beat of the heart. The heart may seem to skip a beat or beat irregularly or very fast or very slowly.

Does Having an Arrhythmia Mean That a Person has Heart Disease?

No, not necessarily. Many arrhythmias occur in people who do not have underlying heart disease.

What Causes Arrhythmias?

Many times, there is no recognizable cause of an arrhythmia. Heart disease may cause arrhythmias. Other causes include: stress, caffeine, tobacco, alcohol, diet pills, and cough and cold medicines.

Are Arrhythmias Serious?

The vast majority of people with arrhythmias have nothing to fear. They do not need extensive exams or special treatments for their condition.

NIH Pub. No. 92-2264 and *FDA Consumer*, October 1992.

In some people, arrhythmias are associated with heart disease. In these cases, heart disease, not the arrhythmia, poses the greatest risk to the patient.

In a very small number of people with serious symptoms, arrhythmias themselves are dangerous. These arrhythmias require medical treatment to keep the heartbeat regular. For example, a few people have a very slow heartbeat (bradycardia), causing them to feel lightheaded or faint. If left untreated, the heart may stop beating and these people could die.

How Common Are Arrhythmias?

Arrhythmias occur commonly in middle-age adults. As people get older, they are more likely to experience an arrhythmia.

What Are the Symptoms of an Arrhythmia?

Most people have felt their heart beat very fast, experienced a fluttering in their chest, or noticed that their heart skipped a beat. Almost everyone has also felt dizzy, faint, or out of breath or had chest pains at one time or another. One of the most common arrhythmias is sinus arrhythmia, the change in heart rate that can occur normally when we take a breath. These experiences may cause anxiety, but for the majority of people, they are completely harmless.

You should not panic if you experience a few flutters or your heart races occasionally. But if you have questions about your heart rhythm or symptoms, check with your doctor.

What Happens in the Heart During an Arrhythmia?

Describing how the heart beats normally helps to explain what happens during an arrhythmia.

The heart is a muscular pump divided into four chambers—two atria located on the top and two ventricles located on the bottom.

Normally each heartbeat starts in the right atrium. Here, a specialized group of cells called the sinus node, or natural pacemaker, sends an electrical signal. The signal spreads throughout the atria to the area between the atria called the atrioventricular (AV) node.

The AV node connects to a group of special pathways that conduct the signal to the ventricles below. As the signal travels through the heart, the heart contracts. First the atria contract, pumping blood into the ventricles. A fraction of a second later, the ventricles contract, sending blood throughout the body.

Usually the whole heart contracts between 60 and 100 times per minute. Each contraction equals one heartbeat.

An arrhythmia may occur for one of several reasons:

- Instead of beginning in the sinus node, the heartbeat begins in another part of the heart.
- The sinus node develops an abnormal rate or rhythm.
- A patient has a heart block.

What is a Heart Block?

Heart block is a condition in which the electrical signal cannot travel normally down the special pathways to the ventricles. For example, the signal from the atria to the ventricles may be (1) delayed, but each one conducted; (2) delayed with only some getting through; or (3) completely interrupted. If there is no conduction, the beat generally originates from the ventricles and is very slow.

What Are the Different Types of Arrhythmias?

There are many types of arrhythmias. Arrhythmias are identified by where they occur in the heart (atria or ventricles) and by what happens to the heart's rhythm when they occur.

Arrhythmias arising in the atria are called atrial or supraventricular (above the ventricles) arrhythmias. Ventricular arrhythmias begin in the ventricles. In general, ventricular arrhythmias caused by heart disease are the most serious.

Different types of arrhythmias are described [below].

Arrhythmia Types

Originating in the Atria

Sinus arrhythmia. Cyclic changes in the heart rate during breathing. Common in children and often found in adults.

Sinus tachycardia. The sinus node sends out electrical signals faster than usual, speeding up the heart rate.

35

Sick sinus syndrome. The sinus node does not fire its signals properly, so that the heart rate slows down. Sometimes the rate changes back and forth between a slow (bradycardia) and fast (tachycardia) rate.

Premature supraventricular contractions or premature atrial contractions (PAC). A beat occurs early in the atria, causing the heart to beat before the next regular heartbeat.

Supraventricular tachycardia (SVT), paroxysmal atrial tachycardia (PAT). A series of early beats in the atria speed up the heart rate (the number of times a heart beats per minute). In paroxysmal tachycardia, repeated periods of very fast heartbeats begin and end suddenly.

Atrial flutter. Rapidly fired signals cause the muscles in the atria to contract quickly, leading to a very fast, steady heartbeat.

Atrial fibrillation. Electrical signals in the atria are fired in a very fast and uncontrolled manner. Electrical signals arrive in the ventricles in a completely irregular fashion, so the heart beat is completely irregular.

Wolff-Parkinson-White syndrome. Abnormal pathways between the atria and ventricles cause the electrical signal to arrive at the ventricles too soon and to be transmitted back into the atria. Very fast heart rates may develop as the electrical signal ricochets between the atria and ventricles.

Originating in the Ventricles

Premature ventricular complexes (PVC). An electrical signal from the ventricles causes an early heart beat that generally goes unnoticed. The heart then seems to pause until the next beat of the ventricle occurs in a regular fashion.

Ventricular tachycardia. The heart beats fast due to electrical signals arising from the ventricles (rather than from the atria).

Ventricular fibrillation. Electrical signals in the ventricles are fired in a very fast and uncontrolled manner, causing the heart to quiver rather than beat and pump blood.

How Does the Doctor Know That I Have an Arrhythmia?

Sometimes an arrhythmia can be detected by listening to the heart with a stethoscope. However, the electrocardiogram is the most precise method for diagnosing the arrhythmia.

An arrhythmia may not occur at the time of the exam even though symptoms are present at other times. In such cases, tests will be done if necessary to find out whether an arrhythmia is causing the symptoms.

Tests for Detecting Arrhythmias

Electrocardiogram (ECG or EKG). A record of the electrical activity of the heart. Disks are placed on the chest and connected by wires to a recording machine. The heart's electrical signals cause a pen to draw lines across a strip of graph paper in the ECG machine. The doctor studies the shapes of these lines to check for any changes in the normal rhythm. The types of ECGs are:

- **Resting ECG.** The patient lies down for a few minutes while a record is made. In this type of ECG, disks are attached to the patient's arms and legs as well as to the chest.

- **Exercise ECG (stress test).** The patient exercises either on a treadmill machine or bicycle while connected to the ECG machine. This test tells whether exercise causes arrhythmias or makes them worse or whether there is evidence of inadequate blood flow to the heart muscle ("ischemia").

- **24-hour ECG (Holter) monitoring.** The patient goes about his or her usual daily activities while wearing a small, portable tape recorder that connects to the disks on the patient's chest. Over time, this test shows changes in rhythm (or "ischemia") that may not be detected during a resting or exercise ECG.

- **Transtelephonic monitoring.** The patient wears the tape recorder and disks over a period of a few days to several weeks. When the patient feels an arrhythmia, he or she telephones a monitoring station where the record is made. If access to a telephone is not possible, the patient has the option

37

of activating the monitor's memory function. Later, when a telephone is accessible, the patient can transmit the recorded information from the memory to the monitoring station. Transtelephonic monitoring can reveal arrhythmias that occur only once every few days or weeks.

- **Electrophysiologic study (EPS).** A test for arrhythmias that involves cardiac catheterization. Very thin, flexible tubes (catheters) are placed in a vein of an arm or leg and advanced to the right atrium and ventricle. This procedure allows doctors to find the site and type of arrhythmia and how it responds to treatment.

What Tests Can Be Done?

First the doctor will take a medical history and do a thorough physical exam. Then one or more tests may be used to check for an arrhythmia and to decide whether it is caused by heart disease. The [list above] gives details about these tests.

How Are Arrhythmias Treated?

Many arrhythmias require no treatment whatsoever.

Serious arrhythmias are treated in several ways depending on what is causing the arrhythmia. Sometimes the heart disease is treated to control the arrhythmia. Or, the arrhythmia itself may be treated using one or more of the following treatments.

Drugs. There are several kinds of drugs used to treat arrhythmias. One or more drugs may be used.

Drugs are carefully chosen because they can cause side effects. In some cases, they can cause arrhythmias or make arrhythmias worse. For this reason, the benefits of the drug are carefully weighed against any risks associated with taking it. It is important not to change the dose or type of your medication unless you check with your doctor first.

If you are taking drugs for an arrhythmia, one of the following tests will probably be used to see whether treatment is working: a 24-hour electrocardiogram (ECG) while you are on drug therapy, an exercise ECG, or a special technique to see how easily the arrhythmia can be caused. Blood levels of antiarrhythmic drugs may also be checked.

Cardioversion. To quickly restore a heart to its normal rhythm, the doctor may apply an electrical shock to the chest wall. Called cardioversion, this treatment is most often used in emergency situations. After cardioversion, drugs are usually prescribed to prevent the arrhythmia from recurring.

Automatic implantable defibrillators. These devices are used to correct serious ventricular arrhythmias that can lead to sudden death. The defibrillator is surgically placed inside the patient's chest. There, it monitors the heart's rhythm and quickly identifies serious arrhythmias. With an electrical shock, it immediately disrupts a deadly arrhythmia.

Artificial pacemaker. An artificial pacemaker can take charge of sending electrical signals to make the heart beat if the heart's natural pacemaker is not working properly or its electrical pathway is blocked. During a simple operation, this electrical device is placed under the skin. A lead extends from the device to the right side of the heart, where it is permanently anchored.

Surgery. When an arrhythmia cannot be controlled by other treatments, doctors may perform surgery. After locating the heart tissue that is causing the arrhythmia, the tissue is altered or removed so that it will not produce the arrhythmia.

How Can Arrhythmias Be Prevented?

If heart disease is not causing the arrhythmia, the doctor may suggest that you avoid what is causing it. For example, if caffeine or alcohol is the cause, the doctor may ask you not to drink coffee, tea, colas, or alcoholic beverages.

Is Research on Arrhythmias Being Done?

The National Heart, Lung, and Blood Institute (NHLBI) supports basic research on normal and abnormal electrical activity in the heart to understand how arrhythmias develop. Clinical studies with patients aim to improve the diagnosis and management of different arrhythmias. These studies will someday lead to better diagnostic and treatment strategies.

Where Can I Find Publications about Heart Disease?

To obtain publications about heart disease, you may want to contact your:

- local American Heart Association chapter.
- local or state health department.

The National Heart, Lung, and Blood Institute also has publications about heart disease. For more information, contact:

NHLBI Communications and Public Information Branch
Building 31, Room 4A21
Bethesda, Maryland 20892

Heart Problems Reported with Two Non-Sedating Allergy Drugs (FDA Consumer, October 1992)

Under certain circumstances, people taking either one of two non-sedating prescription antihistamines may develop life-threatening cardiac arrhythmias, commonly known as abnormal heart rhythms.

For this reason, FDA recently asked Marion Merrell Dow Inc., the manufacturer of Seldane (terfenadine), and Janssen Pharmaceutica, Inc., manufacturer of Hismanal (astemizole), to warn doctors and other health professionals of the problem.

Patients with liver disease are at increased risk from both drugs, because they cannot properly metabolize (process) them. This leads to a drug accumulation in the body that can result in arrhythmias and, in the case of Hismanal, other cardiovascular events, including cardiac arrest and death.

Taking excessive doses of either drug also increases these risks. With Hismanal, the majority of reported cardiovascular events have occurred in patients who greatly exceeded the recommended dose of 10 milligrams (one tablet) a day. However, arrhythmias have occurred at reported doses as low as 20 to 30 milligrams daily. It is important, therefore, that patients not exceed the recommended daily dose.

Patients on Seldane are also at risk if they take the anti-fungal drug Nizoral (ketoconazole) or the antibiotic erythromycin (sold under several brand and generic names) at the same time as Seldane. Studies have shown that Nizoral, also manufactured by Janssen, affects how the body metabolizes Seldane, increasing the blood levels of the allergy drug. Similar studies have not been conducted with erythromycin; however, arrhythmias have occurred in patients taking the antibiotic and Seldane at the same time.

Patients who experience fainting, dizziness or palpitations with either antihistamine should immediately discontinue use and consult their doctors for evaluation, which may include electrocardiographic (ECG) testing.

FDA has asked both companies to revise the physician labeling for these non-sedating antihistamines and develop patient leaflets that reflect the new warnings. FDA is working with Marion Merrell Dow to plan further studies of Seldane metabolism and possible interactions with other drugs and to identify any other patient groups that may be at risk.

In addition, FDA is working with Janssen to warn against the use of Nizoral with Seldane.

Chapter 7

Facts about Heart Failure

What Is Heart Failure?

Heart failure occurs when the heart loses its ability to pump enough blood through the body. Usually, the loss in pumping action is a symptom of an underlying heart problem, such as coronary artery disease.

The term heart failure suggests a sudden and complete stop of heart activity. But, actually, the heart does not suddenly stop. Rather, heart failure usually develops slowly, often over years, as the heart gradually loses its pumping ability and works less efficiently. Some people may not become aware of their condition until symptoms appear years after their heart began its decline.

How serious the condition is depends on how much pumping capacity the heart has lost. Nearly everyone loses some pumping capacity as he or she ages. But the loss is significantly more in heart failure and often results from a heart attack or other disease that damages the heart.

The severity of the condition determines the impact it has on a person's life. At one end of the spectrum, the mild form of heart failure may have little effect on a person's life; at the other end, severe heart failure can interfere with even simple activities and prove fatal. Between those extremes, treatment often helps people lead full lives.

NIH Pub. No. 94-923.

43

But all forms of heart failure, even the mildest, are a serious health problem, which must be treated. To improve their chance of living longer, patients must take care of themselves, see their physician regularly, and closely follow treatments.

Loss of Pumping Action in Heart Failure

Healthy Heart Muscle. Normally, the heart pumps blood by expanding and then contracting its chambers. When the chambers expand, blood comes in; when the chambers contract, blood is pushed out, carrying oxygen and nutrients to the rest of the body.

Weakened Heart Muscle. Heart failure occurs when the heart muscle loses its ability to pump. The chambers cannot expand and contract well. Less blood moves through the chambers and more blood stays in the heart.

Is There Only One Type of Heart Failure?

The term congestive heart failure is often used to describe all patients with heart failure. In reality, congestion (the buildup of fluid) is just one feature of the condition and does not occur in all patients. There are two main categories of heart failure although within each category, symptoms and effects may differ from patient to patient. The two categories are:

- Systolic heart failure—This occurs when the heart's ability to contract decreases. The heart cannot pump with enough force to push a sufficient amount of blood into the circulation. Blood coming into the heart from the lungs may back up and cause fluid to leak into the lungs, a condition known as pulmonary congestion.

- Diastolic heart failure—This occurs when the heart has a problem relaxing. The heart cannot properly fill with blood because the muscle has become stiff, losing its ability to relax. This form may lead to fluid accumulation, especially in the feet, ankles, and legs. Some patients may have lung congestion.

How Common Is Heart Failure?

Between 2 to 3 million Americans have heart failure, and 400,000 new cases are diagnosed each year. The condition is slightly more common among men than women and is twice as common among African Americans as whites.

Heart failure causes 39,000 deaths a year and is a contributing factor in another 225,000 deaths. The death rate attributed to heart failure rose by 64 percent from 1970 to 1990, while the death rate from coronary heart disease dropped by 49 percent during the same period. Heart failure mortality is about twice as high for African Americans as whites for all age groups.

In a sense, heart failure's growing presence as a health problem reflects the Nation's changing population: More people are living longer. People age 65 and older represent the fastest growing segment of the population, and the risk of heart failure increases with age. The condition affects 1 percent of people age 50, but about 5 percent of people age 75.

What Causes Heart Failure?

As stated, the heart loses some of its blood-pumping ability as a natural consequence of aging. However, a number of other factors can lead to a potentially life-threatening loss of pumping activity.

As a symptom of underlying heart disease, heart failure is closely associated with the major risk factors for coronary heart disease: smoking, high cholesterol levels, hypertension (persistent high blood pressure), diabetes and abnormal blood sugar levels, and obesity. A person can change or eliminate those risk factors and thus lower their risk of developing or aggravating their heart disease and heart failure.

Among prominent risk factors, hypertension (high blood pressure) and diabetes are particularly important. Uncontrolled high blood pressure increases the risk of heart failure by about 200 percent, compared with those who do not have hypertension. Moreover, the degree of risk appears directly related to the severity of the high blood pressure.

Persons with diabetes have about a two- to eight-fold greater risk of heart failure than those without diabetes. Women with diabetes having a greater risk of heart failure than men with diabetes. Part of the risk comes from diabetes' association with other heart failure risk

45

factors, such as high blood pressure, obesity, and high cholesterol levels. However, the disease process in diabetes also damages the heart muscle.

The presence of coronary disease is among the greatest risks for heart failure. Muscle damage and scarring caused by a heart attack greatly increase the risk of heart failure. Cardiac arrhythmias, or irregular heartbeats, also raise heart failure risk. Any disorder that causes abnormal swelling or thickening of the heart sets the stage for heart failure.

In some people, heart failure arises from problems with heart valves, the flap-like structures that help regulate blood flow through the heart. Infections in the heart are another source of increased risk for heart failure.

A single risk factor may be sufficient to cause heart failure, but a combination of factors dramatically increases the risk. Advanced age adds to the potential impact of any heart failure risk.

Finally, genetic abnormalities contribute to the risk for certain types of heart disease, which in turn may lead to heart failure. However, in most instances, a specific genetic link to heart failure has not been identified.

What Are the Symptoms?

A number of symptoms are associated with heart failure, but none is specific for the condition. Perhaps the best known symptom is shortness of breath ("dyspnea"). In heart failure, this may result from excess fluid in the lungs. The breathing difficulties may occur at rest or during exercise. In some cases congestion may be severe enough to prevent or interrupt sleep.

Fatigue or easy tiring is another common symptom. As the heart's pumping capacity decreases, muscles and other tissues receive less oxygen and nutrition, which are carried in the blood. Without proper "fuel," the body cannot perform as much work, which translates into fatigue.

Fluid accumulation, or edema, may cause swelling of the feet, ankles, legs, and occasionally, the abdomen. Excess fluid retained by the body may result in weight gain, which sometimes occurs fairly quickly.

Persistent coughing is another common sign, especially coughing that regularly produces mucus or pink, blood-tinged sputum. Some people develop raspy breathing or wheezing.

Because heart failure usually develops slowly, the symptoms may not appear until the condition has progressed over years. The heart hides the underlying problem by making adjustments that delay—but do not prevent—the eventual loss in pumping capacity. The heart adjusts, or compensates, in three ways to cope with and hide the effects of heart failure:

- Enlargement ("dilatation"), which allows more blood into the heart;

- Thickening of muscle fibers ("hypertrophy") to strengthen the heart muscle, which allows the heart to contract more forcefully and pump more blood; and

- More frequent contraction, which increases circulation.

By making these adjustments, or compensating, the heart can temporarily make up for losses in pumping ability, sometimes for years. However, compensation has its limits. Eventually, the heart cannot offset the lost ability to pump blood, and the signs of heart failure appear.

How Do Doctors Diagnose Heart Failure?

In many cases, physicians diagnose heart failure during a physical examination. Readily identifiable signs are shortness of breath, fatigue, and swollen ankles and feet. The physician also will check for the presence of risk factors, such as hypertension, obesity, and a history of heart problems. Using a stethoscope, the physician can listen to a patient breathe and identify the sounds of lung congestion. The stethoscope also picks up the abnormal heart sounds indicative of heart failure.

If neither the symptoms nor the patient's history point to a clear-cut diagnosis, the physician may recommend any of a variety of laboratory tests, including, initially, an electrocardiogram, which uses recording devices placed on the chest to evaluate the electrical activity of a patient's heartbeat.

Echocardiography is another means of evaluating heart function from outside the body. Sound waves bounced off the heart are recorded and translated into images. The pictures can reveal abnormal heart size, shape, and movement. Echocardiography also can be used to calculate a patient's ejection fraction, a measure of the amount of blood pumped out when the heart contracts.

Another possible test is the chest x-ray, which also determines the heart's size and shape, as well as the presence of congestion in the lungs.

The chest x ray also helps rule out other possible causes of a patient's symptoms. For instance, the symptoms of heart failure can result when the heart is made to work too hard, instead of from damaged muscle. Conditions that overload the heart occur rarely and include severe anemia and thyrotoxicosis (a disease resulting from an overactive thyroid gland).

What Treatments Are Available?

Heart failure caused by an excessive workload is curable by treating the primary disease, such as anemia or thyrotoxicosis. Also curable are forms caused by anatomical problems, such as a heart valve defect. These defects can be surgically corrected.

However, for the common forms of heart failure—those due to damaged heart muscle—no known cure exists. But treatment for these forms may be quite successful. The treatment seeks to improve patients' quality of life and length of survival through lifestyle change and drug therapy.

Patients can minimize the effects of heart failure by controlling the risk factors for heart disease. Obvious steps include quitting smoking, losing weight if necessary, abstaining from alcohol, and making dietary changes to reduce the amount of salt and fat consumed. Regular, modest exercise is also helpful for many patients, though the amount and intensity should be carefully monitored by a physician.

But, even with lifestyle changes, most heart failure patients must take medication. Many patients receive two or more drugs. Several types of drugs have proven useful in the treatment of heart failure:

- Diuretics help reduce the amount of fluid in the body and are useful for patients with fluid retention and hypertension.

48

- Digitalis increases the force of the heart's contractions, helping to improve circulation.

- Results of recent studies have placed more emphasis on the use of drugs known as angiotensin converting enzyme (ACE) inhibitors. Several large studies have indicated that ACE inhibitors improve survival among heart failure patients and may slow, or perhaps even prevent, the loss of heart pumping activity.

Originally developed as a treatment for hypertension, ACE inhibitors help heart failure patients by, among other things, decreasing the pressure inside blood vessels. As a result, the heart does not have to work as hard to pump blood through the vessels.

Patients who cannot take ACE inhibitors may get a nitrate and/or a drug called hydralazine, each of which helps relax tension in blood vessels to improve blood flow.

Sometimes, heart failure is life-threatening. Usually, this happens when drug therapy and lifestyle changes fail to control its symptoms. In such cases, a heart transplant may be the only treatment option. However, candidates for transplantation often have to wait months or even years before a suitable donor heart is found. Recent studies indicate that some transplant candidates improve during this waiting period through drug treatment and other therapy, and can be removed from the transplant list.

Transplant candidates who do not improve sometimes need mechanical pumps, which are attached to the heart. Called left ventricular assist devices (LVADs), the machines take over part or virtually all of the heart's blood-pumping activity. However, current LVADs are not permanent solutions for heart failure but are considered bridges to transplantation.

An experimental surgical procedure for severe heart failure is available at a few U.S. medical centers. The procedure, called cardiomyoplasty, involves detaching one end of a muscle in the back, wrapping it around the heart, and then suturing the muscle to the heart. An implanted electric stimulator causes the back muscle to contract, pumping blood from the heart.

Common Heart Failure Medications

Listed below are some of the medications prescribed for heart failure. Not all medications are suitable for all patients, and more than one drug may be needed. Also, the list provides the full range of possible side effects for these drugs. Not all patients will develop these side effects. If you suspect that you are having a side effect, alert your physician.

ACE Inhibitors

These prevent the production of a chemical that causes blood vessels to narrow. As a result, blood pressure drops, and the heart does not have to work as hard to pump blood. *Side effects* may include coughing, skin rashes, fluid retention, excess potassium in the bloodstream, kidney problems, and an altered or lost sense of taste.

Digitalis

Increases the force of the heart's contractions. It also slows certain fast heart rhythms. As a result, the heart beats less frequently but more effectively, and more blood is pumped into the arteries. *Side effects* may include nausea, vomiting, loss of appetite, diarrhea, confusion, and new heartbeat irregularities.

Diuretics

These decrease the body's retention of salt and so of water. Diuretics are commonly prescribed to reduce high blood pressure. Diuretics come in many types, with different periods of effectiveness. *Side effects* may include loss of too much potassium, weakness, muscle cramps, joint pains, and impotence.

Hydralazine

This drug widens blood vessels, easing blood flow. *Side effects* may include headaches, rapid heartbeat, and joint pain.

Nitrates

These drugs are used mostly for chest pain, but may also help diminish heart failure symptoms. They relax smooth muscle and widen blood vessels. They act to lower primarily systolic blood pressure. *Side effects* may include headaches.

Making the Most of Your Doctor Visit

Here are some points you may want to discuss with your doctor. Don't hesitate to ask questions to clarify points. Also, ask your doctor to rephrase a reply you cannot understand. You may want to take a family member or friend to the appointment with you to help you better understand and remember what's said.

- Briefly describe your symptoms, even those you feel may not be important. You may want to keep a list so you will remember them.

- Tell the doctor all of the medications you take—including over-the-counter drugs—and any problems you may be having with them.

- Be sure you understand all of the doctor's instructions—especially for medications. Know what drug to take when, how often, and in what amount.

- Find out what side effects are possible from any drug the doctor prescribes for you.

- Ask the meaning of any medical term you don't understand.

- If, after your appointment, you still have questions or are uncertain about your treatment, call the doctor's office to get the information you need.

A Question for Your Pharmacist

Your pharmacist is a good resource for information about medications. Ask if any drug you're taking interacts badly with certain foods or with other drugs, including nonprescription ones. Your pharmacist also can help you understand product package inserts and label instructions.

51

Can a Person Live with Heart Failure?

Heart failure is one of the most serious symptoms of heart disease. About two-thirds of all patients die within 5 years of diagnosis. However, some live beyond 5 years, even into old age. The outlook for an individual patient depends on the patient's age, severity of heart failure, overall health, and a number of other factors.

As heart failure progresses, the effects can become quite severe, and patients often lose the ability to perform even modest physical activity. Eventually, the heart's reduced pumping capacity may interfere with routine functions, and patients may become unable to care for themselves. The loss in functional ability can occur quickly if the heart is further weakened by heart attacks or the worsening of other conditions that affect heart failure, such as diabetes and coronary heart disease.

Heart failure patients also have an increased risk of sudden death, or cardiac arrest, caused by an irregular heartbeat. To improve the chances of surviving with heart failure, patients must take care of themselves.

Patients must:

- See their physician regularly;
- Closely follow all of their physician's instructions;
- Take any medication according to instructions; and
- Immediately inform their physician of any significant change in their condition, such as an intensified shortness of breath or swollen feet.

Patients with heart failure also should:

- Control their weight;
- Watch what they eat;
- Not smoke cigarettes or use other tobacco products; and
- Abstain from or strictly limit alcohol consumption.

Readying a Q & A for Your Doctor Visit

Going to the doctor can be a nervous time. It may be hard to remember everything you want to ask and everything you hear.

It helps to prepare a list of important questions. [Before your appointment,] list questions you want answered [on a sheet of paper]. Then take this sheet with you to your appointment so you can record the answers.

Before you leave the doctor's office, be sure you understand your condition and its treatment, including any medications.

Even with the best care, heart failure can worsen, but patients who don't take care of themselves are almost writing themselves a prescription for poor health.

The best defense against heart failure is the prevention of heart disease. Almost all of the major coronary risk factors can be controlled or eliminated: smoking, high cholesterol, high blood pressure, diabetes, and obesity.

What Is the Outlook for Heart Failure?

Within the past decade, knowledge of heart failure has improved dramatically but, clearly, much more remains to be learned. The National Heart, Lung, and Blood Institute (NHLBI) supports numerous research projects aimed at building on what is already known about heart failure and at uncovering new knowledge about its process, diagnosis, and treatment. NHLBI research priorities for heart failure include:

- Learning more about basic cellular changes that lead to heart failure;
- Developing tests to detect the earliest signs of heart failure;
- Identifying factors that cause heart failure to worsen;
- Determining how heart failure can be reversed once it starts;
- Understanding better the heart's ability to compensate for lost pumping ability; and
- Developing new therapies, especially those based on early signs of heart failure.

Glossary

Angiotensin converting enzyme (ACE) inhibitor: A drug used to decrease pressure inside blood vessels.

Arrhythmia: An irregular heartbeat.

Cardiomyoplasty: A surgical procedure that involves detaching one end of a back muscle and attaching it to the heart. An electric stimulator causes the muscle to contract to pump blood from the heart.

Congestive heart failure: A heart disease condition that involves loss of pumping ability by the heart, generally accompanied by fluid accumulation in body tissues, especially the lungs.

Diastolic heart failure: Inability of the heart to relax properly and fill with blood as a result of stiffening of the heart muscle.

Dyspnea: Shortness of breath.

Echocardiography: Recording sound waves bounced off the heart to produce images of the heart.

Edema: Abnormal fluid accumulation in body tissues.

Electrocardiogram (EKG or ECG): Measurement of electrical activity associated with heartbeats.

Heart failure: Loss of blood-pumping ability by the heart.

Left ventricular assist device: A mechanical device used to increase the heart s pumping ability.

Pulmonary congestion (or edema): Fluid accumulation in the lungs.

Sudden cardiac death: Cardiac arrest caused by an irregular heartbeat.

Systolic heart failure: Inability of the heart to contract with enough force to pump adequate amounts of blood through the body.

Valves: Flap-like structures that control the direction of blood flow through the heart.

Chapter 8

Congestive Heart Failure: What You Should Know

Congestive heart failure is a condition in which a weakened heart exists along with a buildup of fluid in the body. It can be caused by many forms of heart disease. [For more information about other types of heart failure, see Chapter 7; for information on how the heart functions, see Chapter 1.

There are several things that can cause congestive heart failure. These include: a reduction in the heart muscle's strength leading to weaker contractions; problems that hinder the heart from filling properly with blood; difficulties that cause too much blood to be inside the heart.]

What Happens in Congestive Heart Failure?

When the heart doesn't pump as efficiently as it should, the blood flow slows down and less blood is pumped. Then blood returning to the heart backs up in the veins. This forces fluid from the blood vessels into tissues of the feet and legs. The swelling that follows is called *edema* of the feet, ankles and legs. Sometimes the edema involves the wall of the abdomen and liver, too. (Not all edema results from congestive heart failure—only a doctor is qualified to make this diagnosis.)

Excerpts from American Heart Association Pub. No. 51-1061 (CP). Used by Permission. Editor's comments are bracketed.

The heart's left side receives oxygenated blood from the lungs, then pumps it to the rest of the body. When the heart's left side isn't pumping as well as it should be, blood backs up in the vessels of the lungs. Sometimes fluid is forced out of the lung vessels into the breathing spaces themselves. When this happens it's called *pulmonary edema*; shortness of breath and a lack of stamina often follow.

The kidneys' ability to dispose of sodium (salt) and water is also impaired in cases of congestive heart failure. Sodium that normally would be eliminated in the urine stays in the body and holds water. This makes the excess fluid problem that already exists even worse.

A final problem is that a person who has CHF may feel tired. This happens because not enough blood circulates and tissues and organs don't get as much oxygen and food as they need.

When congestive heart failure is present, the body tries to compensate. One way the heart adjusts is by enlarging. When the heart chamber enlarges, it stretches more and can contract more strongly, so it pumps more blood.

A second way the heart compensates is by developing more muscle mass. This increases the total number of muscle fibers able to contract. More heart muscle fibers means the heart can pump more strongly.

One final way the body compensates is by increasing the stimulation of the heart muscle. This causes the heart to pump more often and improves circulation.

At first these ways of compensating help the heart keep working normally or almost normally. However, when the disease processes worsen, compensation starts to make matters worse. Then it contributes to the deterioration of a person's condition over time.

What Are the Signs of Congestive Heart Failure?

The most common symptom is shortness of breath caused by fluid in the lungs. Breathlessness is most often a problem during exercise, but it can also occur when a person is resting. Sometimes it may come on suddenly at night, making it extremely hard to breathe unless several pillows are used to raise the upper body. Occasionally a person will wake up from sleep.

[Other symptoms may include:

- coughing up blood-tinged phlegm
- excess fluid in the body's tissues
- tiredness, weakness and the inability to exert oneself
- confusion and impaired thinking

Treating Congestive Heart Failure

Congestive heart failure is typically treated with lifestyle modifications, medications, and sometimes surgery. Lifestyle modifications include dietary adjustments to maintain a proper weight and to reduce salt intake. Exercise can also help, but the American Heart Association recommends that congestive heart failure patients get the advice of their doctors before beginning an exercise program. In addition, certain exercises—like weight lifting and isometrics—should be avoided.

Three medications frequently prescribed for congestive heart failure patients are diuretics, digitalis, and vasodilators. Diuretics help the body eliminate excess fluid. Digitalis helps the heart muscle to pump more powerfully. Vasodilators help the heart by expanding blood vessels.

Surgical options include heart valve replacement, coronary bypass surgery, and transplantation. For more information on these procedures, see the related Chapters in Part V of this volume.]

Chapter 9

Facts about
Mitral Valve Prolapse

Mitral valve prolapse is frequently diagnosed in healthy people and is for the most part, harmless. Most people suffer no symptoms whatsoever from mitral valve prolapse. Estimates are that 1 in 10 to 1 in 20 individuals has mitral valve prolapse. It is also called floppy valve syndrome, Barlow's or Reid-Barlow's syndrome, ballooning mitral valve, midsystolic-click-late systolic murmur syndrome, or click murmur syndrome.

Mitral valve prolapse can be present from birth or develop at any age. It occurs in both men and women, but is more common in women. Mitral valve prolapse is one of the most frequently made cardiac diagnoses in the United States.

What Is Mitral Valve Prolapse?

Although in general healthy hearts are structurally similar, like other parts of the body, there are individual variations. The heart's valves work to maintain the flow of blood in one direction, ensuring proper circulation. The mitral valve controls the flow of blood into the left ventricle. Normally when the left ventricle contracts the mitral valve closes and blood flows out through the aortic valve. In mitral valve prolapse the shape or dimensions of the leaflets of the valve are not ideal; they may be too large and fail to close properly or balloon

---

An unnumbered publication of the National Heart, Lung, and Blood Institute.

out, hence the term "prolapse." When the valve leaflets flap, a clicking sound may be heard. Sometimes the prolapsing of the mitral valve allows a slight flow of blood back into the left atrium, which is called "mitral regurgitation," and this may cause a sound called a murmur. Some people with mitral valve prolapse have both a click and a murmur and some have only a click. Many have no unusual heart sounds at all, those who do may have clicks and murmurs which come and go.

Diagnosis

Mitral valve prolapse is commonly diagnosed by listening to the sounds that the heart makes or occasionally is discovered through echocardiographic tests. Sometimes once a physician has heard the characteristic sounds of mitral valve prolapse through a stethoscope, other tests may be ordered. Echocardiography is a common and painless test which uses sound waves of a very high frequency which travel through the layers of the skin and muscle to produce an image of the heart which can be seen on a screen. In this sense it is a technique similar to radar or sonar imaging.

Symptoms

The vast majority of people with mitral valve prolapse have no discomfort whatsoever. Most are surprised to learn that their heart is functioning in any way abnormally. Some individuals report mild and common symptoms such as shortness of breath, dizziness, and either "skipping" or "racing" of the heart. More rarely chest pain is reported. However, these are symptoms which may or may not be related to the mitral valve prolapse.

Treatment

In most cases no treatment is needed. For a small proportion of individuals with mitral valve prolapse, beta-blockers or other drugs are used to control specific symptoms. Serious problems are rare, can easily be diagnosed and if necessary, treated surgically.

Preventing Complications

The overwhelming majority of people with mitral valve prolapse are free of symptoms and never develop any noteworthy problems. However, it is important to understand that in some cases mitral regurgitation, that is, the flow of blood back into the left atrium can occur. Where mitral regurgitation has been diagnosed, there is an increased risk of acquiring bacterial endocarditis, an infection in the lining of the heart. To prevent bacterial endocarditis many physicians and dentists prescribe antibiotics before certain surgical or dental procedures.

Historical Background

It may seem that mitral valve prolapse is becoming more common but actually it has probably always been around and was simply less well recognized. For instance, some historians cite the observation of "soldier's heart" made by Dr. J.M. DaCosta during the Civil War as the first description of mitral valve prolapse. Contemporary understanding of this condition advanced, however, with the work in 1966 of Dr. J.B. Barlow in South Africa when he related the characteristic sounds to the specific anatomical characteristics of the leaflets in mitral valve prolapse. More precise identification became possible as increasingly sophisticated diagnostic tools were available.

The increased visibility of this disorder has also come from one-time or cross-sectional studies of healthy people as well as longitudinal studies which follow individuals over years such as the Framingham Study where routine tests have shown that it is commonly present. No one knew quite how common, and unnoticed, mitral valve prolapse was until 1976 when researchers examined 100 presumably healthy young students at a woman's school. Their finding, that it occurred frequently and that as many as 1 in 10 to 1 in 20 have mitral valve prolapse, was then underscored by findings from the Framingham Study in 1983, as well as by reports from other research.

Clinical Significance

The overwhelming majority of people with mitral valve prolapse are free of symptoms and never develop any noteworthy problems. Whether or not there is any discomfort, health care providers should

61

be notified of the existence of mitral valve prolapse so that recommendations can be made about the advisability of using antibiotics to protect against bacterial endocarditis.

Chapter 10

Facts about Blood Cholesterol

How Serious a Problem Is Coronary Heart Disease in the United States?

More than 6 million Americans have symptoms of coronary heart disease. Every year more than 1 million Americans suffer a heart attack, and over 500,000 die of coronary heart disease.

Most coronary heart disease is due to blockages in the arteries that supply blood to the heart muscle. Cholesterol and fat, circulating in the blood, build up in the walls of these arteries. This buildup narrows the arteries and can slow or block the flow of blood. This process is known as "atherosclerosis." Atherosclerosis is a slow progressive disease that may start very early in life yet might not produce symptoms for many years. Most heart attacks are caused by a clot forming at a narrow part of an artery which supplies blood to the heart muscle.

Blood carries a constant supply of oxygen to the heart. If the flow of blood is slowed or blocked, the oxygen supply may be reduced or cut off. With not enough oxygen to the heart muscle, there may be chest pain ("angina" or "angina pectoris"), and if the oxygen is cut off, there is heart muscle injury and a heart attack.

NIH Pub. No. 90-2696.

Why Should I Care about Blood Cholesterol?

Elevated blood cholesterol is one of the three major controllable risk factors for coronary heart disease (cigarette smoking and high blood pressure are the other two). In other words, the higher your cholesterol level the greater your chance of getting heart disease, especially at levels of 200 mg/dL or more.

More than half the adults 20 years of age or older in the United States have total blood cholesterol levels of 200 mg/dL or more. About one out of every four adults has a blood cholesterol level considered "high," that is, 240 mg/dL or greater.

The risk of heart disease is not limited to those with "high" blood cholesterol. The number of people with heart disease who have blood cholesterol levels below 240 mg/dL is actually greater than the number with levels of 240 mg/dL or above. This is partly a result of the fact that even moderately elevated blood cholesterol levels increase the risk of heart disease, and a large proportion of the population is in this range. The average level in U.S. adults is 210-215 mg/dL. It also results from the influence of risk factors other than elevated blood cholesterol. Fortunately you can do something about elevated blood cholesterol, high blood pressure, and smoking.

Will I Benefit from Lowering My Blood Cholesterol Level?

Lowering your elevated blood cholesterol will slow the fatty buildup in the arteries and in some cases even reverse the process. It will also help reduce your risk of heart disease.

High intakes of saturated fat and dietary cholesterol, and excess calories leading to overweight, all contribute to elevated blood cholesterol. Your usual eating pattern may well be too high in saturated fat, total fat (which may also add too many calories), and cholesterol. Average Americans eat 13 percent of their calories from saturated fat and 36-37 percent of their calories from total fat. The average daily intake of dietary cholesterol is 304 milligrams (mg) for women and 435 mg for men. These intakes are higher than what is recommended for the health of your heart.

The National Cholesterol Education Program recommends that all healthy Americans change their eating patterns to lower their blood cholesterol levels and thus reduce their chances of getting heart disease.

The recommended eating pattern is to eat:

- less than 10 percent of calories from saturated fat,
- an average of 30 percent of calories or less from total fat, and
- less than 300 mg a day of dietary cholesterol.

The saturated fat and total fat recommendations are intended to be achieved as an average intake over several days. Healthy children should also eat this way as they begin to eat with their family, usually at 2 years of age or older. This eating pattern can be achieved by following the guidelines [detailed below].

What Is "Blood Cholesterol?" For That Matter, What Is Cholesterol?

Pure cholesterol is an odorless, white, waxy, powdery substance. You cannot taste it or see it in the foods you eat.

Cholesterol is found in all animal products. Your body needs cholesterol to function normally. It is present in every cell in all parts of the body, including the brain and nervous system, muscle, skin, liver, intestines, heart, and skeleton. Cholesterol is carried from one part of your body to another in blood—"blood cholesterol." Your liver makes enough cholesterol for your body's needs, even if you don't eat any cholesterol—"dietary cholesterol."

How High Is "High" Blood Cholesterol?

A blood cholesterol level of 240 mg/dL or greater is considered "high" blood cholesterol. If your blood cholesterol is 240 mg/dL or greater, you have more than twice the risk of heart disease of someone whose cholesterol is 200 mg/dL, and you need to seek advice from a doctor who should conduct more tests.

But any cholesterol level of 200 mg/dL or more, even in the "borderline-high" category (200-239 mg/dL), increases your risk for heart disease. Levels less than 200 mg/dL put you at lower risk for heart disease. It does not mean "no" risk.

Total Blood Cholesterol Categories

- Less than 200 mg/dL: **Desirable**
- 200 to 239 mg/dL: **Borderline High**
- 240 mg/dL or greater: **High**

Note: These categories apply to anyone 20 years of age or older.

While any single risk factor will increase the likelihood of developing heart-related problems, the more risk factors you have, the more concerned you should be about prevention and treatment. A person with any two risk factors has four times the risk of someone without any risk factors. The presence of all three major controllable risk factors—high blood cholesterol, high blood pressure, and smoking—can raise your risk to eight times that of people who have none of these risk factors. The factors that increase your risk for coronary heart disease are listed [below].

Risk Factors for Coronary Heart Disease

- High blood cholesterol
- Cigarette smoking
- High blood pressure
- Obesity
- Diabetes
- Being a male
- Family history of heart disease before the age of 55
- Low HDL-cholesterol (less than 35 mg/dL)
- Circulation disorders of blood vessels to the legs, arms, and brain

Should I Have My Total Blood Cholesterol Checked?

Yes. The National Cholesterol Education Program recommends that all adults age 20 and over have their total blood cholesterol measured at least once every 5 years. If you do not know your level, ask your doctor to measure it at your next visit.

How Is My Total Blood Cholesterol Measured?

Cholesterol measurement requires a blood sample which may be drawn from a vein in your arm or taken by a fingerprick. If your first measurement is 200 mg/dL or greater, it should be rechecked with a second measurement on blood drawn from your arm. You do not have to fast for a total blood cholesterol measurement.

A second measurement is important. It helps your doctor decide what to do next. Your cholesterol level naturally changes over time. Also, lab errors can affect the number. A second measurement helps your doctor find your average number.

What Are LDL- and HDL-Cholesterol?

LDL and HDL refer to two types of "lipoproteins." These are packages of cholesterol, fat, and protein that are made by the body to carry fat and cholesterol through the blood. They are not in the foods you eat.

LDLs are low density lipoproteins. They carry most of the cholesterol in the blood. If the level of LDL-cholesterol is elevated, cholesterol and fat can build up in the arteries contributing to atherosclerosis. This is why LDL-cholesterol is often called "bad cholesterol."

HDLs are high density lipoproteins. They contain only a small amount of cholesterol. HDLs are thought to carry cholesterol back to the liver. Thus HDLs help remove cholesterol from the blood, preventing the buildup of cholesterol in the walls of arteries. HDL-cholesterol is often called "good cholesterol."

Should I Check My LDL- and HDL-Cholesterol Too?

If the average of your total cholesterol measurements is either "borderline-high" or "high," your doctor should ask you to return for another test. This test will show values for your LDL-cholesterol, HDL-cholesterol, and triglycerides. Your doctor will ask you to fast (except for water or black coffee) for 12 hours before the test.

67

What Do LDL- and HDL-Cholesterol Levels Mean?

LDL- and HDL-cholesterol levels more accurately predict your risk of coronary heart disease than a total cholesterol level alone. A *high* LDL-cholesterol level or a *low* HDL-cholesterol level increases your risk.

If your doctor measured your LDL-cholesterol level, use the chart below to see how your LDL-cholesterol level measures up.

LDL-Cholesterol Categories

- Less than 130 mg/dL: **Desirable**
- 130 to 159 mg/dL: **Borderline-High Risk**
- 160 mg/dL and above: **High Risk**

After evaluating your LDL-cholesterol level and other risk factors for coronary heart disease, your doctor will determine your treatment program. The treatment your doctor will prescribe first is a diet that is low in saturated fat and cholesterol. You may start on a diet that is similar to the recommended eating pattern for all healthy Americans. In general, however, the higher your LDL-cholesterol level the more intensive will be the treatment and followup you receive compared to a person with a lower LDL-cholesterol level. This is because a higher LDL-cholesterol level increases your risk for heart disease.

The lower your HDL-cholesterol level, the greater your risk of coronary heart disease. Any HDL-cholesterol level lower than 35 mg/dL is considered low. Quitting smoking, losing weight if you are overweight, and becoming physically active may help raise your HDL-cholesterol level.

Do Ratios Predict My Risk for Heart Disease?

You may have heard of a cholesterol "ratio." This is actually your total cholesterol or LDL-cholesterol divided by your HDL-cholesterol. Because LDL- and HDL-cholesterol both predict your risk of heart disease, it is more important to know the value for each of these and not combine them into a single number.

What Are Triglycerides?

Triglycerides are the form in which fat is carried through our blood to the tissues. The bulk of your body's fat tissue is in the form of triglycerides. Triglyceride levels less than 250 mg/dL are considered normal.

It is not clear whether high triglycerides alone increase your risk of heart disease. On the other hand, many people with elevated triglycerides also have high LDL-cholesterol or low HDL-cholesterol levels which do influence their doctor's decisions on how to treat high blood cholesterol.

How Does My Cholesterol Level Become Elevated?

Among the factors you can do something about, **what you eat** has the largest effect on your blood cholesterol level. **Saturated fat** raises your blood cholesterol level more than anything else you eat. **Dietary cholesterol** can also increase your blood cholesterol level, but less than saturated fat in most people. Eating in a way that is low in saturated fat and cholesterol will help lower your elevated blood cholesterol.

Being overweight may also increase your blood cholesterol level. Most overweight people with elevated blood cholesterol can help lower their levels by losing weight. Regular physical activity may help control your weight and is associated with a reduced risk of heart disease and lower blood pressure.

Genetic factors affect your blood cholesterol level and can determine how much you can lower your level by diet.

Age and sex also influence blood cholesterol levels. In the United States, blood cholesterol levels in men and women start to rise at about age 20. Women's blood cholesterol levels prior to menopause are lower than those of men of the same age. After menopause, however, the cholesterol level of women usually increases to a level higher than that of men. In men, blood cholesterol generally levels off or declines slightly around age 50. Since the risk of coronary heart disease is especially high in the later decades of life, reducing high blood cholesterol is important in the elderly.

Oral contraceptives and pregnancy can increase blood cholesterol levels in some women. For pregnant women, blood cholesterol levels should return to normal 20 weeks after childbirth.

What Changes Can I Make in the Way I Eat?

Dietary changes that work together to reduce saturated fat, total fat, and cholesterol will work to lower blood cholesterol levels in most people. Whether your level is in the desirable, borderline-high, or high category, making the changes listed in [the guidelines below] will help lower your blood cholesterol. However, if your level is high, you are at greater risk for heart disease and you may need closer followup and nutrition counseling to help lower your blood cholesterol.

Guidelines for Lowering Blood Cholesterol Levels

- Eat fewer foods high in saturated fat.
- Eat fewer high-fat foods.
- Replace part of your saturated fat with unsaturated fat.
- Eat fewer high-cholesterol foods.
- Choose foods high in complex carbohydrates (starch and fiber).
- Lose weight, if you are overweight.

These guidelines are also consistent with the "Dietary Guidelines for Americans" developed by the U.S. Department of Agriculture and the U.S. Department of Health and Human Services.

Eat Fewer High-Fat Foods

There are two major types of dietary fat—**saturated** and **unsaturated**. Unsaturated fats are further classified as either **polyunsaturated** or **monounsaturated** fats. Together, saturated, polyunsaturated, and monounsaturated fats equal total fat. All foods containing fats have a mixture of these types.

One of the goals in lowering your blood cholesterol level is to eat less total fat, especially saturated fat. Because fat (all types) is the richest source of calories, eating less fat will help you cut calories to lose weight if you are overweight. If you are not overweight and want to maintain your weight, choose more often foods high in complex carbohydrates and eat less frequently foods high in fat. While your calorie level remains the same, the percent of calories from fat decreases and the percent of calories from carbohydrates increases.

70

Eat Fewer Foods High in Saturated Fat

Saturated fat raises your blood cholesterol level more than anything else in your eating plan. The best way to reduce your blood cholesterol level is to reduce the amount of saturated fat that you eat.

Animal products as a group are a major source of saturated fat in the typical American diet. The fat in whole-milk dairy products (like butter, cheese, whole milk, ice cream, and cream) contains high amounts of saturated fat. Skim-milk, low-fat, and nonfat dairy products can be substituted for the higher fat products.

Saturated fat is also concentrated in the fat that surrounds meat and in the white streaks of fat in the muscle of meat (marbling). Well-trimmed cuts from the "round" cuts of the animal are lower in saturated fat than well-marbled, untrimmed meat. In general, poultry, especially when the skin is removed, is lower in saturated fat than meat. Fish is generally lower in saturated fat than poultry and meat.

A few vegetable fats—coconut oil, palm kernel oil, and palm oil—are high in saturated fat. Although recently the food industry has largely discontinued the use of these fats in many foods, they may be used for commercial deep fat frying and in foods such as cookies and crackers, whipped toppings, coffee creamers, cake mixes, and even frozen dinners. Because you can not see these vegetable fats in foods it is important for you to read food labels. The label may tell you what type of fat or how much saturated fat a food contains. This information will help you choose foods lowest in saturated fats.

Replace Part of Your Saturated Fat with Unsaturated Fat

Replacing unsaturated fat for saturated fat helps lower blood cholesterol levels. Use fats and oils that contain primarily unsaturated fats whenever possible.

Polyunsaturated fats are found in greatest amounts in safflower, corn, soybean, cottonseed, sesame, and sunflower oils, which are common cooking oils. Polyunsaturated fats are also found in most salad dressings.

Olive and canola oil are examples of oils that are high in monounsaturated fats. Like other vegetable oils, these oils are used in cooking as well as in salad dressings.

Not all salad dressings are made with oils that contain primarily unsaturated fats. Some could be high in saturated fats. Read the labels to find out.

Eat Fewer High-Cholesterol Foods

Dietary cholesterol is the cholesterol found in some of the foods we eat. It can also raise your blood cholesterol level, but less than saturated fat in most people.

Although you can not see cholesterol, it is found in all foods that come from animals, including egg yolks, meat, fish, poultry, and dairy products. Egg yolks and organ meats (liver, kidney, sweetbread, brain) are particularly rich sources of cholesterol. Egg whites and foods that come from plants, like fruits, nuts, vegetables, grains, cereals and seeds, have no cholesterol.

Since cholesterol is not a fat, you can find it in both high-fat and low-fat animal foods. In other words, even if a food is low in fat, it may be high in cholesterol. For instance, organ meats, like liver, are low in fat but are high in cholesterol.

Choose Foods High in Complex Carbohydrates (Starch and Fiber)

Breads, pasta, rice, cereals, dry peas and beans, fruits, and vegetables are good sources of complex carbohydrates (starch and fiber) and contain little or no saturated fat and no cholesterol. They are excellent substitutes for foods that are high in saturated fat and cholesterol.

Contrary to popular belief, high-carbohydrate foods (like pasta, rice, potatoes) are lower in calories than foods high in fat. What adds calories to these foods is the addition of butter, rich sauces, whole milk, cheese, or cream, which are high in fat, especially saturated fat.

Lose Weight, If You Are Overweight

People who are overweight tend to have higher blood cholesterol levels than people of desirable weight. You can reduce your weight by eating fewer calories and by increasing your physical activity on a regular basis. By reducing the amount of fat in your diet, you will be cutting down on the richest source of calories. Fat has more than twice the calories as the same amount of protein or carbohydrate. Substituting foods that are high in complex carbohydrates for high-fat foods is a good way to help you lose weight.

Are the Recommended Changes in Eating Safe?

Yes. Eating patterns designed to lower blood cholesterol can be as high in nutritional quality as, or higher than, other diets. The special needs of women for nutrients such as calcium, iron, and zinc can be met in these patterns. Eating a variety of foods helps to assure nutritional adequacy. This also applies to children and teenagers.

Calories are necessary to maintain growth, and it is important that children and adolescents get enough calories. An eating pattern low in saturated fat, total fat, and cholesterol is not necessarily a low-calorie way of eating. On the other hand, many young children pass through a phase when they are more selective and more independent about food; desire for food becomes erratic and the variety of foods selected may become limited. During this phase what the child does eat should be as nutritious as possible.

Pregnant or breastfeeding women and many patients with diabetes, kidney, heart or liver disease may need special counseling from an expert in nutrition such as a registered dietitian.

Can I Really Lower My Blood Cholesteron Level?

Generally your blood cholesterol level should begin to drop 2 to 3 weeks after you start with a cholesterol-lowering eating pattern. Over time, the average reduction in blood cholesterol level will be about 10-15 percent. Also, the higher your blood cholesterol level is to begin with, the greater reduction you can expect.

How much you reduce your blood cholesterol levels depends on:

- how well you follow your new way of eating;
- how much saturated fat and how much cholesterol you were eating before starting to eat the cholesterol-lowering way;
- how much weight you lose, if you are overweight;
- and how responsive your body is to your changed way of eating.

73

How Do I Change?

Look at your overall eating pattern and begin to plan. You don't have to cut out all the high-saturated fat and high-cholesterol foods that you eat. Try to substitute one or two low-saturated fat or low-cholesterol foods each day, and soon you will reach your goal of a low-saturated fat, low-cholesterol way of eating.

If you are eating few foods high in saturated fat, an occasional high-saturated fat food won't raise your blood cholesterol level. If you expect a high-saturated fat, high-cholesterol day, have especially low-saturated fat, low-cholesterol days before and after.

Lean Cuts of Meat

Beef: Round, Sirloin, Chuck, Loin
Veal: All trimmed cuts
Pork: Tenderloin, Leg (fresh), Shoulder (arm or picnic)
Lamb: Leg, Arm, Loin

You should eat a variety of foods each day to get the nutrients you need. One way to do this is to choose, using the tips below, heart healthy foods from different food groups—meat, poultry, fish, and shellfish; dairy products; eggs; fats and oils; fruits and vegetables; breads, cereals, pasta, rice, and dry peas and beans; and sweets and snacks. Foods are grouped by the nutrients they provide. Sweets and snacks often are high in saturated fat, cholesterol, and calories. The number and size of the portions should be adjusted to reach and maintain your desirable weight.

The following tips will help you choose foods low in saturated-fat and cholesterol within groups:

Meat, Poultry, Fish, and Shellfish

Buying tips:

- Choose fish, poultry, lean cuts of meat, and eat moderate portions (about 6 oz. a day). Choose fish and poultry without the skin more often. They are, in general, lower in saturated fat than meat.

- "Select" grades of meat are lower in fat than "choice." "Choice" grades are lower in fat than "prime" grades.

- Shellfish generally has less saturated fat than meat, poultry, and fish, but its cholesterol content varies—some are relatively high and some are low.

- Cholesterol is found in high amounts in organ meats (liver, kidney, sweetbread, brain).

- Processed meats, like bacon, bologna, salami, hot dogs, and sausage, are high in fat; they should be eaten infrequently.

- "Lean," "lite," "leaner," and "lower fat" generally refer to foods containing less fat. They may not be "low" in fat. Read label information for grams of fat.

- Goose, duck, and many processed poultry products, like chicken or turkey bologna and hot dogs, are very high in saturated fat and should be limited.

Preparation tips:

- Trim fat from meat and remove skin from poultry before cooking and eating.

- Bake, broil, roast, poach or braise instead of frying to reduce the fat.

Dairy Products

Buying tips

- Drink skim and 1% milk rather than 2% and whole milk.

- Substitute low-fat and imitation cheeses whenever possible for natural, processed, and hard cheeses which are higher in saturated fat.

- Instead of hard cheese choose low-fat cottage cheese, farmer cheese or pot cheese which are lower in saturated fat. Choose low-fat cheeses that have between 2 and 6 grams of fat per ounce.

- Substitute low-fat or nonfat yogurt for sour cream in recipes or as toppings.

Eggs

Buying tips

- The egg yolks you eat include those hidden in processed foods and many baked goods.

Preparation tips

- Egg whites contain no cholesterol; substitute two whites for each whole egg in recipes.

Fats and Oils

Buying tips

- Choose liquid vegetable oils that are highest in unsaturated fat such as canola, safflower, sunflower, corn, olive, sesame, and soybean oils, in cooking and in salad dressings.

- The vegetable oils from palm kernel, coconut, and palm, as well as cocoa fat, which are used in some commercial products, contain large amounts of saturated fat.

- Read labels of commercially prepared foods to find out what type of fat or how much saturated fat they contain.

Preparation tips

- In your cooking, limit your use of butter, lard, fatback, and solid shortenings.

- When using fats and oils, use only small amounts and replace those high in saturated fat with those that contain mostly unsaturated fat.

- Use margarine instead of butter as a spread.

Fruits and Vegetables

Buying tips

- Fruits and vegetables—fresh, frozen or canned—contain no cholesterol and are almost always very low in saturated fat.

Preparation tips

- Use fruits as a snack or dessert.

- Prepare vegetables as snacks and side dishes. Limit use of cream, cream cheese, cheese, and butter or other animal fats in preparing and serving them.

Breads, Cereals, Pasta, Rice, and Dry Peas and Beans

Buying tips

- Cereals are usually low in saturated fat, except for granola-type cereals.

- Breads and most rolls are low in saturated fat; however, many other types of commercially baked goods such as croissants, doughnuts, muffins, biscuits, and butter rolls are made with large amounts of fat, especially saturated fats.

Preparation Tips

- Try pasta, rice, and dry peas and beans (like split peas, lentils, kidney beans, and navy beans) as main dishes, casseroles, soups, or other one-dish meals with low-fat sauces.

- Extend meat with pasta or vegetables for hearty dishes.

- Bake your own muffins and quick breads using unsaturated vegetable oils, and substitute two egg whites for each egg yolk.

Sweets and Snacks (Avoid Too Many Sweets)

Buying tips

- Commercial cakes, pies, cookies, cheese crackers, and some types of chips are high in saturated fat, cholesterol, and calories. Read labels carefully.

- Try angel food cake, fig bars, and ginger snaps as substitutes for commercial baked goods high in saturated fat.

- Try frozen desserts like ice milk, low-fat or nonfat yogurt, sorbets, and popsicles which are low in saturated fat, instead of ice cream which contains considerably more saturated fat and cholesterol.

Preparation tips

- Try a piece of fruit, some vegetables, or a low-fat snack like unbuttered popcorn or breadsticks.

What Do I Look for on Food Labels?

Look for the amount of saturated fat, total fat, and cholesterol given with the nutrition information provided per serving. Use this information to compare and choose products lower in total fat, saturated fat, and cholesterol.

In addition, food labels include a list of ingredients. The ingredient in the greatest amount is listed first. The ingredient in the least amount is listed last. To avoid too much fat, saturated fat, and cholesterol go easy on products that list first any ingredient higher in saturated fat or cholesterol. Some examples of these ingredients include animal fats like bacon, beef fat, butter, and lard; coconut, coconut oil, palm kernel or palm oil; and egg and egg yolk solids.

Will I Be Able to Eat Out?

Yes. Whether you are eating on the run or sitting down to a full course meal, you can make choices that are low in saturated fat and cholesterol. Choose restaurants that have low-fat, low-cholesterol items on their menus; or call ahead to find out if special requests will be honored. Ask how menu items are prepared. Ask about the availability of foods not on the menu. Select meat, poultry or fish that is broiled, grilled baked, steamed, or poached rather than fried. If the portion served is large, take home the extra. Choose lean deli meats such as fresh turkey instead of higher fat cut such as salami or bologna. Look for vegetables seasoned with herbs or spices rather than butter, sour cream, or cheese. Try sharing dessert with a friend or order a light dessert such as sherbet, fruit ice, or sorbet.

How Much Saturated Fat and Cholesterol Are There in Different Foods?

There are higher and lower saturated-fat foods within each of the food groups. The tips in this fact sheet will help you select and prepare lower saturated-fat and cholesterol foods.

Prepared dishes which are made from a combination of foods will vary in saturated fat content. How much they vary depends on the type and amount of fat-containing ingredients. Addition of fat during frying or basting may add to the saturated fat content of the final meal. Prepared foods include recipes made at home takeout food, restaurant food, and commercial prepackaged items.

Chapter 11

Facts about
High Blood Pressure

It's Important to Know about High Blood Pressure

High blood pressure, also called hypertension, is a risk factor for heart and kidney diseases and stroke. This means that having high blood pressure increases your chance (or risk) of getting heart or kidney disease, or of having a stroke. This is serious business: Heart disease is the number one killer in the United States, and stroke is the third most common cause of death.

About one in every four American adults has high blood pressure. High blood pressure is especially dangerous because it often gives no warning signs or symptoms. Fortunately, though, you can find out if you have high blood pressure by having your blood pressure checked regularly. If it is high, you can take steps to lower it. Just as important, **if your blood pressure is normal, you can learn how to keep it from becoming high. This fact sheet will tell you how.**

The National Heart, Lung, and Blood Institute—part of the National Institutes of Health—sponsors a nationwide education program to help people avoid the ill effects of high blood pressure, and to help prevent high blood pressure altogether.

NIH Pub. No. 94-3281.

81

What Is Blood Pressure—and What Happens When II Is High?

Since blood is carried from the heart to all of your body's tissues and organs in vessels called arteries, blood pressure is the force of the blood pushing against the walls of those arteries. In fact, each time the heart beats (about 60-70 times a minute at rest), it pumps out blood into the arteries. Your blood pressure is at its greatest when the heart contracts and is pumping the blood. This is called **systolic pressure**. When the heart is at rest, in between beats, your blood pressure falls. This is the **diastolic pressure**.

Blood pressure is always given as these two numbers, systolic and diastolic pressures. Both are important. Usually they are written one above or before the other, such as 120/80 mm Hg, with the top number the systolic, and the bottom the diastolic.

Different actions make your blood pressure go up or down. For example, if you run for a bus, your blood pressure goes up. When you sleep at night, your blood pressure goes down. These changes in blood pressure are normal.

Some people have blood pressure that stays up all or most of the time. Their blood pushes against the walls of their arteries with higher-than-normal force. If untreated this can lead to serious medical problems like these:

Arteriosclerosis ("hardening of the arteries"). High blood pressure harms the arteries by making them thick and stiff. This speeds the build up of cholesterol and fats in the blood vessels like rust in a pipe, which prevents the blood from flowing through the body, and in time can lead to a heart attack or stroke.

Heart attack. Blood carries oxygen to the body. When the arteries that bring blood to the heart muscle become blocked, the heart cannot get enough oxygen. Reduced blood flow can cause chest pain (angina). Eventually, the flow may be stopped completely, causing a heart attack.

Enlarged Heart. High blood pressure causes the heart to work harder. Over time, this causes the heart to thicken and stretch. Eventually the heart fails to function normally causing fluids to back up into the lungs. Controlling high blood pressure can prevent this from happening.

Kidney damage. The kidney acts as a filter to rid the body of wastes. Over a number of years, high blood pressure can narrow and thicken the blood vessels of the kidney. The kidney filters less fluid and waste builds up in the blood. The kidneys may fail altogether. When this happens, medical treatment (dialysis) or a kidney transplant may be needed.

Stroke. High blood pressure can harm the arteries, causing them to narrow faster. So, less blood can get to the brain. If a blood clot blocks one of the narrowed arteries, a stroke (thrombotic stroke) may occur. A stroke can also occur when very high pressure causes a break in a weakened blood vessel in the brain (hemorrhagic stroke).

Who's Likely to Develop High Blood Pressure?

Anyone can develop high blood pressure, but some people are more likely to develop it than others. For example, high blood pressure is more common—it develops earlier and is more severe—in African-Americans than in whites.

In the early and middle adult years, men have high blood pressure more often than women. But as men and women age, the reverse is true. More women after menopause have high blood pressure than men of the same age. And the number of **both** men and women with high blood pressure increases rapidly in older age groups. More than half of all Americans over age 65 have high blood pressure. And older African-American women who live in the Southeast are more likely to have high blood pressure than those in other regions of the United States.

In fact, the southeastern states have some of the highest rates of death from stroke. High blood pressure is the key risk factor for stroke. Other risk factors include cigarette smoking and overweight. These 11 states—Alabama, Arkansas, Georgia, Indiana, Kentucky, Louisiana, Mississippi, North Carolina, South Carolina, Tennessee, and Virginia—have such high rates of stroke among persons of all races and in both sexes that they are called the "Stroke Belt States."

Finally, heredity can make some families more likely than others to get high blood pressure. If your parents or grandparents had high blood pressure, your risk may be increased. While it is mainly a disease of adults, high blood pressure can occur in children as well. Even if everyone is healthy, be sure you and your family get your blood pressure checked. Remember high blood pressure has no signs or symptoms.

How Is Blood Pressure Checked?

Having your blood pressure checked is quick, easy, and painless. Your blood pressure is measured with an instrument called a sphygmomanometer (sfig'-mo-ma-nom-e-ter).

It works like this: A blood pressure cuff is wrapped around your upper arm and inflated to stop the blood flow in your artery for a few seconds. A valve is opened and air is then released from the cuff and the sounds of your blood rushing through an artery are heard through a stethoscope. The first sound heard and registered on the gauge or mercury column is called the **systolic** blood pressure. It represents the maximum pressure in the artery produced as the heart contracts and the blood begins to flow. The last sound heard as more air is released from the cuff is the **diastolic** blood pressure. It represents the lowest pressure that remains within the artery when the heart is at rest.

What Do the Numbers Mean?

Blood pressure is always expressed in two numbers that represent the systolic and diastolic pressures. These numbers are measurements of millimeters (mm) of mercury (Hg). The measurement is written one above or before the other, with the systolic number on the top and the diastolic number on the bottom. For example, a blood pressure measurement of 120/80 mm Hg is expressed verbally as "120 over 80." See the [table on the top of the next page] which shows categories for blood pressure levels in adults.

If your blood pressure is less than 140/90 mm Hg it is considered normal. However, a blood pressure below 120/80 mm Hg is even better for your heart and blood vessels. People use to think that low blood pressure (for example, 105/65 mm Hg in an adult) was unhealthy. Except for rare cases, this is not true. High blood pressure or "hypertension" is classified by stages and is more serious as the numbers get higher.

84

CATEGORIES FOR BLOOD PRESSURE LEVELS IN ADULTS		
(AGE 18 YEARS AND OLDER)		
	Blood Pressure Level (mm Hg)	
Category	Systolic	Diastolic
Normal	<130	<85
High normal	130-139	85-89
Hypertension*		
Stage 1	140-159	90-99
Stage 2	160-179	100-109
Stage 3	180-209	110-119
Stage 4	≥210	≥120

*Note: "Hypertension" is the medical term for high blood pressure. These categories are from the National High Blood Pressure Education Program, JNCV Report.

(<=less than   >=greater than or equal to)

Figure 11.1.

What Causes High Blood Pressure?

For most people, there is no single known cause of high blood pressure. This type of high blood pressure is called "primary" or "essential" hypertension. This type of blood pressure can't be cured, although in most cases it can be controlled. That's why it's so important for everyone to take steps to reduce their chances of developing high blood pressure.

In a few people, high blood pressure can be traced to a known cause like tumors of the adrenal gland, chronic kidney disease, hormone abnormalities, use of birth control pills, or pregnancy. This is called "secondary hypertension." Secondary hypertension is usually cured if its cause passes or is corrected.

How Can You Prevent High Blood Pressure?

Everyone—regardless of race, age, sex, or heredity—can help lower their chance of developing high blood pressure. Here's how:

1. Maintain a healthy weight, lose weight if you are over-weight,

2. Be more physically active,

3. Choose foods lower in salt and sodium, and

4. If you drink alcoholic beverages, do so in moderation.

These rules are also recommended for treating high blood pressure, although medicine is often added as part of the treatment. It is far better to keep your blood pressure from getting high in the first place.

Another important measure for your health is to not smoke: While cigarette smoking is not directly related to high blood pressure, it increases your risk of heart attack and stroke.

Let's look more closely at the four rules to prevent high blood pressure and for keeping a healthy heart:

Rule 1: Maintain a Healthy Weight, Lose Weight If You Are Overweight

As your body weight increases, your blood pressure rises. In fact, being overweight can make you two to six times more likely to develop high blood pressure than if you are at your desirable weight. Keeping your weight in the desirable range is not only important to prevent high blood pressure but also for your overall health and well being.

It's not just **how much** you weigh that's important: It also matters **where** your body stores extra fat. Your shape is inherited from your parents just like the color of your eyes or hair. Some people tend to gain weight around their belly; others, around the hips and thighs. "Apple-shaped" people who have a pot belly (that is, extra fat at the waist) appear to have higher health risks than "pear-shaped" people with heavy hips and thighs.

No matter where the extra weight is, you can reduce your risk of high blood pressure by losing weight. Even small amounts of weight loss can make a big difference in helping to prevent high blood pressure. Losing weight, if you are overweight and already have high blood pressure, can also help lower your pressure.

To lose weight, you need to eat fewer calories than you burn. But **don't** go on a crash diet to see how quickly you can lose those pounds. The healthiest and longest-lasting weight loss happens when you do it slowly, losing 1/2 to 1 pound a week. By cutting back by 500 calories a day by eating less and being more physically active, you can lose about 1 pound (which equals 3,500 calories) in a week.

Losing weight and keeping it off involves a new way of eating and increasing physical activity for life. Here's how to eat and get on your way to a lower weight:

Choose foods low in calories and fat. Naturally, choosing low-calorie foods cuts calories. But did you know that choosing foods low in fat also cuts calories? Fat is a concentrated source of calories, so eating fewer fatty foods will reduce calorie intake. Some examples of fatty foods to cut down on are: butter, margarine, regular salad dressings, fatty meats, skin of poultry, whole-milk dairy foods like cheese, fried foods, and many cookies, cakes, pastries and snacks.

Choose foods high in starch and fiber. Foods high in starch and fiber are excellent substitutes for foods high in fat. They are lower in calories than foods high in fat. These foods are also good sources of vitamins and minerals.

Limit serving sizes. To lose weight, it's not just the **type** of foods you eat that's important, but also the **amount**. To take in fewer calories, you need to limit your portion sizes. Try especially to take smaller helpings of high calorie foods like high fat meats and cheeses. And try not to go back for seconds.

Here's a good tip to help you control or change your eating habits: Keep track of what you eat, when you eat, and why, by writing it down. Note whether you snack on high fat foods in front of the television, or if you skip breakfast and then eat a large lunch. Once you see your habits, you can set goals for yourself: Cut back on TV snacks and, when you do snack, have fresh fruit, unsalted air-popped popcorn, or unsalted pretzels. If there's no time for breakfast at home, take a low fat muffin, bagel (skip the cream cheese), or cereal with you to eat at work. Changing your behavior will help you change your weight for the better.

Increase physical activity. There's more to weight loss than just eating less. Another important ingredient is increasing physical activity, which burns calories. Cutting down on fat and calories combined with regular physical activity can help you lose more weight and keep it off longer than either way by itself. Check the [table below] to see how many calories you can burn during different activities.

CALORIES BURNED DURING PHYSICAL ACTIVITIES

Activity	Calories Burned Up Per Hour*	
	Man**	Woman**
Light activity:	300	240
Cleaning house		
Playing baseball		
Playing golf		
Moderate activity:	460	370
Walking briskly (3.5 mph)		
Gardening		
Cycling (5.5 mph)		
Dancing		
Playing basketball		
Strenuous activity:	730	580
Jogging (9 min./mile)		
Playing football		
Swimming		
Very strenuous activity:	920	740
Running (7 min./mile)		
Racquetball		
Skiing		

* May vary depending on a variety of factors including environmental conditions.
**Healthy man, 175 pounds; healthy woman, 140 pounds.

Source: Dietary Guidelines for Americans, U.S. Department of Agriculture, U.S. Department of Health and Human Services, Third edition, 1990 (adapted from McArdle, et al., "Exercise Physiology," 1986).

Figure 11.2.

Rule 2: Be More Physically Active

Besides losing weight, there are other reasons to be more active: Being physically active can reduce your risk for heart disease, help lower your total cholesterol level and raise HDL-cholesterol (the "good" cholesterol that does not build up in the arteries), and help lower high blood pressure. And people who are physically active have a lower risk of getting high blood pressure—20 to 50 percent lower—than people who are not active. You don't have to be a marathon runner to benefit from physical activity. Even light activities, if done daily, can help lower your risk of heart disease. So you can fit physical activity into your daily routine in small but important ways.

More vigorous exercise has added benefits. It helps improve the fitness of the heart and lungs. And that in turn protects you more against heart disease. Activities like swimming, brisk walking, running, and jumping rope are called "aerobic." This means that the body uses oxygen to make the energy it needs for the activity. Aerobic activities can condition your heart and lungs if done at the right intensity for at least 30 minutes, three to four times a week. But if you don't have 30 minutes for a break, try to find two 15-minute periods or even three 10-minute periods. Try to do some type of aerobic activity in the course of a week.

Most people don't need to see a doctor before they start exercising, since a gradual, sensible exercise program has few health risks. But if you have a health problem like high blood pressure; if you have pains or pressure in the chest or shoulder area; if you tend to feel dizzy or faint; if you get very breathless after a mild workout; or are middle-age or older and have not been active, and you are planning a vigorous exercise program, you should check with your doctor first. Otherwise, get out, get active, and get fit—and help prevent high blood pressure. The sample walking program [on the next two pages] can help you get started.

Rule 3: Choose Foods Lower in Salt and Sodium

Americans eat more salt (sodium chloride) and other forms of sodium than they need. And guess what? They also have higher rates of high blood pressure than people in other countries who eat less salt.

Often, if people with high blood pressure cut back on salt and sodium, their blood pressure falls. Cutting back on salt and sodium also prevents blood pressure from rising. Some people like African-Ameri-

A SAMPLE WALKING PROGRAM

	Warm up	Target zone exercising*	Cool down time	Total
Week 1				
Session A	Walk normally 5 min.	Then walk briskly 5 min.	Then walk normally 5 min.	15 min.
Session B	Repeat above pattern			
Session C	Repeat above pattern			

Continue with at least three exercise sessions during each week of the program. If you find a particular week's pattern tiring, repeat it before going on to the next pattern. You do not have to complete the walking program in 12 weeks.

	Warm up	Target zone exercising*	Cool down time	Total
Week 2	Walk 5 min.	Walk briskly 7 min.	Walk 5 min.	17 min.
Week 3	Walk 5 min.	Walk briskly 9 min.	Walk 5 min.	19 min.
Week 4	Walk 5 min.	Walk briskly 11 min.	Walk 5 min.	21 min.
Week 5	Walk 5 min.	Walk briskly 13 min.	Walk 5 min.	23 min.
Week 6	Walk 5 min.	Walk briskly 15 min.	Walk 5 min.	25 min.
Week 7	Walk 5 min.	Walk briskly 18 min.	Walk 5 min.	28 min.
Week 8	Walk 5 min.	Walk briskly 20 min.	Walk 5 min.	30 min.
Week 9	Walk 5 min.	Walk briskly 23 min.	Walk 5 min.	33 min.
Week 10	Walk 5 min.	Walk briskly 26 min.	Walk 5 min.	36 min.
Week 11	Walk 5 min.	Walk briskly 28 min.	Walk 5 min.	38 min.
Week 12	Walk 5 min.	Walk briskly 30 min.	Walk 5 min.	40 min.

Week 13 on:

Check your pulse periodically to see if you are exercising within your target zone. As you get more in shape, try exercising within the upper range of your target zone. Gradually increase your brisk walking time to 30 to 60 minutes, three or four times a week. Remember that your goal is to get the benefits you are seeking and enjoy your activity.

Figure 11.3(a)

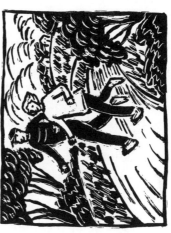

* Here's how to check if you are within your target heart rate zone:

1) Right after you stop exercising, take your pulse: Place the tips of your first two fingers lightly over one of the blood vessels on your neck, just to the left or right of your Adam's apple. Or try the pulse spot inside your wrist just below the base of your thumb.

2) Count your pulse for 10 seconds and multiply the number by 6.

3) Compare the number to the right grouping below: Look for the age grouping that is closest to your age and read the line across. For example, if you are 43, the closest age on the chart is 45; the target zone is 88-131 beats per minute.

AGE	Target HR Zone
20 years	100-150 beats per minute
25 years	98-146 beats per minute
30 years	95-142 beats per minute
35 years	93-138 beats per minute
40 years	90-135 beats per minute
45 years	88-131 beats per minute
50 years	85-127 beats per minute
55 years	83-123 beats per minute
60 years	80-120 beats per minute
65 years	78-116 beats per minute
70 years	75-113 beats per minute

SOURCE: *Exercise and Your Heart*, National Heart, Lung, and Blood Institute and the American Heart Association, NIH Publication No. 93-1677.

Figure 11.3(b)

cans and the elderly are more affected by sodium than others. Since there's really no practical way to predict exactly who will be affected by sodium, it makes sense to limit intake of salt and sodium to help prevent high blood pressure.

All Americans, especially people with high blood pressure, should eat no more than about 6 grams of salt a day, which equals about 2,400 milligrams of sodium. That's about 1 teaspoon of table salt. But remember to keep track of **ALL** salt eaten—including that in processed foods and added during cooking or at the table. Americans eat 4,000 to 6,000 milligrams of sodium a day, so most people need to cut back on salt and sodium.

You can teach your taste buds to enjoy less salty foods. Here are a few tips:

- Check food labels for the amount of sodium in foods. Choose those lower in sodium most of the time. *Look for products that say "sodium free," "very low sodium," "low sodium," "light in sodium," "reduced or less sodium," or "unsalted," especially on cans, boxes, bottles, and bags.*

- Buy fresh, plain frozen, or canned with "no salt added" vegetables. Use fresh poultry, fish and lean meat, rather than canned or processed types.

- Use herbs, spices, and salt-free seasoning blends in cooking and at the table instead of salt. See the [list titled "Spice It Up"] on ways to spice up your foods.

- Cook rice, pasta, and hot cereals without salt. Cut back on instant or flavored rice, pasta, and cereal mixes because they usually have added salt.

- Choose "convenience" foods that are lower in sodium. Cut back on frozen dinners, mixed dishes like pizza, packaged mixes, canned soups or broths, and salad dressings which often have a lot of sodium.

- When available, buy low- or reduced-sodium, or "no-salt-added" versions of foods like these: canned soup, dried soup mixes, bouillon; canned vegetables and vegetable juices;

cheeses, lower in fat; margarine; condiments like catsup, soy sauce; crackers and baked goods; processed lean meats; and snack foods like chips, pretzels, nuts.

- Rinse canned foods like tuna to remove some sodium.

Spice It Up

It's easy to make foods tasty without using salt. Try these foods with the suggested flavorings, spices, and herbs:

MEAT, POULTRY AND FISH

- **Beef:** Bay leaf, marjoram, nutmeg, onion, pepper, sage, thyme
- **Lamb:** Curry powder, garlic, rosemary, mint
- **Pork:** Garlic, onion, sage, pepper, oregano
- **Veal:** Bay leaf, curry powder, ginger, marjoram, oregano
- **Chicken:** Ginger, marjoram, oregano, paprika, poultry seasoning, rosemary, sage, tarragon, thyme
- **Fish:** Curry powder, dill, dry mustard, lemon juice, marjoram, paprika, pepper

VEGETABLES

- **Carrots:** Cinnamon, cloves, marjoram, nutmeg, rosemary, sage
- **Corn:** Cumin, curry powder, onion, paprika, parsley
- **Green Beans:** Dill, curry powder, lemon juice, marjoram, oregano, tarragon, thyme
- **Greens:** Onion, pepper
- **Peas:** Ginger, marjoram, onion, parsley, sage
- **Potatoes:** Dill, garlic, onion, paprika, parsley, sage
- **Summer Squash:** Cloves, curry powder, marjoram, nutmeg, rosemary, sage
- **Winter Squash:** Cinnamon, ginger, nutmeg, onion
- **Tomatoes:** Basil, bay leaf, dill, marjoram, onion, oregano, parsley, pepper

Rule 4: If You Drink Alcoholic Beverages, Do So in Moderation

Drinking too much alcohol can raise your blood pressure. It may also lead to the development of high blood pressure. So to help prevent high blood pressure, if you drink alcohol, limit how much you drink to no more than 2 drinks a day. The "Dietary Guidelines for Americans" recommend that for overall health women should limit their alcohol to no more than 1 drink a day.

This is what counts as a drink:

- 1-1/2 ounces of 80-proof or 1 ounce of 100-proof whiskey,
- 5 ounces of wine, or
- 12 ounces of beer (regular or light).

You may have heard that some alcohol is good for your heart health. Some news reports suggest that people who consume a drink or two a day have lower blood pressure and live longer than those who consume no alcohol or those who consume excessive amounts of alcohol. Others note that wine raises the "good" blood cholesterol that prevents the build up of fats in the arteries. While these news stories may be correct they don't tell the whole story: Too much alcohol contributes to a host of other health problems, such as motor vehicle accidents, diseases of the liver and pancreas, damage to the brain and heart, an increased risk of many cancers, and fetal alcohol syndrome. Alcohol is also high in calories. So you should limit how much you drink.

What Else Might Prevent High Blood Pressure?

Other things also may help prevent blood pressure. Here's a roundup of what's being said about them—and whether it's true or false.

Dietary Supplements—Potassium, Calcium, Magnesium, Fish Oils

Potassium. Eating foods rich in potassium appears to protect some people from developing high blood pressure. You probably can get enough potassium from your diet, so a supplement isn't necessary.

Many fruits, vegetables, dairy foods, and fish are good sources of potassium.

Calcium. Populations with low calcium intakes have high rates of high blood pressure. However, it has not been proven that taking calcium tablets will prevent high blood pressure. But it is important to be sure to get at least the recommended amount of calcium—800 milligrams per day for adults (pregnant and breastfeeding women need more)—from the foods you eat. Dairy foods like, low fat selections of milk, yogurt, and cheese are good sources of calcium. Low fat and nonfat dairy products have even more calcium than the high fat types.

Magnesium. A diet low in magnesium may make your blood pressure rise. But doctors don't recommend taking extra magnesium to help prevent high blood pressure—the amount you get in a healthy diet is enough. Magnesium is found in whole grains, green leafy vegetables, nuts, seeds, and dry peas and beans.

Fish oils. A type of fat called "omega-3 fatty acids" is found in fatty fish like mackerel and salmon. Large amounts of fish oils may help reduce high blood pressure, but their role in prevention is unclear. But taking fish oil pills is not recommended because high doses can cause unpleasant side effects. The pills are also high in fat and calories. Of course, most fish if not fried or made with added fat are low in saturated fat and calories and can be eaten often.

Other Factors

Fats, Carbohydrates, and Protein. Varying the amount and type of fats, carbohydrates, and protein in the diet has little, if any, effect on blood pressure. But for overall heart health, it is crucial to limit the amount of fat in your diet, especially the saturated fat found in foods like fatty meats and whole milk dairy foods. Saturated fats raise your blood cholesterol level, and a high blood cholesterol level is another risk factor for heart disease. Foods high in fat are also high in calories. Remember, foods high in complex carbohydrate (starch and fiber) are low in fat and calories—so eating these foods in moderate amounts instead of high fat foods can help you to lose weight if you are overweight or to prevent you from gaining weight.

Caffeine. The caffeine in drinks like coffee, tea, and sodas may cause blood pressure to go up, but only temporarily. In a short time your blood pressure will go back down. Unless you are sensitive to caffeine and your blood pressure does not go down, you do not have to limit caffeine to prevent developing high blood pressure.

Garlic or Onions. Increased amounts of garlic and onions have not been found to affect blood pressure. Of course, they are tasty substitutes for salty seasonings and can be used often.

Stress Management. Stress can make blood pressure go up for a while and over time, may contribute to the cause of high blood pressure. So it's natural to think that stress management techniques like biofeedback, meditation, and relaxation would help prevent high blood pressure. But this doesn't seem to be the case: the few studies that have looked at this have not shown that stress management helps to prevent high blood pressure. Of course, stress management techniques are helpful if they help you feel better or stick to a weight-loss and/or exercise program.

Here's a Recap

After going through all the things that may affect blood pressure, it's worth noting again the things that are sure to help you prevent high blood pressure:

1. Maintaining a healthy weight—losing weight if you are overweight,

2. Being more physically active,

3. Choosing foods low in salt and sodium, and

4. If you drink alcoholic beverages, doing so in moderation.

By following these guidelines, you can help reduce or prevent high blood pressure for life—and, in turn, lower your risk for heart disease and stroke.

Want to Know More?

For more information on either high blood pressure or weight and physical activity, contact:

National Heart, Lung, and Blood Institute Information Center
P.O. Box 30105
Bethesda, MD 20824-0105
(301) 251-1222

Chapter 12

Aneurysms and Other Vascular Disorders

Aneurysms

An aneurysm is a bulging, balloon-like sac that occurs on the wall of a blood vessel (artery or vein) or the heart. When an aneurysm ruptures spontaneously, internal bleeding occurs. Three common types of aneurysms are aortic aneurysms, peripheral artery aneurysms, and berry aneurysms.

Although aneurysms occur in many places in the body, the most common place for one to occur is on the abdominal aorta below the renal (kidney) arteries. The abdominal aorta is the large blood vessel that carries blood from the heart into other arteries. Thoracic aneurysms, another type of aortic aneurysm, develop on the aorta in the chest by the heart.

An aortic aneurysm's risk for rupture increases with the size of the aneurysm. Aortic aneurysms less than two inches in diameter do not often rupture, but patients with untreated aortic aneurysms

This chapter summarizes the content of several information packets available from the National Heart, Lung, and Blood Institute and reproduces the text from "Aneurysm Clips and MRI," *FDA Consumer*, July-August 1993 and "Stent Approved for Unclogging Leg Arteries" *FDA Consumer*, January-February 1992. To receive one of the NHLBI's packets on aneurysms, leg ulcers, thrombophlebitis, pulmonary embolisms, deep vein thrombosis, or information on other cardiovascular disorders contact the NHLBI Information Center at P.O. Box 30105, Bethesda, MD 20824-0105. Phone (301) 251-1222; fax (301) 251-1223.

greater than two and a half inches face a 90 percent chance of dying within five years. According to a 1992 report in *FDA Consumer*, ruptured aortic aneurysms were the ninth leading killer of American men over the age of 55.

Peripheral artery aneurysms occur in the femoral (down the leg) and popliteal (behind the knee) arteries. Peripheral artery aneurysms in the groin area are more likely to burst than those behind the knee. Those behind the knee, however, can interfere with blood circulation in the lower leg which, if untreated, can result in the need for amputation.

Berry aneurysms occur in arteries at the base of the brain and look like berries. When berry aneurysms rupture they cause hemorrhagic strokes. This type of stroke strikes approximately 30,000 people in the U.S. each year. Approximately 50 percent of the victims die immediately and many more suffer longer-term fatal complications from recurring bleeding and irreversible brain damage.

Several causes contribute to the development of aneurysms including hardening of the arteries (atherosclerosis), high blood pressure, cigarette smoking, congenital defects, heredity, injuries, diabetes, syphilis, and cocaine use.

Symptoms

People with abdominal aneurysms may experience lower back pain or abdominal pain, but for nearly 75 percent of patients, there are no symptoms. Abdominal aneurysms may be discovered during routine physical examinations if the physician sees or feels a throbbing mass. Peripheral artery aneurysms can also sometimes be seen or felt upon examination.

Symptoms associated with thoracic aneurysms can include pain in the shoulder, lower back, neck and abdomen, a persistent dry cough (described as "brassy"), hoarseness, and loss of voice. Thoracic aneurysms can also be discovered on chest x-rays. A complication of a thoracic aneurysm called a dissecting aortic aneurysm results when the artery wall is separated. This can result in a tearing chest pain that is sometimes mistaken for a heart attack.

Berry aneurysms frequently present no symptoms until the aneurysm ruptures. Warning signs, present in only ten percent of cases, include headaches, nausea and neck stiffness. A ruptured berry aneurysm can cause a severe headache, nausea, vomiting, and temporary or permanent loss of consciousness. Other symptoms may include blurred vision, paralysis on one side of the body, difficulty walking or talking, seizures, or personality changes.

Treatment

Aortic aneurysms less than two inches are usually treated with drugs (for example, beta blockers) to lower blood pressure and the aneurysm is carefully monitored. Large aortic aneurysms can be treated by surgically replacing the affected blood vessel with a special man-made material, however, the operation is a difficult procedure. For peripheral artery aneurysms the affected portion of the artery can be replaced using part of the leg vein.

Berry aneurysms can be diagnosed using an angiogram (an x-ray procedure using a dye to make the blood vessels more visible) and a CT scan (another special x-ray-type procedure). Berry aneurysms that are diagnosed before rupturing are typically removed if they are causing pain or other symptoms or if they are larger than two-fifths of an inch. Ruptured berry aneurysms can sometimes be repaired using special metal clips that help recreate a passageway through which blood flow can be restored.

Aneurysm Clips and MRI (FDA Consumer, 7-8/93)

Physicians should exercise caution when ordering or performing magnetic resonance imaging (MRI) scans on patients who have aneurysm clips, FDA urges.

Aneurysm clips are spring devices surgically implanted to take pressure off a blood-filled ballooning, or aneurysm, that can occur on artery walls. MRI, a commonly used diagnostic technique, can induce a magnetic force on some clips that could dislodge the clip or cause hemorrhage.

FDA is alerting doctors about the possible hazard through an article in the *FDA Medical Bulletin.* The action follows a recent MRI-related death of a patient with an aneurysm clip implanted in the brain.

To help prevent an MRI mishap, FDA suggests that doctors give patients information about their particular implants and urge patients to carry an alert card or wear a medical bracelet or necklace identifying the implant. In addition, physicians and MRI facilities should carefully screen patients for metallic implants.

The agency stresses there is no way presently to ensure that a person with an implanted clip can be MRI-scanned safely. No established method exists to test the magnetic properties of aneurysm clips. Also, published safety studies are unreliable because they were conducted with a limited number of a particular model of clips and may not represent a company's entire production of that model, which may have changed over time. Of particular concern are steel or steel-alloy clips, as well as those made before MRI's advent in the mid-1980s.

Scans should be performed only when there are substantial medical benefits that cannot be achieved by other methods and when the implanted clip and its probable magnetic properties can be identified. But even with these precautions, FDA warns that there still are risks from possible magnetic effects.

Varicose Veins

Varicose veins occur when veins in the leg become distended. This may happen as a result of weakness in the walls of the blood vessels or as a result of valve malfunction. Factors that place individuals at risk for developing varicose veins include obesity, pregnancy, the use of birth control pills, the wearing of constricting clothing, and heredity. Varicose veins are a common condition and usually do not require medical treatment.

Symptoms

Varicose veins appear on the leg as discolored, bulging veins. Most patients with varicose veins have no other symptoms. When circulation is sufficiently obstructed, however, they may experience swelling in the foot and ankle, nocturnal leg and foot cramps, discomfort, itching, scaling, and in serious, untreated cases, skin ulcers.

Treatment

Elevating the affected leg and exercising are sometimes effective in treating varicose veins. Special elastic stockings can also be worn to help maintain circulation. Surgery can be performed to remove affected veins for cosmetic reasons or to help alleviate symptoms.

A procedure called sclerotherapy can also be used to treat varicose veins. Sclerotherapy involves injecting a solution into the vein which causes it to be destroyed and disappear. Blood flow is not affected because other unaffected veins can take over for the lost vein. After injection, the leg is wrapped with a compression bandage for several days (typically two to seven depending on the size and type of blood vessel involved). A reported 85 to 90 percent of patients experience relief of symptoms for a year following sclerotherapy. After three or four years, however, symptoms may return necessitating additional treatment.

Leg Ulcers

Leg ulcers are chronic lesions on the lower legs and feet that do not heal. They are a common problem. According to one estimate, two percent of the population will develop leg ulcers. Older people are more susceptible. Arterial lesions occur as a result of abnormal blood flow through the leg arteries. Venous lesions occur as a result of high pressure in the veins near the skin. Leg ulcers can also occur as a result of diseases other than arterial and vascular disorders. These include diabetes, infection, infestation, blood diseases, cellular disorders, lymphatic diseases, trauma, cancer, and as a side-effect from certain drugs.

Symptoms

Leg ulcers appear as lesions on the lower legs or feet. They can cause pain and are frequently accompanied by an unpleasant odor. The ulcers often restrict mobility. When pain is present upon exertion but can be relieved by rest, an arterial disease may be involved. Pain that is unrelated to exertion and that can be relieved by elevating the leg for extended periods of time may be related to a venous disease.

Treatment

Treating the actual wound site will include attempts to improve blood supply and clear up any infection that may be present. Treatment of the underlying cause of the ulcer may include efforts to lower blood pressure, reduce tissue swelling (edema), and improve circulation. Compression bandages or stockings may be used to help reduce pressure in the veins. A device called a compression pump can also be

used to improve blood flow. Exercise and weight control may help reduce instances of recurrence.

Stent Approved for Unclogging Leg Arteries (FDA Consumer, 1-2/92)

An implantable tube-shaped device was approved Sept. 27, 1991,
for unclogging iliac arteries in the pelvis when they are blocked with
fibrous deposits called plaque. The iliac arteries supply blood to the
legs, where severe blockage can lead to amputation.

FDA approved the Palmaz Balloon-Expandable Stent for use in
some patients when balloon angioplasty has failed to unclog their iliac
arteries.

In iliac balloon angioplasty, a balloon-tipped catheter is threaded
through a puncture in the thigh to the iliac artery. When the balloon
reaches the blockage, it's inflated to compress the plaque against the
artery walls. The balloon is then deflated, and the catheter withdrawn.

Implanting the Palmaz Stent also requires an angioplasty balloon. Collapsed over the deflated balloon at insertion, the device's
stainless-steel mesh "scaffold" expands with inflation of the balloon
and then remains in place to hold the artery open after the balloon is
removed.

Surgeons perform some 60,000 iliac balloon angioplasties each
year, according to the stent's manufacturer, Johnson & Johnson
Interventional Systems Company, of Warren, N.J. One study showed
that within six months, about 46 percent of these patients needed further treatment, such as repeat angioplasty, blood vessel surgery, or
even amputation, the firm said. By contrast, the firm's data on 202 patients implanted with the Palmaz Stent to treat iliac blockage after
angioplasty showed that only 5 percent required further treatment
during an 18-month follow-up.

On Feb. 5, 1991, the Center for Devices and Radiological Health
had approved the device to treat blockages of major bile ducts when
other techniques don't work. The stent is named for its inventor, Julio
Palmaz, M.D., of the University of Texas Health Science Center at San
Antonio.

Thrombophlebitis

Thrombophlebitis is a condition in which blood clots are formed as a result of the inflammation of a vein near the skin. Vein inflammation, called phlebitis, is typically the result of an infection or injury. Untreated thrombophlebitis can result in blood poisoning or deep-vein thrombosis.

Symptoms

Thrombophlebitis frequently causes pain, redness, tenderness, itching, and a cord-like swelling along the affected vein. Fever may also be present.

Treatment

According to The American Medical Association's *Family Medical Guide*, thrombophlebitis often clears up in approximately one week if it is not accompanied by an infection. Aspirin can help ease the pain and zinc oxide ointment can help reduce itching. Sometimes anti-inflammatory drugs are used to treat thrombophlebitis. When an infection is also present, antibiotics are often prescribed.

Deep Vein Thrombosis

While thrombophlebitis affects the veins near the skin, deep vein thrombosis affects veins deeper within the legs and arms. The condition results in approximately 300,000 hospitalizations annually. The primary danger of deep vein thrombosis is that it can lead to pulmonary embolism.

Symptoms

Deep vein thrombosis may cause pain or tenderness and redness or swelling of the whole limb. To diagnose deep vein thrombosis a doctor may use an ultrasound test or take an x-ray after injecting a dye into the veins.

Treatment

Deep vein thrombosis is typically treated by elevating the affected extremity (usually the leg) and with anticoagulants such as heparin and warfarin. Surgery, either to tie off a vein or to insert a filter, may be performed to prevent a clot from becoming dislodged and working its way into the lungs.

Pulmonary Embolism

An embolism is a clot of material, most often blood, that clogs an artery. Although an embolism can block any artery in any part of the body, the area most often affected is the lungs. An embolism in the lungs is called a pulmonary embolism. Pulmonary embolism is a common cardiopulmonary illness. According to one estimate, as many as 95 percent of all pulmonary emboli termed clinically significant originated from thrombosis in the leg veins (see thrombophlebitis and deep vein thrombosis).

Approximately ten percent of patients experiencing a pulmonary embolism die within the first hour. For the remaining 90 percent, however, prognosis for recovery is good.

Risk factors for developing a pulmonary embolism include prolonged periods of inactivity, stroke, heart attack, obesity, and leg or hip fractures.

Symptoms

A pulmonary embolism may cause shortness of breath, sudden chest pain, anxiety, sweating, blood-streaked sputum, and low grade fever. These symptoms can sometimes be mistaken for pneumonia. A massive embolism can result in loss of consciousness. To diagnose pulmonary embolism a physician may use a lung scan and an angiography.

Treatment

Pulmonary embolism is treated with anticoagulants such as heparin, dextran, and warfarin. Medication may be used to dissolve existing clots or to help prevent future clots. Aspirin, however, has not been demonstrated to be helpful in preventing embolism development, according to a document made available by The National Institutes of Health Office of Medical Applications of Research.

Chapter 13

Facts about Raynaud's Phenomenon

What is Raynaud's Phenomenon?

Raynaud's Phenomenon is a disorder of the small blood vessels that feed the skin. During an attack of Raynaud's, these arteries contract briefly, limiting blood flow. This is called a vasospasm. Deprived of the blood's oxygen, the skin first turns white then blue. The skin turns red as the arteries relax and blood flows again. Extremities—hands and feet—are most commonly affected, but Raynaud's can attack other areas such as the nose and ears.

What Are the Symptoms?

Symptoms include changes in skin color (white to blue to red) and skin temperature (the affected area feels cooler). Usually there is no pain, but it is common for the affected area to feel numb or prickly, as if it has fallen asleep.

What Causes Raynaud's?

Doctors do not completely understand the cause of Raynaud's, but they believe the body's blood vessels overreact to cold.

NIH Pub. No. 93-2263.

When the body is exposed to cold, the hands and feet lose heat rapidly. To conserve heat, the body reduces the amount of blood flowing to these areas by narrowing the small arteries that supply them with blood. In persons with Raynaud's, these small blood vessels over-respond to cold. For example, reaching into a refrigerator may trigger an attack.

Cold temperatures are more likely to provoke an attack when the individual is physically or emotionally stressed. For some persons, exposure to cold is not even necessary; stress alone causes vessels to narrow.

Who Is Affected?

Women between the ages of 15 and 50 are most often affected, but anyone can have the problem. It is not known for sure how many people suffer from these symptoms, but Raynaud's is a common problem.

How Is Raynaud's Diagnosed?

An attack is usually temporary, so the doctor relies on the patient's description to diagnose the problem. The doctor will also determine whether the patient has Raynaud's alone (called primary Raynaud's phenomenon) or if another disease or some aspect of the patient's lifestyle is causing the symptoms. If the problem is caused by another disease or risk factor, the patient is said to have secondary Raynaud's phenomenon.

Is Primary Raynaud's Different from Secondary Raynaud's?

Yes. Primary Raynaud's usually affects both hands and both feet, and the cause is not known for certain. Secondary Raynaud's usually affects either both hands or both feet. Causes of secondary Raynaud's can be identified. Smoking is one cause. Some drugs may also cause this form of Raynaud's phenomenon. These include:

- Some heart and blood medications.
- Migraine headache medications.

Other medical conditions that may cause secondary Raynaud's phenomenon include:

- *Scleroderma*: a thickening and hardening of the skin and other body tissues.

- *Systemic lupus erythematosus*: a chronic inflammation of the skin and organ systems.

- *Rheumatoid arthritis*: a chronic inflammation and swelling of tissue in the joints.

- *Blood flow reduction*: problems that slow or stop blood flow in a vessel. These include inflammation and hardening of the arteries (arteriosclerosis).

- *Nerve problems*: problems that affect the nerves supplying the muscles.

- *Pulmonary hypertension*: a condition in which the blood pressure rises in the blood vessels of the lungs.

Injuries may also cause Raynaud's phenomenon. They can result from frostbite, surgery, or other causes. For example, regular use of machinery such as chain saws and vibrating drills can hurt blood vessels. Other activities that may aggravate the phenomenon are regular typing and piano playing.

What Are the Treatments for Raynaud's?

Patients with primary Raynaud's are taught how to prevent attacks (see below). In patients with secondary Raynaud's, doctors first treat the underlying cause. Vasodilators—drugs that help relax artery walls to improve blood flow—may be prescribed for patients with secondary Raynaud's or primary Raynaud's that resists other forms of therapy.

Are There Ways to Prevent Attacks?

Yes. People suffering from Raynaud's should protect themselves from cold and keep all parts of their body warm—not just their extremities. Outdoors in winter, they should wear scarves, warm socks and boots, and mittens or gloves under mittens because gloves alone allow heat to escape. People with Raynaud's should also wear wristlets to close the space between the sleeve and mitten. Indoors, people should wear socks and comfortable shoes. When taking food out of the refrigerator or freezer, they should wear mittens, oven mitts, or pot holders.

Patients with Raynaud's should guard against cuts, bruises, and other injuries to the affected areas. Activities such as sewing may have to be limited.

Patients who smoke should quit. Doctors may also adjust medications if the drugs appear to be responsible for the symptoms.

After several sessions of training, patients can often prevent or stop attacks using biofeedback, a technique in which patients are taught to "think" their fingers or toes warm.

It is important for persons who suspect they have Raynaud's to talk with their personal physicians. The doctor can give advice on the best ways to manage and treat the problem.

What Is the Prognosis?

Between 40 to 60 percent of patients with primary Raynaud's respond to management techniques. A rare but serious complication of primary Raynaud's is dry gangrene, or dead flesh. This may occur if the arteries stay contracted so that blood cannot bring oxygen to the area.

In most people with secondary Raynaud's, the problem does not get worse. All patients with Raynaud's should discuss any questions about their prognosis with their doctor.

Is More Information Available on Raynaud's Phenomenon?

Yes. For more information, you may wish to contact:

Arthritis Foundation
1314 Spring Street
Atlanta, GA 30309
(404) 872-7100

United Scleroderma Foundation, Inc.
P.O. Box 350
Watsonville, CA 95077-0350
(408) 728-2202

American Lupus Society
23751 Madison Street
Torrance, CA 90505
(213) 373-1335

Chapter 14

Primary Pulmonary Hypertension

Introduction

Primary, or unexplained, pulmonary hypertension (PPH) is a rare lung disorder in which the blood pressure in the pulmonary artery rises far above normal levels for no apparent reason. The pulmonary artery is the blood vessel carrying oxygen-poor blood from the right ventricle, one of the pumping chambers of the heart, to the lungs. In the lungs, the blood picks up oxygen and then flows to the left side of the heart, where it is pumped by the left ventricle to the rest of the body through the aorta.

Hypertension is the medical term for an abnormally high blood pressure. Normal mean pulmonary-artery pressure is approximately 14 mmHg at rest. In the PPH patient, the mean blood pressure in the pulmonary artery is greater than 25 mmHg at rest and 30 mmHg during exercise. This abnormally high pressure (pulmonary hypertension) is associated with changes in the small blood vessels in the lungs, resulting in an increased resistance to blood flowing through the vessels.

This increased resistance, in turn, places a strain on the right ventricle, which now has to work harder than usual against the resistance to move adequate amounts of blood through the lungs.

NIH Pub. No. 92-3291.

Incidence

The true incidence of primary pulmonary hypertension is unknown. The first reported case occurred in 1891, when E. Romberg, a German doctor, published a description of a patient who, at autopsy, showed thickening of the pulmonary artery but no heart or lung disease that might have caused the condition. In 1951, when 39 cases were reported by Dr. D.T. Dresdale in the United States, the illness received its name.

Between 1967 and 1973, a 10-fold increase in unexplained pulmonary hypertension was reported in central Europe. The rise was subsequently traced to aminorex fumarate, an amphetamine-like drug introduced in Europe in 1965 to control appetite. Only about 1 in 1,000 people who took the drug developed PPH. When they stopped taking the drug, some improved considerably; in others, the disease kept getting worse. Once aminorex was removed from the market, the incidence of primary pulmonary hypertension went down to normal levels.

In the United States it has been estimated that 300 new cases of PPH are diagnosed each year; the greatest number are reported in women between the ages of 21 and 40. Indeed, at one time the disease was thought to occur among young women almost exclusively; we now know, however, that males and females in all age ranges, from very young children to elderly people, can get PPH. Apparently it also affects people of all race and ethnic origins equally.

Cause

There may be one or more causes of PPH; however, all remain unknown. The low incidence makes learning more about the disease extremely difficult. Studies of PPH also have been difficult because no animal model of the disease has been available. However, a strain of rats was recently identified in which pulmonary hypertension develops spontaneously. These rats may prove useful for the study of the causes and disease processes of PPH.

One thought is that some people with PPH may be hyperreactors. This means they are unusually susceptible to agents that cause constriction, or narrowing, of blood vessels. Indeed, people with Raynaud's disease, a condition in which the fingers and toes easily turn blue when cold because of an extreme reaction of the blood vessels in their fingers and toes to cold, seem to be more likely than others to get PPH.

PPH sometimes occurs among close family members, suggesting there may be some inherited tendency toward hyperreactivity. But even among brothers and sisters with PPH, the areas of the lung affected and the course of the disease may differ greatly.

Course of the Disease

Researchers believe that one of the ways PPH starts is with injury to the layer of cells (the endothelial cells) that line the small blood vessels of the lungs. This injury, which occurs for unknown reasons, may bring about changes in the way the endothelial cells interact with smooth muscle cells in the vessel wall. As a result, the smooth muscle contracts more than normal and thereby narrows the vessel.

The process eventually results in the development of extra amounts of tissue in the walls of the pulmonary arteries. The amount of muscle increases in some arteries, and muscle appears in the walls of arteries that normally have no muscle. With time, scarring, or fibrosis, of the arteries takes place, and they become stiff as well as thickened. Some vessels may become completely blocked. There is also a tendency for blood clots to form within the smaller arteries.

In response to the extra demands placed on it by PPH, the heart muscle gets bigger, and the right ventricle expands in size. Overworked and enlarged, the right ventricle gradually becomes weak and loses its ability to pump enough blood to the lungs. Eventually, the right side of the heart may fail completely, resulting in death.

Symptoms

In general, researchers find there is no correlation between the time PPH is thought to have started, the age at which it is diagnosed, and the severity of symptoms. In some patients, especially children, the disease progresses fairly rapidly.

The first symptom is frequently tiredness, with many patients thinking they tire easily because they are simply out of shape. Difficulty in breathing (dyspnea), dizziness, and even fainting spells (syncope) are also typical early symptoms. Swelling in the ankles or legs (edema), bluish lips and skin (cyanosis), and chest pain (angina) are among other symptoms of the disease.

Patients with PPH may also complain of a racing pulse; many feel they have trouble getting enough air. Palpitations, a strong throbbing sensation brought on by the increased rate of the heartbeat, can also cause discomfort.

Some people with PPH do not seek medical advice until they can no longer go about their daily routine. The more severe the symptoms, the more advanced the disease. In these more advanced stages, the patient is able to perform only minimal activity and has symptoms even when resting. The disease may worsen to the point where the patient is completely bedridden.

Diagnosis

PPH is rarely picked up in a routine medical examination. Even in its later stages, the signs of the disease can be confused with other conditions affecting the heart and lungs. Thus, much time can pass between the time the symptoms of PPH appear and a definite diagnosis is made.

PPH remains a diagnosis of exclusion. This means that it is diagnosed only after the doctor finds pulmonary hypertension and excludes or cannot find other reasons for the hypertension, such as a chronic obstructive pulmonary disease (chronic bronchitis and emphysema), pulmonary emboli, or some forms of congenital heart disease.

The first tests for PPH help the doctor determine how well the heart and lungs are performing. If the results of these tests do not give the doctor enough information, the doctor must perform a cardiac catheterization. The procedure, discussed below, is the way the doctor can make certain that the patient's problems are due to PPH and not to some other condition.

Electrocardiogram. The electrocardiogram (ECG) is a record of the electrical activity produced by the heart. An abnormal ECG may indicate that the heart is undergoing unusual stress.

In addition to the usual ECG performed while the patient is at rest, the doctor may order an exercise ECG. This ECG helps the doctor evaluate the performance of the heart during exercise. For example, walking a treadmill in the doctor's office.

Echocardiogram. In an echocardiogram, the doctor uses sound waves to map the structure of the heart by placing a slim device that looks like a microphone on the patient's chest. The instrument sends sound waves into the heart, which then are reflected back to form a moving image of the beating heart's structure on a TV screen. A record is made on paper or videotape. The moving pictures show how well the heart is functioning. The still pictures permit the doctor to measure the size of the heart and the thickness of the heart muscle; in the patient with severe pulmonary hypertension, the still pictures will show that the right heart is enlarged, while the left heart is either normal or reduced in size.

Pulmonary Function Tests. A variety of tests called pulmonary function tests (PFTs) evaluate lung function. In these procedures, the patient, with a nose clip in place, breathes in and out through a mouthpiece. The patient's breathing displaces the air held in a container suspended in water. As the container rises and falls in response to the patient's breathing, the movements produce a record, or spirogram, that helps the doctor measure lung volume (how much air the lungs hold) and the air flow in and out of the lungs. Some devices measure air flow electronically.

A mild restriction in air movement is commonly seen in patients with PPH. This restriction is thought to be due, in part, to the increased stiffness of the lungs resulting from both the changes in the structure and the high blood pressure in the pulmonary arteries.

Perfusion Lung Scan. A perfusion lung scan shows the pattern of blood flow in the lungs; it can also tell the doctor whether a patient has large blood clots in the lungs. In the perfusion scan, the doctor injects a radioactive substance into a vein. Immediately after the injection, the chest is scanned for radioactivity. Areas in the lung where blood clots are blocking the flow of blood will show up as blank or clear areas.

Two patterns of pulmonary perfusion are seen in patients with PPH. One is a normal pattern of blood distribution; the other shows a scattering of patchy abnormalities in blood flow. A major reason for doing a perfusion scan is to distinguish patients with PPH from those whose pulmonary hypertension is due to blood clots in the lungs.

Right-Heart Cardiac Catheterization. In right-heart cardiac catheterization, the doctor places a thin, flexible tube, or catheter, through an arm, leg, or neck vein in the patient, and then threads the

117

catheter into the right ventricle and pulmonary artery. Most important in terms of PPH is the ability of the doctor to get a precise measure of the blood pressure in the right side of the heart and the pulmonary artery with this procedure. It is the only way to get this measure, and must be performed in the hospital by a specialist.

During catheterization, the doctor can also evaluate the right heart's pumping ability; this is done by measuring the amount of blood pumped out of the right side of the heart with each heartbeat.

Functional Classification. Once PPH is diagnosed, most doctors will classify the disease according to the functional classification system developed by the New York Heart Association. It is based on patient reports of how much activity they can comfortably undertake.

- Class 1: Patients with no symptoms of any kind, and for whom ordinary physical activity does not cause fatigue, palpitation, dyspnea, or anginal pain.

- Class 2: Patients who are comfortable at rest but have symptoms with ordinary physical activity.

- Class 3: Patients who are comfortable at rest but have symptoms with less-than-ordinary effort.

- Class 4: Patients who have symptoms at rest.

Treatment

Some patients do well by taking medicines that make the work of the right ventricle easier. Anticoagulants, for example, can decrease the tendency of the blood to clot, thereby permitting blood to flow more freely. Diuretics decrease the amount of fluid in the body, further reducing the amount of work the heart has to do.

Until recently, nothing more could be done for people who have primary pulmonary hypertension. However, today doctors can choose from a variety of drugs that help lower blood pressure in the lungs and improve the performance of the heart in many patients.

Some patients also require supplemental oxygen delivered through nasal prongs or a mask if breathing becomes difficult; some need oxygen around the clock. In severely affected cases, a heart-lung, single lung, or double lung transplantation may be appropriate.

Drugs

Doctors now know that PPH patients respond differently to the different medicines that dilate, or relax, blood vessels and that no one drug is consistently effective in all patients. Because individual reactions vary, different drugs have to be tried before chronic or long-term treatment begins. During the course of the disease, the amount and type of medicine may also have to be changed. To find out which medicine works best for a particular patient, doctors evaluate the drugs during cardiac catheterization. This way they can see the effect of the medicine on the patient's heart and lungs. They can also adjust the dose to reduce the side effects that may occur—for example, systemic low blood pressure (hypotension); nausea; angina; headaches; or flushing.

To determine whether a drug is improving a patient's condition, both the pulmonary pressure and the amount of blood being pumped by the heart (the cardiac output) must be evaluated. A decrease in pulmonary pressure alone, for example, does not necessarily mean that the patient is recovering; cardiac output must either increase or remain unchanged. The most desirable response is a decrease in pressure and an increase in cardiac output. Once the patient has reached a stable condition, he or she can go home, returning every few weeks or months to the doctor for followup.

At present, results with calcium channel blocking drugs are encouraging. By relaxing the smooth muscle in the walls of the heart and blood vessels, these calcium blockers improve the ability of the heart to pump blood.

A new vasodilator, prostacycline, is helping some severely ill patients. The drug, which is now being studied in clinical trials, imitates the natural prostacycline that the body produces on its own to dilate blood vessels. Prostacycline also seems to help prevent blood clots from forming.

Prostacycline is administered intravenously by a portable, battery-operated syringe pump. The pump is worn attached to a belt around the waist or carried in a small shoulder pack. The medicine is then slowly and continuously pumped into the body through a catheter placed in a vein in the neck.

Prostacycline seems to improve pulmonary hypertension and permit more physical activity. Currently limited in supply, it is sometimes used as a bridge to help those patients waiting for a transplant. It may become long-term treatment for more patients once it is released for general distribution.

Transplantation

The first heart-lung transplant was performed in this country in 1981. Many of these operations were performed for patients with primary pulmonary hypertension. The survival rate is the same as for other patients with heart-lung transplants, about 60 percent for 1 year, and 37 percent for 5 years.

Meanwhile, the single lung transplant is becoming another method of transplant used in cases of PPH. This newer procedure, in which one lung—either the left or right—is replaced, was first performed in 1983 in patients with pulmonary fibrosis. Double lung transplants have also been done to treat PPH, but are less common than the single lung transplant for treatment of PPH.

There are fewer complications with the single lung transplant than with the heart-lung transplant, and the survival rate is on the order of 70 to 80 percent for 1 year. A surprising finding is the remarkable ability of the right ventricle to heal itself. In patients with lung transplants, both the structure and function of the right ventricle markedly improve.

The Primary Pulmonary Hypertension Patient Registry (1981-1988)

In 1981, the National Heart, Lung, and Blood Institute (NHLBI) established the first PPH-patient registry in the world. The registry followed 194 people with PPH; over a period of at least 1 year and, in some cases, for as long as 7.5 years. Much of what we know about the illness today stems from this study.

At the time the patients enrolled in the registry, 75 percent were in functional classes 3 or 4. They had an average mean pulmonary artery pressure three times the normal, an abnormally high pressure in the right side of the heart, and a reduced cardiac output. In making the diagnosis of PPH, investigators found no complications arising from cardiac catheterization.

The study findings show that pulmonary artery pressure in patients who had symptoms for less than 1 year was similar to that in patients who had symptoms for more than 3 years. Researchers also found that patients whose only symptom was difficulty in breathing upon exercise already had very high pulmonary artery pressure. This suggests that the pulmonary artery pressure rises to high levels early in the course of the disease.

No correlations could be found between the cause of PPH and cigarette smoking, occupation, place of residence, pregnancy, use of appetite suppressants, or use of prescription drugs, including oral contraceptives. This study was designed to serve only as a registry, so it was not possible to evaluate the effectiveness of treatment.

Because we still do not understand the cause or have a cure for PPH, NHLBI remains committed to supporting basic and clinical studies of this illness. Basic research studies are focusing on the possible involvement of immunologic and genetic factors in the cause and progression of PPH, looking at agents that cause narrowing of the pulmonary blood vessels, and identifying factors that cause growth of smooth muscle and formation of scar tissue in the vessel walls. Most important is finding a reliable way to diagnose PPH early in the course of the disease and that does not require cardiac catheterization.

Living with Primary Pulmonary Hypertension

With the cause of primary pulmonary hypertension still unknown, there is at present no known way to prevent or cure this disease. However, many patients report that by changing some parts of their lifestyle, they can go about many of their daily tasks. For example, they do relaxation exercises, try to reduce stress, and adopt a positive mental attitude.

People with PPH go to school, work at home or outside the home part-time or fulltime, and raise their children. Indeed, most patients with PPH do not look sick, and some feel perfectly well much of the time as long as they do not strain themselves physically.

Walking is good exercise for many patients; others choose swimming. Some patients with advanced PPH carry portable oxygen when they go out; patients who find walking too exhausting may use a wheelchair or motorized scooter. Others stay busy with activities that are not of a physical nature.

For the patient who lives at a high altitude, a move to a lower altitude—where the air is not so thin, and thus the amount of oxygen is higher—can be helpful. Medical care is important, preferably by a doctor who is a pulmonary vascular specialist. These specialists are usually located at major research centers.

PPH patients can also help themselves by following the same sensible health measures that everyone should observe. These include eating a healthy diet, not smoking, and getting plenty of rest. Pregnancy is not advised because it puts an extra load on the heart. Oral contraceptives are not recommended, and other methods of birth control should be used.

Most doctors and patients agree that it is important for both patient and family to be as informed as possible about PPH. In this way everyone can understand the illness and apply that information to what is happening. In addition to family and close friends, support groups can help the PPH patient.

For More Information

If you are interested in receiving more information on primary pulmonary hypertension, contact:

Office of the Director
Division of Lung Diseases
National Heart, Lung, and Blood Institute
National Institutes of Health
Bethesda, MD 20892
(301) 496-7208

Part Two

Statistical and Demographic Data

Chapter 15

U. S. Cardiovascular Disease Risk Factors

Overview

The National Heart, Lung, and Blood Institute (NHLBI) sponsored a Cardiovascular Disease Risk Factor Supplement to the September 1989 Current Population Survey conducted by the Census Bureau. This Supplement was added to collect data on the three major modifiable risk factors for cardiovascular disease including 1) the prevalence of cigarette smoking and 2) the awareness and treatment of high blood pressure and high blood cholesterol.

The Current Population Survey is a national probability sample of households in the United States. Interviews are conducted in approximately 55,000 households; information is collected on all members of the household (approximately 115,000 individuals). Household members aged 15 years and older were asked the NHLBI supplemental questions. The Supplement included questions concerning the respondents' smoking behavior; the length of time since their blood pressure was last measured and whether or not they were ever told it was high; whether or not they ever had their blood cholesterol measured, if they were told their level, and whether or not they were told their level was high. These data, which are based on interviews, are intended to measure public awareness and health behavior rather than actual blood pressure or cholesterol levels.

An unnumbered publication of the National Heart, Lung, and Blood Institute dated May 1992.

125

The large sample size and unique cluster design allow for reliable state-specific estimates to be made according to demographic characteristics.

NHLBI has prepared a series of Data Fact Sheets which present these data for the United States as a whole and for each State individually.

The state-specific data will be useful to State health departments and community-based organizations in planning their own cardiovascular disease risk factor education programs. Furthermore, since the Current Population Survey data are presented according to demographic variables including age, sex, race, and Hispanic origin, the States can use these data to determine specific targets for intervention.

This Data Fact Sheet presents estimates of the prevalence of cigarette smoking and awareness of high blood pressure and high blood cholesterol for the adult population 18 years of age and older in the United States according to age, sex, race, and Hispanic origin.

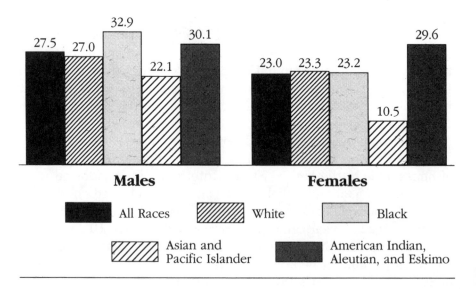

Figure 15.1. Percent of adults who are current smokers, according to sex and race

Cigarette Smoking

The major objectives of the NHLBI Smoking Education Program are to increase the number and effectiveness of state and community-based education programs on smoking cessation in preventing and controlling cardiovascular and pulmonary disease. Data in support of a continued emphasis on smoking prevention and health promotion related to smoking are necessary in order to emphasize the magnitude of the problem to State and community health officials, and other public health program planners.

[Figure 15.1] presents the percent of United States adults who are current smokers according to sex and race, and [Figure 15.2] presents the percent of current smokers according to sex and Hispanic origin. The definition of a current smoker is one who has smoked 100 cigarettes and smokes now. The definition of a former smoker is one who has smoked 100 cigarettes but does not smoke now.

[Figure 15.3] presents the percent of United States adults who are current or former smokers according to sex and age. [Figure 15.4] presents the percent of current United States smokers by the number of cigarettes they smoke each day according to sex and race. [Figure 15.5] presents the percent of current United States smokers by the number of cigarettes they smoke each day according to sex and Hispanic origin.

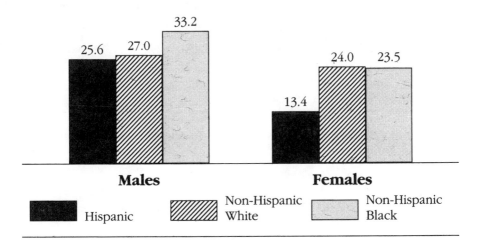

Figure 15.2. Percent of adults who are current smokers, according to sex and Hispanic origin.

127

	Males		Females	
	Current	Former	Current	Former
Total	27.5	27.6	23.0	18.0
18-24 yrs	21.5	7.5	21.7	7.5
25-44 yrs	31.6	20.2	26.7	16.8
45-64 yrs	30.4	38.7	25.2	22.8
65+ yrs	15.2	51.5	12.0	22.1

Figure 15.3. *Percent of adults who are current or former smokers, according to sex and age.*

	Males					Females				
No. of Cigs/Day	All Races	White	Black	Asian & PI	Amer. Ind. +	All Races	White	Black	Asian & PI	Amer. Ind. +
1-14	26.7	23.3	45.6	52.7	28.1	36.3	32.8	59.6	59.9	46.7
15-24	43.6	44.4	40.7	26.6	47.4	44.6	46.7	30.3	28.9	42.6
25+	29.7	32.3	13.7	20.7	24.5	19.1	20.5	10.1	11.2	10.7

+ *Includes American Indian, Aleutian, and Eskimo*

Figure 15.4. *Percent of smokers by number of cigarettes smoked per day, according to sex and race.*

	Males			Females		
No. of		Non-Hispanic			Non-Hispanic	
Cigs/Day	Hispanic	White	Black	Hispanic	White	Black
1-14	56.5	20.7	45.9	61.2	31.5	59.6
15-24	29.5	45.5	40.4	29.7	47.5	30.4
25+	14.0	33.8	13.7	9.1	21.0	10.0

Figure 15.5. Percent of smokers by number of cigarettes smoked per day, according to sex and Hispanic origin.

Hypertension

The National High Blood Pressure Education Program's objectives are to maintain the steady increase in the awareness, treatment, and control rates for high blood pressure and to increase the number of hypertensives who stay on therapy. The data collected by the Current Population Survey describe the awareness of hypertension.

Hypertension awareness begins with detection and requires continued surveillance. Health professionals are encouraged to measure blood pressure at each patient visit, and State health departments are continuing to find it necessary to conduct mass screening. [Figure 15.6] presents the percent of adults in the United States distributed by how long it has been since they had their blood pressure measured according to sex and race. [Figure 15.7] presents the same data according to sex and Hispanic origin.

According to the second National Health and Nutrition Examination Survey (1976-1980), approximately 30 percent of the adult population have high blood pressure, defined as a blood pressure >140/90 or taking antihypertensive medication. This is based on actual blood pressure measurement and interview.

This Supplement collected data on the percent of the population who are aware hypertensives. Aware hypertensives are defined as those who have been told by a doctor or other health professional that they have high blood pressure or hypertension. [Figures 15.8 and 15.9] present the percent of adults in the United States who are aware hypertensives according to sex and Hispanic origin. [Figure 15.10] presents the percent of adults who are aware hypertensives according to sex and age.

	Males					Females				
	All Races	White	Black	Asian & PI	Amer. Ind. +	All Races	White	Black	Asian & PI	Amer. Ind. +
Less Than 6 Months	53.6	54.0	54.9	39.1	55.2	64.9	65.2	66.9	48.9	64.6
6 Months to 1 Year	20.6	20.6	20.2	21.7	14.4	19.2	19.2	18.2	24.0	16.2
1 Year to 5 Years	16.6	16.8	14.1	18.8	17.5	11.0	11.1	9.1	14.0	15.2
5 Years or More	3.2	3.2	2.4	4.1	5.1	1.7	1.7	1.5	2.7	0.2
Never Had Checked	1.8	1.7	1.6	5.7	2.3	0.8	0.7	0.9	3.8	1.3
Don't Know	4.2	3.7	6.8	10.6	5.5	2.4	2.1	3.4	6.6	2.5

+ *Includes American Indian, Aleutian, and Eskimo*

Figure 15.6. Percent of adults by amount of time since blood pressure was last checked, according to sex and race

	Males			Females		
	Hispanic	Non-Hispanic White	Non-Hispanic Black	Hispanic	Non-Hispanic White	Non-Hispanic Black
Less Than 6 Months	39.2	55.4	54.9	55.6	65.9	67.3
6 Months to 1 Year	18.6	20.8	20.5	19.0	19.2	18.1
1 Year to 5 Years	19.2	16.6	13.9	14.8	10.8	8.8
5 Years or More	4.7	3.1	2.4	2.1	1.7	1.5
Never Had Checked	9.8	0.9	1.6	3.9	0.5	0.9
Don't Know	8.5	3.2	6.7	4.6	1.9	3.4

Figure 15.7. Percent of adults by amount of time since blood pressure was last checked, according to sex and Hispanic origin

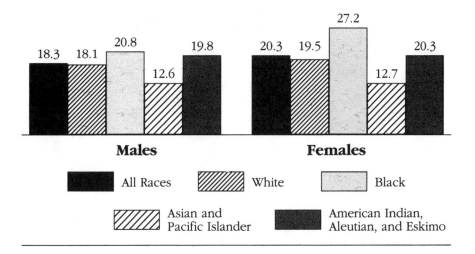

Figure 15.8. *Percent of adults who have ever been told they have hypertension, according to sex and race.*

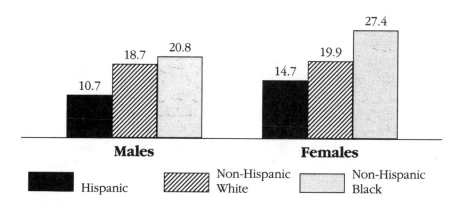

Figure 15.9. *Percent of adults who have ever been told they have hypertension, according to sex and Hispanic origin*

	Males	**Females**
Total	18.3	20.3
18-24 yrs	3.7	4.8
25-44 yrs	11.0	9.9
45-64 yrs	28.4	28.4
65+ yrs	37.8	45.1

Figure 15.10. Percent of adults who have ever been told they have hypertension, according to sex and age

High Blood Cholesterol

Among the objectives of the National Cholesterol Education Program are to increase the proportion of Americans who have their blood cholesterol measured, to increase the proportion of Americans who know their blood cholesterol level, to encourage people identified as having high blood cholesterol to seek professional advice, and to increase the proportion of people with high blood cholesterol who adhere to their cholesterol-lowering regimen of diet, weight control, exercise, and taking prescribed medications.

State health departments take an important role in cholesterol education and work to increase the general public's awareness about the importance of having their blood cholesterol level checked and knowing what their blood cholesterol level is.

[Figure 15.11] presents the percent of adults in the United States who have ever had their blood cholesterol level measured according to sex and race. [Figure 15.12] presents the percent of adults in the United States who have ever had their blood cholesterol level measured according to sex and Hispanic origin. [Figure 15.13] presents the percent of adults who have had their blood cholesterol level measured according to sex and age. [Figures 15.14 and 15.15] present the percent of adults who were told their blood cholesterol level according to sex and race, and according to sex and Hispanic origin. [Figure 15.16] presents this according to sex and age.

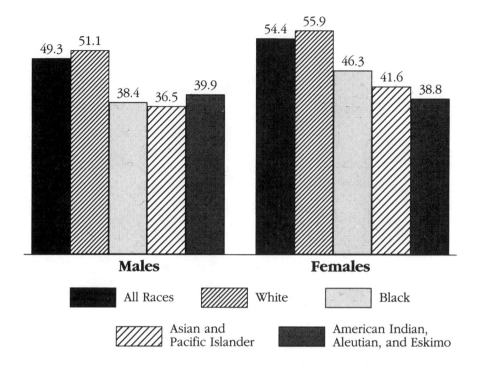

Figure 15.11. Percent of adults who have ever had their blood cholesterol level checked, according to sex and race

Recent reports from the National Health and Nutrition Examination Survey (1976-1980) estimate that in the United States, 27 percent of adults have high blood cholesterol, defined as a serum total cholesterol level of 240 mg/dL or greater. On the basis of LDL-cholesterol levels together with the presence of other CHD risk factors, a total of 36 percent of adults are candidates for medical advice or intervention to lower their cholesterol levels. This estimate is derived from actual blood cholesterol measurements and personal interviews.

[Figures 15.17 and 15.18] present the percent of adults in the United States who were told by a physician or other health professional that their blood cholesterol level is high according to sex and race, and according to sex and Hispanic origin. [Figure 15.19] presents the percent of adults who have been told that their cholesterol level is high according to sex and age.

133

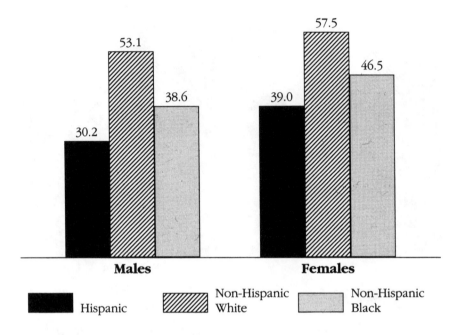

Figure 15.12. *Percent of adults who have ever had their blood cholesterol level checked, according to sex and Hispanic origin*

	Males	**Females**
Total	49.3	54.4
18-24 yrs	20.4	26.3
25-44 yrs	41.9	47.0
45-64 yrs	66.0	68.2
65+ yrs	72.1	73.5

Figure 15.13. *Percent of adults who have ever had their bood cholesterol level checked, according to sex and age.*

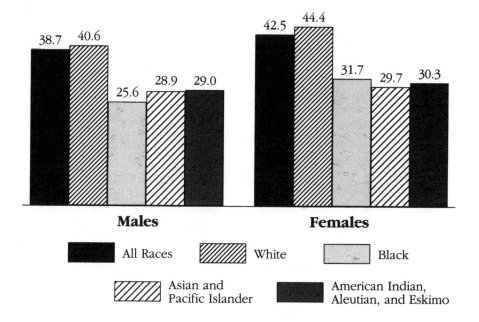

Figure 15.14. *Percent of adults who have ever been told their blood choles-terol level, according to sex and race*

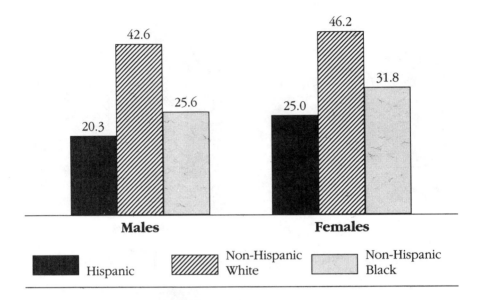

Figure 15.15. *Percent of adults who have ever been told their blood cholesterol level, according to sex and Hispanic origin*

	Males	**Females**
Total	38.7	42.5
18-24 yrs	13.6	17.3
25-44 yrs	33.4	37.3
45-64 yrs	53.5	55.8
65+ yrs	54.3	55.0

Figure 15.16. *Percent of adults who have ever been told their blood cholesterol level, according to sex and age*

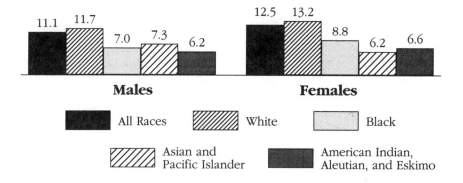

Figure 15.17. *Percent of adults who have ever been told their blood cholesterol level was high, according to sex and race*

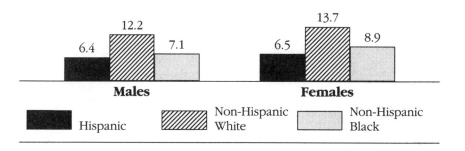

Figure 15.18. *Percent of adults who have ever been told their blood cholesterol level was high, according to sex and Hispnaic origin*

	Males	**Females**
Total	11.1	12.5
18-24 yrs	1.5	2.5
25-44 yrs	7.7	6.0
45-64 yrs	19.0	20.9
65+ yrs	17.1	23.4

Figure 15.19. *Percent of adults who have ever been told their blood cholesterol level was high, according to sex and age*

The data collected in this Supplement will allow the National Cholesterol Education Program to evaluate its progress by estimating the proportion of the population who have had their blood cholesterol measured, who have been told their blood cholesterol level, and who have been told their blood cholesterol level was high.

Chapter 16

Workplace Facts on Heart Disease and Stroke

The purpose of this fact sheet is to provide health professionals, program planners, and decision-makers at the workplace with information about cardiovascular disease (CVD) among workers, its impact on business, and programs to help improve the health of the workforce.

Overview

More people die from cardiovascular disease, which includes heart disease and stroke, than from any other single cause of death—almost 1 million Americans annually. Most employees in the United States have at least one of the three major risk factors for cardiovascular disease—high blood pressure, high blood cholesterol, and cigarette smoking. The impact of cardiovascular disease on employers is enormous. The annual costs of cardiovascular disease exceed those for any other category of illness and are 18 percent of the cost of all illness. Recognizing the extent of this problem, many businesses have initiated health promotion programs that encourage employees to control their blood pressure, adopt heart-healthy diets, and stop smoking, among other activities. Nationally, more than two-thirds of worksites with 50 or more employees have at least one health promotion activity. Their reasons for sponsoring programs include health care cost

An unnumbered publication of the National Heart, Lung, and Blood Institute dated July 1990.

containment, improved employee health, increased productivity, enhanced company image, and improved employee morale. Most employers offering these programs believe that the benefits outweigh any costs involved.

Workers At Risk

Most employees have at least one of the three major risk factors for cardiovascular disease—high blood pressure, high blood cholesterol, and cigarette smoking.

High Blood Pressure

Adults with uncontrolled high blood pressure are three to four times more likely to have heart disease and seven times more likely to have a stroke than are those with normal blood pressure. However, when high blood pressure is controlled, the risk of heart disease and stroke approaches that of persons with normal blood pressure. Blacks are more likely to have high blood pressure (38 percent) than whites (29 percent). In addition, blacks tend to get high blood pressure at younger ages and have more severe high blood pressure. They also are much more likely to die of a stroke.

High Blood Cholesterol

Adults with high blood cholesterol are twice as likely to have heart disease than those with desirable blood cholesterol levels. The good news for people with high blood cholesterol is that for every 1-percent reduction in blood cholesterol there is a corresponding 2-percent reduction in the risk of cardiovascular disease.

Cigarette Smoking

Compared with nonsmokers, smokers are 10 times more likely to die of lung disease and 2 times more likely to suffer heart attacks and strokes. When smokers quit, however, they substantially reduce their risk of dying from coronary heart disease and their risk of stroke. For example, death rates for coronary heart disease are significantly lowered in ex-smokers 2 years after quitting. In addition, the risk for stroke in ex-smokers 5 years after quitting is no greater than the risk for people who never smoked. Cigarette smoking remains the largest avoidable cause of premature death and disability in the United States.

Extent of the Problem

More people die from cardiovascular disease than from any other single cause of death—almost 1 million Americans annually. This represents 46 percent of all deaths. Heart disease is the leading cause of death, and stroke is the third leading cause. Contrary to the popular belief that heart disease strikes mostly men, it is estimated that almost half of the coronary heart disease deaths and two-thirds of the stroke deaths occur among women.

The Impact on Employers

The economic impact of cardiovascular disease on employers is staggering. The annual costs of cardiovascular disease exceed those of any other single category of illness—$127 billion in medical expenses and lost productivity. This is 18 percent of the cost of all illness.

In addition:

- About 29 million workdays a year are lost due to cardiovascular disease-related illness. This translates into $1.5 billion in earnings lost to American business.

- Ten times as many employees die from cardiovascular disease than from industrial accidents.

- The average smoker of more than one pack of cigarettes per day may cost his or her employer $336 to $601 per year (in January 1980 dollars) more in lost time and medical benefits than a comparable nonsmoker.

- Absenteeism rates for smokers are approximately 50 percent higher than for nonsmokers. The number of job-related accidents among smokers is twice that among nonsmokers.

What Businesses Can Do to Promote Worker Health

Recognizing the enormous impact that cardiovascular disease has on their companies' bottom line, many employers have initiated health promotion programs. They help employees control their blood pressure, learn to eat heart-healthy foods, and stop smoking, among other activities.

High Blood Pressure Programs

Most workers with high blood pressure are aware they have it, but they don't have it under control. Younger people and men tend to be less aware and have it under less control than older people and women. Workplace programs can screen and monitor employees with high blood pressure and help them keep it under control.

Cholesterol Education

Almost 60 percent of adults report having their blood cholesterol level checked, up from 35 percent 5 years earlier. However, only 17 percent know their cholesterol level. Workplace programs can screen employees to identify those with high blood cholesterol, offer counseling to lower their cholesterol, and educate all employees about heart-healthy eating.

Stop Smoking Activities

Most smokers—77 percent—say they want to quit smoking, and more than 30 percent try to quit each year. However, because smoking is addictive, only 8 percent of all the smokers who try to quit stay off for more than 3 months. Programs at the workplace can use coworker support to help smokers quit. No-smoking policies also help by creating an environment supportive of the quitting smoker.

Blue-Collar Smokers: Taking Extra Risks

Smoking rates among some workers have decreased. For example, smoking among white-collar men dropped from 37 percent in 1976 to 26 percent in 1985. However, smoking rates for blue-collar workers remain substantially higher than those for white-collar workers. A recent survey estimates that among blue-collar workers, 42 percent of men and 35 percent of women smoke cigarettes; among white-collar workers, 26 percent of men and 28 percent of women smoke.

What National Surveys Show

Surveys of companies and unions nationwide show that health promotion programs are widespread. A 1985 national survey of more than 1,300 worksites sponsored by the U.S. Public Health Service showed that more than two-thirds of worksites with 50 or more employees had at least one health promotion activity. In companies with more than 750 workers, about half offered these programs.

The employers surveyed gave the following reasons for sponsoring health promotion activities:

- Health care cost containment
- Improved employee health
- Increased productivity
- Enhanced company image
- Improved employee morale.

The survey also showed that most employers with health promotion programs believe the benefits outweigh the costs.

Another national survey of more than 660 companies conducted in 1986 by the Bureau of National Affairs found that 59 percent had smoking policies or were considering one.

In a 1985 survey of 25 international unions representing more than 12 million workers, more than half reported that a health promotion program was available to their members. Cardiovascular disease risk reduction programs were among the most common programs. Blood pressure testing was offered by 62 percent of the unions, exercise and fitness activities by 39 percent, diet and nutrition education by 23 percent, and weight control programs by 15 percent.

Promoting Health Around the Nation

Businesses and unions around the country offer cardiovascular disease risk reduction programs. Here is a sampling of these programs.

143

DuPont (Memphis, Tennessee)

In 1980, the Memphis DuPont plant offered its mostly male, middle-aged employees tests to determine their blood cholesterol and triglyceride levels. Individuals with elevations received counseling about diet, exercise, and smoking. As a result, 75 percent of the participants decreased their blood cholesterol levels an average of 13 percent and the smoking rate in the plant dropped from 31 percent to 24 percent in 3 years. In addition, a high blood pressure control program and a Weight Watchers program were brought to the plant. Since the start of the program, heart attacks and stroke have decreased dramatically and disability days have been cut in half.

GTE-Northwest (Everett, Washington)

GTE-Northwest offered all 5,000 blue- and white-collar employees over a five-state area several smoking cessation options when it decided to go smoke-free. One option, the "Free and Clear" self-help smoking cessation program, was offered free to every employee who smoked. This program includes I year's worth of telephone counseling. Of 73 employees who received the full set of phone calls, 27 percent were smoke-free at 1 year. A similar program, "Stop Smoking For Life," also included a year of telephone counseling and had quit rates of close to 50 percent at 1 year.

United Auto Workers/General Motors Corporation (Michigan)

Four General Motors plants in Michigan experimented with various approaches to engage and maintain blue-collar workers in smoking cessation, weight loss, high blood pressure control, fitness, and stress management programs. The project was a joint effort of the United Auto Workers of America, General Motors Corporation, and The University of Michigan. While health improvement occurred at all four plants, the two sites that utilized wellness counselors, consistent followup, and peer group support produced higher participation and overall success rates.

AT&T Communications (Nationwide)

The Cholesterol/Nutrition Program is one module of "Total Life Concept," which is a national health promotion program for AT&T

employees. This module includes cholesterol screening and a health risk appraisal. Followup strategies for cholesterol management include small group sessions and an employee-led, self-learning course. About 80,000 AT&T employees have completed the health risk appraisal and 40 percent of these had cholesterol followup. Program participants experienced an average blood cholesterol drop of 23 mg/dL at 1-year followup.

Baltimore Gas and Electric Company (Baltimore, Maryland)

Since 1976, the medical department of the Baltimore Gas and Electric Company has provided a high blood pressure screening and education program. Employees with elevated blood pressure readings are referred to a physician for evaluation and treatment or are offered treatment through the company—and are also invited to participate in followup activities. Almost 1,900 employees—21 percent of the workforce—are now in the followup system. The rate of control for participants in the followup program has consistently been over 80 percent. In addition, the participants have less absenteeism than other employees.

Chapter 17

Morbidity from Coronary Heart Disease in the United States

Coronary heart disease (CHD) is the leading cause of death in the United States. The two major components of coronary heart disease are heart attacks (or myocardial infarctions) and angina pectoris (chest pain). Despite major declines in mortality, CHD still causes over 500,000 deaths annually.

While mortality is relatively easy to measure and to monitor over time, it is much more difficult to gauge the degree of morbidity from CHD in the U.S. The toll from CHD is described below in terms of its prevalence, hospitalizations for the condition, physician visits, and resulting disability. The economic costs to the nation are also addressed.

Prevalence

Based on data from the 1988 National Health Interview Survey, conducted by the National Center for Health Statistics, about 3.1 percent of Americans report having coronary heart disease. Overall, about 7 million Americans have CHD.

As shown in [Figure 17.1], prevalence increases dramatically with age, especially among women. Prevalence rates are higher among men than women, especially in the group 45-64 years of age. In most age groups, prevalence of coronary heart disease is greater in the white than the black populations. For total heart disease, however,

An unnumbered publication of the National Heart, Lung, and Blood Institute, reprinted May 1992.

Figure
17.1

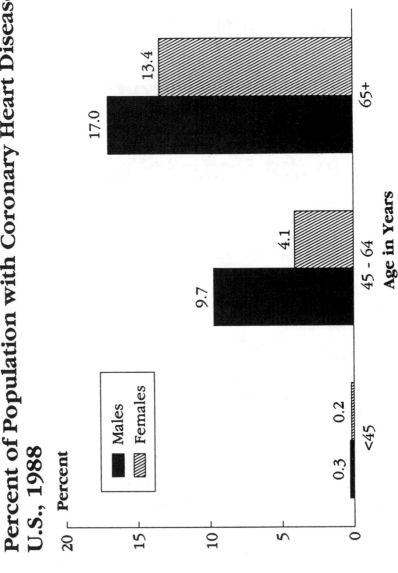

Percent of Population with Coronary Heart Disease, U.S., 1988

Source: National Health Interview Survey

prevalence is greater in blacks under 65 years of age than in whites of that age group.

Hospitalizations

Data from the National Hospital Discharge Survey, sponsored by the National Center for Health Statistics, indicate that the hospital discharge rate for acute myocardial infarctions (heart attacks) increases substantially with age. In 1987, the rate was 61.5 per 10,000 persons aged 45-64 years, compared to 145.0 per 10,000 persons aged 65 and over. It is also much higher among men than women (40.7 vs. 22.6 per 10,000 population, respectively).

Trend data show that hospitalizations for heart attacks have fluctuated over the past decade, but generally increased. Among persons 45-64 years of age, the hospital discharge rate for heart attacks was 53.0 per 10,000 population in 1970 and 61.5 per 10.000 in 1987. Among those 65 years and older, it rose from 122.0 per 10,000 to 145.0 per 10.000 ([Figure 17.2]).

Data from the National Hospital Discharge Survey indicate that, in 1987, there were over 2.2 million hospital discharges for coronary heart disease in the United States, up from 1.7 million in 1977. On the other hand, as shown in [Figure 17.3], the average hospital length of stay for coronary heart disease has dropped over the past ten years, from 10.4 to 6.5 days. Because of this decline in length of stay, the total number of hospital days for coronary heart disease has actually declined (from 17.7 million to 14.2 million), despite the increase in the number of discharges. [Figure 17.4] graphically shows the actual number of hospital days for coronary heart disease from 1977 to 1987. It also shows a projection of expected hospital days, assuming the average length of stay did not change since 1977. The expected number of hospital days in 1987 is 59 percent greater than the actual number, representing an estimated cost savings of $6.3 billion.

Physician Visits

Data on physician visits for coronary heart disease are estimated using the National Disease and Therapeutic Index, a data base sponsored by IMS America, Ltd., of Plymouth Meeting, Pennsylvania. In 1989, there were an estimated 27.7 million physician visits for coronary heart disease. The majority of visits were made by older persons.

149

Rate of Hospitalizations for Acute Myocardial Infarction, Ages 45 - 64 and 65 and Over, U.S., 1970 - 1987

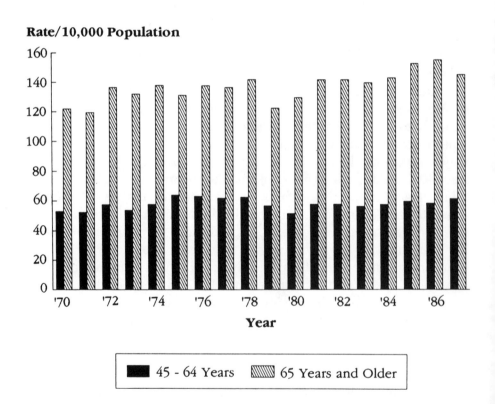

Source: National Hospital Discharge Survey

Figure 17.2

Average Hospital Length of Stay for Coronary Heart Disease, U.S., 1977 - 1987

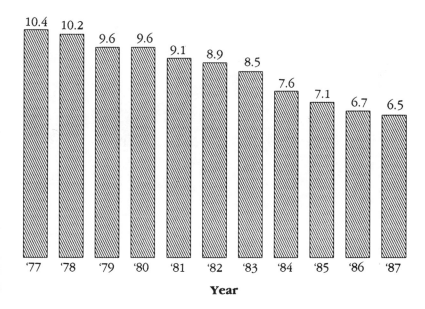

Source: *National Hospital Discharge Survey*

Figure 17.3

151

Number of Hospital Days for Coronary Heart Disease, U.S., 1977 - 1987

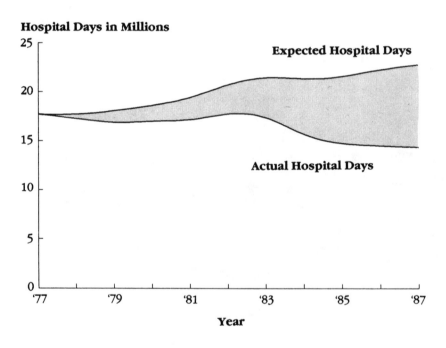

Hospital Days in Millions

Source: *National Hospital Discharge Survey*

Figure 17.4

For example, only about 1 percent of these visits were made by patients 20-39 years of age, 17 percent were among those 40-59 years of age, 13 percent were among those 60-64 years of age, and 69 percent were among patients 65 and older. Among men, 43 percent of visits were made by persons 40-64 years of age and 61 percent were made by persons 65 and older. On the other hand, among women, these per-

Physician Visits for Coronary Heart Disease, by Patient Age and Sex, U.S., 1989

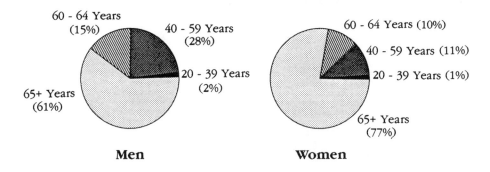

Men   **Women**

Source: National Disease and Therapeutic Index

Figure 17.5

centages were 21 percent and 77 percent, respectively. (See [Figure 17.5]).

Disability

As shown in [Figure 17.6], during the time period 1983-1985, diseases of the heart was the third leading chronic condition causing limitation of activity. If coronary heart disease, a subset of diseases of the heart, was considered separately, it would rank as the fifth leading

Prevalence of Leading Chronic Conditions Causing Limitation of Activity, U.S., 1983 - 1985

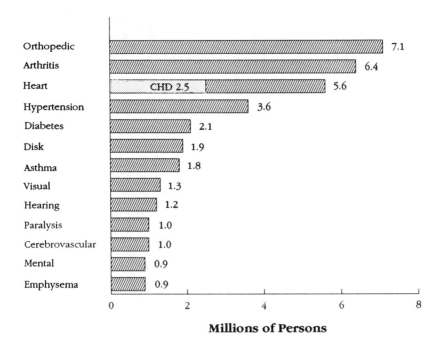

Millions of Persons

Source: National Health Interview Survey

Figure 17.6

chronic condition. Thirty-six percent of persons with CHD are limited in activity. This percentage is similar for men and women, bu most 58 percent for blacks as compared with 35 percent for wh

[Figure 17.7] presents data from the National Health Int Survey on restricted activity associated with heart conditions (ing rheumatic and hypertensive heart disease). In 1983, peop heart conditions had an average of 18.7 days of restricted acti sociated with this disease. Men with heart disease were somewhat more likely to have restricted activity days than women (22 vs. 16 days per year, respectively). Fewer days of restricted activity were reported among people under 45 years of age. Between 45 and 64 years of age, there were an average of 25 days of restricted activity for each person with heart disease, with no differences by sex. Among older Americans, men with heart disease reported a substantially greater proportion of restricted activity days than did women. It also has been reported (1979-1981 National Health Interview Survey) that annual restricted activity days per condition for heart disease and for the subset coronary heart disease are greater in the black than in the white populations.

Economic Impact

The total economic impact of coronary heart disease amounted to an estimated $43 billion in 1987, 42.5 percent of which can be attributed to direct and indirect costs of illness. Direct costs (i.e., hospital stays, emergency room visits, physicians visits, surgery, drugs, nursing home care, etc.) amounted to an estimated $15.3 billion in 1987, representing about 35 percent of the total economic impact of CHD. Indirect morbidity costs (i.e., lost earnings based on work-loss days, days lost due to illness by homemakers, and lost earnings by those unable to work or in long-term institutions) totaled an additional $3.1 billion, or 7 percent of the total. To complete the picture, indirect mortality costs (representing the lost income from future earnings) were estimated to be $24.9 billion, or 58 percent of the economic impact of CHD. Direct costs, indirect morbidity costs, and indirect mortality costs are graphically depicted in [Figure 17.8].

Days of Restricted Activity Associated With Heart Conditions (Excluding Rheumatic and Hypertensive), U.S., 1983

Days Per Person With Condition Per Year

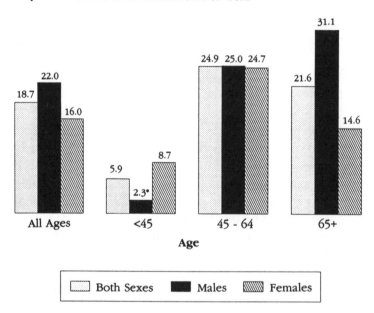

Estimate does not meet standards of reliability

Source: *National Health Interview Survey*

Figure 17.7

Economic Impact of Coronary Heart Disease, U.S., 1987

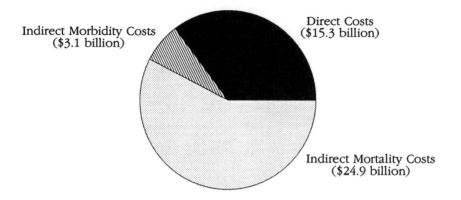

Source: *NHLBI estimates based on data from the National Center for Health Statistics and the Health Care Financing Administration*

Figure 17.8

Chapter 18

Heart Disease Data for Various Racial/Ethnic Groups

Data on Black Americans

In 1989, the difference in life expectancy between all U.S. males (71.8 years) and black males (64.8 years) was 7.0 years; the difference in life expectancy between all U.S. females (78.6 years) and black females (73.5 years) was 5.1 years.

[Figure 18.1] shows the five leading causes of death in blacks in 1989. Approximately 36 percent of total deaths in blacks were due to diseases of the heart and cerebrovascular disease.

[Figure 18.2] presents the prevalence of selected cardiovascular disease risk factors for the black population.

According to the 1989 Current Population Survey, the prevalence of current smokers who were black men was 32.9 percent compared with 27.5 percent of all men in the U.S. population. The rate for black women (23.2 percent) was the same as the rate for the total U.S. female population.

The National Health and Nutrition Examination Survey (1976-80) found that 37.9 percent of black males and 38.6 percent of black females had hypertension, compared with 33 percent of all U.S. males and 26.8 percent of all U.S. females.

National Heart, Lung, and Blood Institute, May 1992.

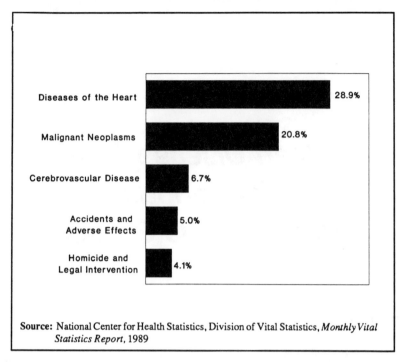

Figure 18.1. *Percent of all deaths due to the five leading caues of death for blacks, 1989.*

About 24 percent of black male and female adults had high blood cholesterol (greater than or equal to 240 mg/dL). This was slightly lower than the rate for the total population (27 percent).

Overweight is common in black women. The prevalence of overweight in black females was 43.8 percent compared with 27.1 percent of the total U.S. female population.

The prevalence of diabetes in blacks, as estimated by the National Health and Nutrition Examination Survey, is 1.6 times that of the total population (19 percent versus 12 percent).

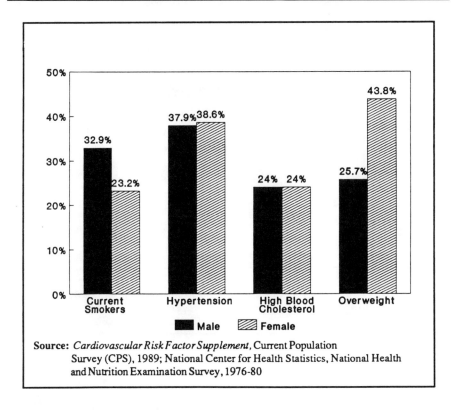

Figure 18.2. *Prevalence of smoking (1989), hypertension, high blood choles-terol, and overweight (1976-80) in blacks.*

Data on American Indians

[Figure 18.3 on the next page] shows the five leading causes of death among American Indians and Alaska Natives in 1988. Approximately 28 percent of total deaths in these populations were due to diseases of the heart and cerebrovascular disease.

[Figure 18.4] presents the risk factor profile for the American Indian population, based on 1989 Current Population Survey data and the 1987 National Medical Expenditure Survey.

The reported prevalence of current smokers among American Indian men was 30.1 percent compared with 27.5 percent of all men in the U.S. population. The rate for American Indian women was 29.6 percent compared with 23.2 percent for all women in the U.S. population.

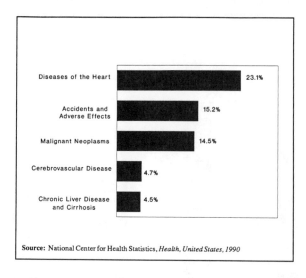

Figure 18.3. Percent of all deaths due to the five leading causes of death for American Indians, 1988.

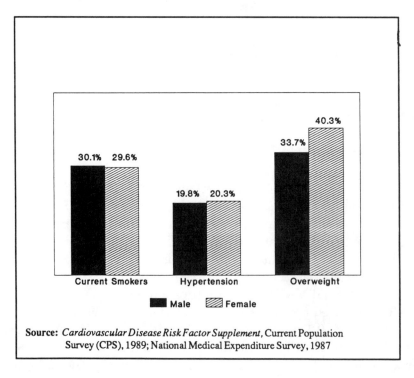

Figure 18.4. Percent of American Indian adults who are current smokers (1989), who have been told they have hypertension, or report they are overweight (1987), by sex

About 19.8 percent of American Indian males had been told by a doctor they have hypertension. This was slightly higher than that for the total U.S. male population (18.3 percent). The percent of American Indian females who had been told they have hypertension was the same as that of the total U.S. female population (20.3 percent).

Diabetes, a risk factor for heart disease, is prevalent among American Indians. In 1987, the age-adjusted prevalence rate of previously diagnosed diabetes for those aged 19 years and older was 13 percent compared with 5 percent of the general population. Differences in prevalence rates among tribes were also reported.

The magnitude of the obesity problem in American Indians is not well documented. Prevalence studies on obesity have been based on limited population surveys of specific tribes. In the 1987 National Medical Expenditure Survey, an estimated 33.7 percent of American Indian males and 40.3 percent of American Indian females were overweight, based on their self-reported weight and height. This is significantly greater than the total U.S. prevalence of overweight, which is 24.1 percent among men and 25.0 percent among women.

Data on Hispanic Americans

In 1989, the difference in life expectancy between all U.S. males (71.8 years) and Hispanic males (69.6 years) was 2.2 years; the difference in life expectancy between all U.S. females (78.6 years) and Hispanic females (77.1 years) was 1.5 years.

[Figure 18.5] shows the five leading causes of death among Hispanics in 1989. Approximately 30 percent of total deaths in Hispanics were due to diseases of the heart and cerebrovascular disease.

[Figure 18.6] presents the prevalence of selected cardiovascular disease risk factors for the Hispanic population.

According to the 1989 Current Population Survey, 25.6 percent of Hispanic men and 13.4 percent of Hispanic women were current smokers, compared with 27.5 percent of men and 23.2 percent of women in the total U.S. population.

This Hispanic Health and Nutrition Examination Survey (1982-1984) found that the prevalence of high blood cholesterol (greater than or equal to 240 mg/dL) is lower among Hispanic men and women (17-23 percent) than among non-Hispanic men (24-25 percent) and women (25-28 percent) in 1976-80.

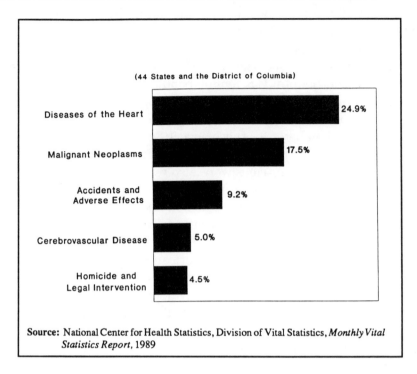

(44 States and the District of Columbia)

- Diseases of the Heart — 24.9%
- Malignant Neoplasms — 17.5%
- Accidents and Adverse Effects — 9.2%
- Cerebrovascular Disease — 5.0%
- Homicide and Legal Intervention — 4.5%

Source: National Center for Health Statistics, Division of Vital Statistics, *Monthly Vital Statistics Report*, 1989

Figure 18.5. *Percent of all deaths due to the five leading causes of death for Hispanics, 1989.*

The prevalence of diabetes in adults 45-74 years of age was twice as high for Mexican Americans and Puerto Ricans (24 and 26 percent in 1982-84) as for non-Hispanic Whites (12 percent in 1976-80).

[Figure 18.6] also presents the percent of Hispanic adult males, by ethnic group, who had hypertension; the highest percent of hypertension was found in Cuban males (22.8 percent) and females (15.5); Mexican American males (16.8) and females (14.1) were second and Puerto Rican males (15.6) and females (11.5) had the lowest percent of hypertension.

Overweight is common among Hispanics, especially women; the highest percent of overweight was found in Mexican American females (42.3) and Cuban females (38.2) had the lowest percent of overweight. Among Hispanic males, the highest percent of overweight was in Cuban males (34.0) and the lowest was in Puerto Rican males (31.3).

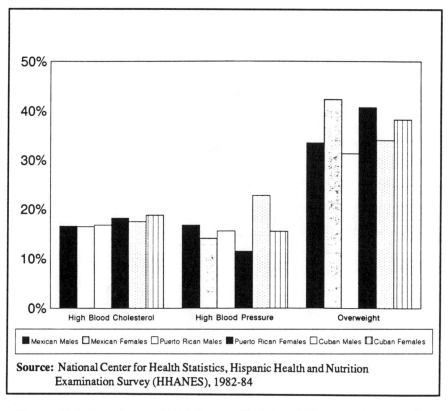

Figure 18.6. *Prevalence of High Serum Cholesterol, Hypertension, and Overweight in Hispanics*

Data on Asian/Pacific Islanders

[Figure 18.7 on the next page] shows the five leading causes of death among Asian/Pacific Islanders in 1988. Approximately 36 percent of total deaths in Asian/Pacific Islanders were due to diseases of the heart and cerebrovascular disease.

[Figure 18.8] presents the risk factor profile of the Asian/Pacific Islander population and is based on 1989 Current Population Survey data.

The reported prevalence of current smokers among Asian men was 22.1 percent compared with 27.5 percent of men in the U.S. population. The rate for Asian women was 10.5 percent compared with 23.3 percent for all women in the U.S. population.

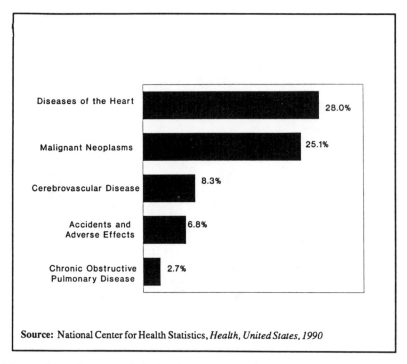

Source: National Center for Health Statistics, *Health, United States, 1990*

Figure 18.7. *Percent of all deaths due to the five leading causes of death for Asians and Pacific Islanders, 1988.*

Other studies have shown the variation in the smoking rates of this diverse group. Among California immigrant groups, the rate of smoking among men was: 92 percent of Laotians, 71 percent of Cambodians, and 65 percent of Vietnamese. No data was available for women in these groups.

The percent of Asian/Pacific Islanders who had been told they have hypertension was approximately 13 percent for both males and females, compared with 18.3 percent for all U.S. males and 20.3 percent for all U.S. females.

The percent of Asian/Pacific Islander males who had been told they have high blood cholesterol was 7.3 percent compared with 11.1 percent for all U.S. males. The percent of Asian/Pacific Islander females who had been told they have high blood cholesterol was 6.2 percent, compared with 12.5 percent for all U.S. females.

Native Hawaiians, one group of the Pacific Islanders, have a high prevalence of overweight among men (65.5 percent) and women (62.6 percent.)

166

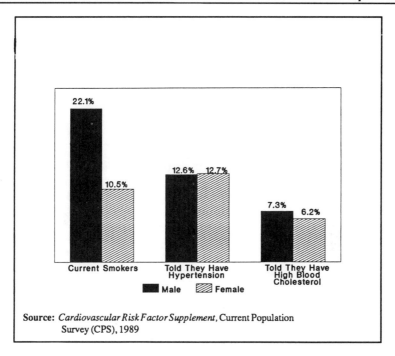

Figure 18.8. *Percent of Asian and Pacific Islander adults who are current smokers and percent who have been told they have hyptertension or high blood cholesterol, by sex, 1989.*

Chapter 19

Minority Health Issues

Higher Poverty Rates, Mortality Among Minorities Defy Simple Solutions

Louis Sullivan, M.D.
Secretary, Department of Health and Human Services
Washington, D.C.

Over the past 20 years, the Nation has made much progress in the prevention of coronary heart disease. "We're saving more lives," Sullivan said. "Death rates from stroke for black men and women dropped between 1979 and 1988."

But these death rates are still higher for blacks than for whites, a fact that continues to cause concern among minorities and health care professionals nationwide.

Changes in Minority Health Since 1975

When the first National Minority Health Forum was held in 1975, hypertension was the key issue. Now the list of critical issues in-

---

Excerpts from Proceedings of the 4th National Forum on Cardiovascular Health, Pulmonary Disorders, and Blood Resources, sponsored by The National Heart, Lung, and Blood Institute (NHLBI), The NHLBI Ad Hoc Committee on Minority Populations and The National Medical Association; June 26-27, 1992.

cludes cardiovascular and pulmonary diseases, blood resources, and bone marrow donation.

According to Sullivan, the growth of interest in minority health has led to positive developments: more research into minority populations, more effective targeting of educational materials to minorities, more researchers recruited to study pulmonary disease.

But these efforts haven't addressed the basic problems in the minority community, including:

- **Poverty.** "As stated in *Healthy People 2000*, a national plan for health promotion and disease prevention, poverty and near-poverty appear as underlying elements of many health problems," Sullivan said.

- **Risk factors** (hypertension, high blood cholesterol, diabetes, smoking, obesity, heavy drinking, and lack of exercise). "Minorities are overrepresented in most of these areas."

- **Asthma.** In 1979, blacks were twice as likely to die from asthma as whites. In 10 years that ratio has risen from 2 to 1 to approximately 3 to 1.

Great Strides in Bone Marrow Transplants

While other minority health problems have remained unchanged or have gotten worse in recent years, the availability of bone marrow donors has greatly increased. Due to the collaborative educational efforts of the NHLBI and the National Marrow Donor Program, the number of minority bone marrow donors has increased tenfold on the national registry—to a level of 80,000 donors—since 1989.

"As a result, four times as many minority patients have received transplants," Sullivan reported, "most of them within the past year."

Sullivan's Five-Point Plan

To address other problems in minority health care, the Department of Health and Human Services has adopted a five-point, $150 million plan designed to "improve access through prevention research and education efforts."

Sullivan outlined the broad goals of the plan as follows:

- To increase access to appropriate primary and preventive health care in urban and rural areas.
- To increase the number of health professionals in under-served areas.
- To encourage early preventive care for children.
- To improve health to enhance learning.
- To prevent complications from hypertension through enhanced research and education.

Of the $150 million allotted for the program, over $24 million will be used by the lead agency in the hypertension effort—the NHLBI—to pursue four major initiatives:

- A 9-year program to prevent obesity in young American Indians.
- Comparative trials of antihypertensive drug treatments.
- Care programs for inner-city residents with hypertension.
- Phase II of the Strong Heart Study and other assessment of cardiovascular disease in American Indians.

Increased Efforts by the NHLBI

In addition, the NHLBI is doing more to promote minority health issues, according to Sullivan. He recognized the importance of the NHLBI's efforts through its grant programs which "encourage more members of minority communities to pursue careers in biomedical research."

Sullivan also elaborated on one of the key goals of *Healthy People 2000*: "To expand minority representation in health and related fields."

Specifically, one goal of *Healthy People 2000* is to increase the proportion of all health-related degrees awarded to minorities by the following percentages: blacks, from 5 to 8 percent; Hispanics, from 3 to 6 percent; American Indians and Alaska Natives, from 0.3 to 0.6 percent.

More Minority Professionals Serving Minorities

In Sullivan's view, increasing the number of minorities in health care can only improve the overall health outlook for the Nation's minority groups.

"Minority health professionals are more willing to establish their practices in medically underserved areas," he said. "They can significantly improve access to quality care for disadvantaged communities."

In addition, minority professionals can help solve the national glut of specialists and the shortage of primary care givers. "Minority physicians tend to more frequently choose primary care specialties such as family practice, internal medicine, and pediatrics."

But in order to reach these goals, Sullivan emphasized, the United States needs an organized effort. "We need the commitment that you and your organizations can make to a stronger, healthier America for all," he said. "Your efforts are essential for our success."

CVD Mortality Among Harlem's Black Males Higher Than in Third World

Charles Francis, M.D.
Director, Department of Medicine
Harlem Hospital Center
New York, New York

Although Charles Francis has seen some improvement in the minority health picture in recent years, he is still appalled by one statistic. According to a study published in the *New England Journal of Medicine*, CVD mortality rates for black males living in Harlem, New York City, is currently higher than that of third-world Bangladesh.

"That is totally unacceptable," Francis said. "A long list of reasons explains why, but poverty is the prime culprit."

As director for the Department of Medicine, Harlem Hospital Center, Francis keeps close watch on developments in minority health and is aware of the major trends affecting minorities—one of which is their growing status as a majority: "By the year 2065, whites will probably not be the majority in this country," he said. "This is something that we as a society are going to have to confront."

Along the way, the United States must face other issues in minority health—namely, the disparity between the health status of the majority and the poorer health of minorities. Francis outlined several specific problems in need of attention, including:

- Higher mortality among nonwhite women as compared to white women.

- Falling rates of life expectancy for black men and women.

- Strokes as the third leading cause of death among blacks.

- The unusually high incidence of diabetes among Hispanics.

- Increased death rates from hypertension in blacks. "Comparing black women and men to the total population, you see nearly a twofold difference in death rates," Francis said.

- A ten- to seventeen-fold difference in end-stage renal disease among blacks.

But considering the prevalence of hypertension, diabetes, and adverse lifestyles among minority groups, Francis is surprised that there isn't more illness—especially CVD.

He identified some factors that must be addressed in order to improve minority health over the coming years.

- **Better data on minorities.** "There is a great scarcity of data on minority populations. We need not only epidemiologic data but also mechanistic data, treatment data, and long-term prognostic data," he said.

- **Genetic factors.** "There is a great deal of information that will help our understanding of racial and ethnic differences as we learn more about genetic coding," he said.

- **Environment.** "This is what most of us feel has made the most significant difference in the decline in CVD rates in this country: improving our lifestyle."

- **Smoking.** "A major problem," he said. "The tobacco industry has targeted minority and low-income populations . . . the young people as well."

- **Obesity.** "There have been some interesting studies on black teenage girls. Why do we tend to be more obese? What is it about our diet and exercise patterns which impact on this?"

- **Increase in blood pressure in response to stress among blacks.** "Why is it that there is this difference in vascular reactivity, and what impact does it have?"

- **Common increases in left-ventricular (LV) mass among blacks.** "There might be some independent factor which leads to increased LV mass."

But by far the largest impact on minority health is poverty, according to Francis. "At our hypertension clinic, we're actually finding our control rates are not as good as they used to be," he reported. "Compliance seems to be a major problem. Patients may not have access to care. Or they may have difficulty getting into the health care system. The culprit underlying all of this is poverty."

In Francis' view, because of their low-income status, patients aren't getting two important resources that could lead to improved health outcomes: insurance and education.

"Of the uninsured in this country, 22 percent are black. We need a very comprehensive universal coverage system to get these people covered," he reported. "Also, some diseases hit blacks at a higher rate than whites. Education ought to be changing eating, drinking, and smoking habits to help reduce the incidence of these diseases. That is our challenge."

Exploding Myths about Health Superiority of Asian Americans

Samuel Lin, M.D., Ph.D.
Assistant Surgeon General
Acting Deputy Assistant Secretary
Office of Minority Health
Public Health Service
Rockville, Maryland

As the highest ranking Asian and Pacific Islander American in the Department of Health and Human Services (DHHS), Samuel Lin is well acquainted with the stereotypes surrounding Asian Americans: "The images are familiar," he quoted from a recent news article. Armed with little more than the will to succeed, they open stores where no other entrepreneur will venture. They streak to the top of the technical world of computers and mathematics. Their workers are the most dedicated and tireless. Their children are the smartest. They are wealthy and self-sufficient.

"This is a bit flattering; unfortunately, it is not real," he said. In truth, Asian Americans have a bimodal demographic and health distribution. They do have higher median family incomes, but they also suffer from a higher poverty rate. Asian Americans are also credited with a higher level of overall health, Lin reported, which is another misperception. The reason for this misperception, according to Lin, is the inadequate and misleading health data on Asian Americans.

"States with high concentrations of Asian people, like New York, Illinois, and Texas, collect birth and death data only as white and nonwhite," he reported. "Such methods forget or ignore differences between those born in the United States and abroad, and differences between very diverse groups."

In order to clear up some of the misconceptions, Lin set forth some facts that *are* known about the Asian American/Pacific Islander American health picture:

- Knowledge of cardiovascular risks and morbidity in Asian Americans is based on a handful of studies conducted in Hawaii, California, and New York. Most of this work was done with Americans of Chinese, Japanese, and Filipino ancestry— the largest segment of the Asian ethnic population in the United States.

- Except for Japanese American men, aged 18 to 49, hypertension is reported to be lower than for white Americans; and yet Filipino Americans, as a group, have higher rates of hypertension, close to that of African Americans.

- Among Southeast Asian Americans, heart disease risk factors are similar to that of the United States as a whole.

- In a 1979 California hypertension study, hypertension was poorly controlled among Asian American ethnic groups undergoing treatment.

- In comparison to most Americans, Asian and Pacific Islander Americans are less likely to be aware of hypertension or to be undergoing treatment.

- In a study of Cambodian, Laotian, and Vietnamese immigrants, 94 percent had no knowledge of what blood pressure was.

- Southeast Asian American males, including Laotian and Vietnamese Americans, have smoking rates ranging from 35 to 72 percent.

- Hypercholesterolemia may be a problem. Japanese American, Hawaiian, Filipino American, and possibly Vietnamese American males are likely to have high levels of serum cholesterol.

Before the health community can address these problems, Lin believes that more knowledge is needed of the ethnic health situation: "We must convince the NHLBI, Centers for Disease Control and Prevention (CDC), and appropriate State and health officials that these are the issues that are worth an investment of their time, energy, and effort."

In addition, Lin outlined other measures to improve ethnic health:

- "We need scientifically valid disease prevention and health promotion programs that are culturally, ethnically, and linguistically appropriate."

- "We need to aim these programs toward strengthening community capacity to identify and address health problems that damage the well-being of our communities."

- "We must target efforts at the local level, where minority citizens are *subtle* victims of alcohol and tobacco advertising and *overt* victims of violence and substance abuse."

Finally, Lin wants to see communities involved in these efforts at the grassroots level: "Build real partnerships," he said. "Involve local people in advising, planning, and decision-making sessions."

As an example of this kind of grassroots cooperation, Lin cited a healthy-heart video series developed for an Asian American community in Ohio: "They were distributed in the same grocery stores that rented Asian movies to Southeast Asian immigrants. And they worked."

Heart Disease Now Ranked As Number One Killer of American Indians

Everett Rhoades, M.D.
Assistant Surgeon General
Director, Indian Health Service
Rockville, Maryland

Once a rarity, heart disease is the leading cause of deaths among American Indians. It accounts for nearly a quarter of all American Indian deaths.

"Only recently have American Indians been able to die of old age, in contrast to dying at an average age of 46 years," said Everett Rhoades. "We have not had to worry about ischemic heart disease in American Indian communities until this decade."

Rhoades reported other recent findings about the American Indian and Alaska Native communities, some of which go against the stereotypes:

- The total number of individuals in the American Indian and Alaska Native communities is now 2 million or more.

- In contrast to some minority groups, there is a national system of health care delivery for American Indian people.

- Many communities are still extremely isolated. Three out of four Navajo households have no telephone. Often patients are several hundred miles from their physicians.

- Some American Indian populations are among the most obese in the entire world.

- Some American Indian populations have the highest rates of diabetes ever encountered.

- A greater proportion of the American Indian population is under age 20 as compared to the United States as a whole.

- Heart disease has not been a problem in the American Indian community until recently. Now it is the number one killer.

- Fifteen years ago, the leading cause of death was injury.

- The third leading cause of death is cancer. Cancer is the number two killer in the general population.

- The rate of tuberculosis is six times greater than in the general population.

- Otitis media (middle-ear infection) is the second leading cause of doctor visits.

- Childbirth is the number one cause of hospitalizations. The American Indian fertility rate is nearly twice that of the United States as a whole.

One surprising but encouraging finding, according to Rhoades, is the relatively lower incidence of ischemic heart disease among the American Indian population. "Even when they have enormous rates of obesity and diabetes," he said. "There may be a relationship to decreased metabolism, decreased manufacture of low density lipoproteins, and a different ratio between low- and high-density types. This may, in fact, be protective for American Indian people."

Rhoades emphasized the need for more information about this phenomenon, so that these differences can be understood and applied to the treatment of CVD.

CVD Death Rate 50 Percent Higher Among Blacks

Michael Horan, M.D.
Director, Division of Heart and Vascular Diseases
National Heart, Lung, and Blood Institute
National Institutes of Health
Bethesda, Maryland

When Michael Horan looks at trends in CVD among minorities, he is alarmed not only by the prevalence of the disease but also by the high prevalence of risk factors.

That is one reason why Horan wants to see more analysis of minority epidemiologic data. The second reason is scientific. "When we observe differences in disease frequency or severity, this provides clues which can be studied scientifically," he explained. "The end result is that we will come up with better mechanisms for advancing the health of minorities and a better overall understanding of CVD."

In terms of trends in CVD and CVD mortality in minorities, Horan had little good news to report. "One of the first things to call to your attention is that, overall, blacks have the highest mortality rate," he said.

Horan listed other trends related to CVD mortality, including:

- **Heart failure death rates.** Blacks die of heart failure 2.5 times more frequently than whites and seven times more frequently than Asians.

- **Stroke death rates.** Blacks die of stroke three times more frequently than whites.

- **CHD prevalence by age.** Blacks have a higher prevalence at younger ages than whites but a lower prevalence at older ages.

- **Atherosclerosis.** Blacks have less epicardial or large coronary artery atherosclerosis.

- **Hypertension.** Black women have the highest prevalence—almost 39 percent.

- **Cholesterol.** Hispanics have a substantially lower prevalence of high blood cholesterol. Blacks and whites are nearly the same.

- **Smoking.** Hispanics have the highest prevalence. Black men have a higher prevalence than white men.

- **Obesity.** This is higher among both blacks and Hispanics than whites.

179

Judging from the trends, Horan finds ample cause for concern about the current state of minority health. But what is doubly worrisome, he feels, is the excessive level of some health trends. "We're talking about excess prevalence of hypertension in *both* black men and women," he said. "Also, excess stroke death, excess CHD death, and excess heart failure death."

Horan emphasized the need to understand the reason for these excesses, particularly in hypertension. "Is the higher prevalence of morbidity and mortality associated with hypertension in blacks genetic? Is it environmental? Or is it the result of genetic predisposition interacting with environment?"

By examining physiological characteristics among minorities and nonminorities, Horan believes that it may be possible to derive hypotheses for the causes of hypertension. He outlined numerous characteristics of minority groups, including:

- **Blood pressure.** Among adults, blacks have higher blood pressures than whites.

- **Obesity.** Among the hypertensive population, 44 percent suffer from obesity. Among black hypertensives, 54 percent are obese. Overall, blacks have 50 percent higher prevalence than whites.

- **Diabetes.** Black men have a 50 percent higher prevalence than white men. Black women have a 100 percent higher prevalence.

- **Left ventricular mass.** Blacks have 80 percent excess prevalence as compared to whites. "People with increased left heart size tend to die sooner because of cardiovascular causes."

- **Cardiovascular reactivity.** Compared to whites, blacks tend to react to mental and physical stressors less with increases in pulse and more with increases in blood pressure.

- **Kidney factors.** Compared to whites, blacks have blunted sodium excretion, increased blood pressure sensitivity to sodium challenge, decreased renal blood flow, and higher renal vascular resistance.

- **Endocrine factors.** Compared to whites, blacks have increased serum parathyroid hormone levels, increased serum 1,25 dihydroxy vitamin D levels, increased urinary kallikrein, and increased blood pressure response to infused norepinephrine.

- **Drug response.** Blacks respond well to diuretics but not as well to beta blockers and angiotensin converting enzyme (ACE) inhibitors compared to whites.

- **Potassium intake.** Compared to whites, blacks have a lower potassium intake.

- **Bypass recovery.** Functional recovery from bypass surgery is lower among blacks than whites.

- **Thrombolytic therapy.** Blacks appear to be more sensitive to tissue plasminogen activator (+-PA) than whites.

- **Smoking.** Approximately 30 percent more blacks than whites smoke.

- **Lipoprotein (a) [LP(a)] levels.** Blacks have higher levels of LP(a)—a lipoprotein found to be directly proportional to risk of CHD—than whites.

With these characteristics established, Horan believes that certain hypotheses can be suggested. In his view, hypertension in blacks could be:

- A membrane disorder, resulting from insufficient handling of sodium and calcium by vascular smooth muscle
- A renal or kidney problem, with inability to efficiently excrete a sodium load
- A metabolic problem, with high blood pressure as a response to increased peripheral vascular resistance.

In order to test these hypotheses, Horan wants to see more research focused on CVD in minorities. "Given this state of affairs, in

1990 we developed an RFA (request for applications) setting aside special monies for special research in order to study hypertension in blacks."

For the future, Horan will be overseeing more research into this troublesome area. "In fiscal year 93, we will be committing almost $19 million to the completion of these studies and, in fiscal year 94, almost $26 million."

Research Cuts Through Myths about Hypertension in Blacks and Whites

John M. Flack, M.D., M.P.H.
Assistant Professor, Divisions of Medicine and Epidemiology
Director, Division of General Internal Medicine
University of Minnesota
Minneapolis, Minnesota

One widely held belief challenged by John Flack is the idea that ethnicity has some dramatic effect on the relationship between high blood pressure and CVD.

"There may be differences in the absolute level of risk at a given blood pressure, but the shape of the relationship is the same: the higher the blood pressure, the higher the risk," Flack said.

Flack outlined some of the known facts about hypertension and the relationship between hypertension and ethnicity, including:

- **Prevalence.** At some point in life 70 to 75 percent of the population, both black and white, becomes hypertensive.

- **Causes.** In a study of 438 black women, researchers found strong correlations between age, obesity, income, and hypertension. "For every 10-year increase in age, we saw an increase in systolic pressure of about 5.5 mm," Flack reported. "Income was also negatively related to blood pressure. The higher your income, the lower your pressure."

- **Degree of control through medication.** "People on medication are not necessarily taking their medications, and not everybody who takes their medication has adequate control," he said.

- **Isolated systolic hypertension (ISH).** One of the particularly lethal forms of hypertension, ISH occurs mainly in people over the age of 60. The prevalence of the disease is virtually identical in both black and white men, according to Flack.

Over the years, beliefs about the relationship between systolic and diastolic pressure have changed. Flack outlined some of the common perceptions of the past, including:

- The idea that diastolic blood pressure is more important in assessing risk than is systolic
- The idea that increases in systolic blood pressure don't matter if diastolic pressure remains normal.

In fact, according to Flack, systolic pressure appears to be the key to predicting risk for CVD and death. "Clearly, for all causes of CVD, death is higher in people with normal diastolic pressures of less than 90, but with ISH," he reported.

Flack made it clear that he wants to dispel these myths about the systolic/diastolic relationship. He then outlined two other myths that have long been regarded as fact:

- The elderly don't benefit from hypertensive treatment. An increase in blood pressure as people age is normal. "One problem with that is that not every society in the world has an increase in blood pressure with age."

- Because of their unique circulatory physiology, treating patients with ISH is too risky.

As proof that both of these beliefs are false, Flack cited several past and recent studies of hypertension in the elderly:

Medical Research Council Study (MRC Study). "The blood pressure differential between active treatment and placebo was 15/8 mm. The reduction in stroke and coronary events did not attain statistical significance, but was certainly in the right direction," he said.

183

Systolic Hypertension in the Elderly Program (SHEP). "This was a diuretic-based treatment regimen which led to significant drops in blood pressure, fatal stroke, and CHD."

Treatment of Mild Hypertension Study (TOMHS). This trial involved four different clinical centers and men and women, ages 45 to 69, who were mildly hypertensive, 18 to 19 percent black, mildly overweight, and light drinkers. Patients received five different drug regimens. A sixth group received placebo. All groups received intensive intervention for weight loss, sodium reduction, alcohol reduction, and exercise increase. Flack outlined the results of the study as follows:

- At 24 months, the nondrug group showed similar positive changes in condition for both the under- and over-60 age groups.

- At 48 months, both black and white hypertensives, drug and nondrug groups, experienced a substantial decrease in systolic pressure.

- Diastolic pressure was lowered virtually the same in all groups, black and white.

- When nondrug therapy was added to a drug regimen, a greater decrease in systolic pressure resulted.

- Young and old responded similarly to drug therapy.

- LV mass dropped in all groups.

- Compliance to therapy by drug groups was higher in older patients than in younger patients. "That really goes against the idea that older patients won't take their medication," Flack said.

Compliance and Renal Disease

To deal effectively with hypertension in the future, Flack believes that physicians will have to find a way to deal with problems such as compliance in younger patients, renal disease, and other issues, including:

- Noncompliance to drug therapy in young hypertensive black males. "This is a particular problem because they end up showing up in emergency departments with malignant hypertension, and then they're on their way to dialysis, which can cost $30,000 to $40,000 per year."

- Sexual dysfunction in men on diuretic drug therapy. "If people present to you with sexual dysfunction, I would consider this a reason probably not to use the diuretics," he said.

- Steep increase in prevalence of end-stage renal disease in blacks later in life. "Most people who develop renal disease develop hypertension," he reported. "Sometimes you don't know which one preceded the other."

According to Flack, renal disease is an important issue because of the way it affects the black population. Blacks have a much harder time getting renal transplants than whites. This has an impact on black health issues as well as national economic issues. "Medicare is paying for most of this, and the costs are nearly $3 billion a year," he said.

In addition to these issues, there are therapeutic considerations physicians must keep in mind in treating hypertensive patients. They include:

- **Cost.** "You can prescribe the best, most potent drugs, but if the patient can't afford them, they will be taking their medicine every couple of days to stretch it out."

- **Coexisting medical conditions** such as arrhythmias and hyperthyroidism, orthostatic hypotension, diabetes and glucose intolerance, constipation, conduction system abnormalities, hyponatremia, depression, salt sensitivity, and general drug therapy side effects.

"There is a very high likelihood of coexisting medical conditions in all the elderly, the black elderly particularly," Flack said. "The potential benefits of CVD risk reduction are probably greater in blacks than whites because of the greater absolute risk in the former. This is an extrapolation of what we're seeing from younger populations. The major thing we can hang our hats on right now regarding preservation of renal function in humans is blood pressure control, blood pressure control, blood pressure control...."

How to Factor Aging into Antihypertensive Therapy

Elijah Saunders, M.D.
Associate Professor of Medicine
Head, Hypertension Division
Clinical Director, Hypertension Center
University of Maryland School of Medicine
Baltimore, Maryland

As the population ages, more physicians will have to learn how to factor old age into drug and nondrug hypertension interventions, according to Elijah Saunders.

"By the year 2030, 21.8 percent of the population will be over the age of 65, and the minority elderly will represent 25 percent of this population," he said.

For an aging population, hypertension is an extremely important disease because it's a disease that increases steadily with age. It is also a condition that disproportionately affects blacks.

Because the incidence of hypertension in the population can only increase over time, Saunders believes it is time for the health care industry to learn how to treat the elderly and how to balance the special considerations that arise, such as changes in physiology.

"As people get older, these physiologic functions decrease: nerve conduction, basal metabolic rate, the amount of water in the body and cells, cardiac output, renal flow and function, liver function, and so on," he said. "What is the importance of this? This has a tremendous impact on what happens to the drugs you put in people's bodies."

Saunders outlined several conditions and special circumstances physicians must be aware of in treating older patients:

- Antihypertensive drugs dilate arteries, and many will reduce LV hypertrophy. "We think this is beneficial, but we need more data," he said.

- How the drug is distributed in blood plasma.

- Hypertension and diabetes. "There are drugs such as beta blockers that do have some impact upon the diabetic state," he said. "We have to keep in mind that the impact may not be favorable."

- The benefit to keeping systolic pressure under 140 to 160 is now clear. "Insurance companies knew it for a long time," he said. "The SHEP program showed the benefit of treating isolated systolic hypertension."

- Decreased elastic tissue in cardiac output. "The ventricle becomes stiffer as people get older. The effect upon drug disposition is that the drugs are not cleared as well; therefore, they have an increased half-life."

- Changes in gastrointestinal (GI) tract. "The GI motility is down; acid is also down. The secretory activity of the gastric mucosa is down. Therefore, the effect will be an altered breakdown of drugs and decreased transport."

- Liver problems. "If you have a bad liver, there may be an increase in the half-life of a drug because it's getting into the system slower and peaking later and staying around for a longer period of time."

- Kidney problems. "Again, the half-life is increased because the drug is around longer."

Elderly Hypertension Responds to Therapy

Despite the difficulties of treating the elderly, Saunders cited numerous ways in which the elderly benefit from antihypertensive therapy. He quoted from several studies that have proven these benefits:

- **Hypertension Detection and Followup Program (HDFP).** "We broke down the results of this study in terms of younger, middle, and older groups," Saunders said. "We compared people we treated in our clinics with those we treated in the community. We saw, in every class of individuals in the study, some benefit, better with stroke, but also some benefit from coronary disease."

- **SHEP.** "We were able to show that the control groups [without treatment] did worse," he reported.

- **European Working Party on High Blood Pressure in the Elderly.** "We showed that total mortality was reduced by 38 percent and fatal myocardial infarction (MI) by 60 percent.This was a high-risk population—elderly people with MI's—and it was reduced by 60 percent."

Drug Therapy in Old Versus Young Patients

Although drug therapy has proven effective in most patients, Saunders sees the value in nondrug therapy for elderly patients. "This approach may be more important to older people than younger. If you are advising them in nonpharmacologic means—salt restriction, weight loss, reasonable exercise—they are much more likely to follow your advice than younger people."

In treating the elderly patient with drug therapy, Saunders offered several known facts about drug action in older patients versus younger patients:

- **Beta blockers, ACE inhibitors.** "Should have a better efficacy profile in younger individuals," he said.

- **Diuretics.** "In blacks, diuretics often work better, especially in older people. However, hypokalemia is more likely. Older people tend to be on much more restricted diets (e.g., low in citrus), probably because of economic factors."

- **Calcium channel blockers.** "Preliminary studies suggest equitable benefits in older and younger people." However, more studies are necessary to confirm the degree of benefit in older people.

In addition to specific drug guidelines, Saunders also had general advice for physicians treating elderly patients:

- **Ask about other drugs.** "Tell them to bring all their medicines in with them. But you better have a big table around when they do. I have a ball throwing this stuff out."

- **Discuss high blood pressure.** "People become very suspicious, especially older people. You see them every 2 or 3 months and collect the fee, and they wonder if you're just taking their money. Discuss with them what high blood pressure is all about."

- **Communicate with the family.** "Selecting the right drug is one thing, but the biggest challenge with elderly people is handling all of these other problems, other than just the hypertension."

CVD Rates Highest Among American Indians in the Northern Plains

Thomas Welty, M.D., M.P.H.
Medical Epidemiologist
Aberdeen Area Indian Health Service
Principal Investigator, Strong Heart Study
Rapid City, South Dakota

When researchers began studying the rate of CVD among American Indians for the Strong Heart Study, they weren't sure what they would find.

The only thing the investigators knew going into the study was that CVD rates were increasing among Indian people, and that CVD had surpassed injuries as the number one killer of American Indians.

What they found, according to Thomas Welty, was a dramatic difference between CVD rates in Northern Plains and Arizona Indians. "There is a large difference. The Arizona Indians have quite low rates—about half the rate of heart disease found among the Northern Plains Indians," Welty said.

Welty is the principal investigator of the South and North Dakota three-center, multitribe, ongoing study. So far, researchers have completed the first phase or first examination of 1,500 participants from three different areas: North and South Dakota, Oklahoma, and Arizona. Tribes involved in the study include the Oglala Sioux, Cheyenne

River Sioux, Devil's Lake Sioux, Kiowa, Apache, Comanche, Caddo Wichita, Delaware, Fort Sill Apache, Maricopa, and Salt River and Gila River Pima Indians.

The following is a summary of the first-phase findings:

- **Smoking** is common in Northern Plains Indians, ranging from 40 to 58 percent. Southwestern Indians have lower rates, as low as 10 percent among women. Oklahoma Indians have intermediate rates.

- **High cholesterol.** Between 30 and 40 percent of all Indians studied had cholesterols higher than 200. LDL levels are highest among Northern Plains Indians and lowest among Arizona Indians. "Elevated cholesterol levels, combined with smoking, may be the two most important risk factors that lead to the higher rates of heart disease," he said.

- **Hypertension.** The rate of hypertension is lower among Northern Plains Indians than among Arizona Indians and Oklahoma Indians.

- **Diabetes.** "This is really the most striking finding. All groups had a prevalence rate of more than 30 percent. In some places, it exceeds 60 percent," Welty noted.

- **Body mass index (BMI).** "The ideal would be between 20 and 25," he said. "The mean we found is closer to 30, with women a little bit heavier than men."

- **Binge drinking.** "We know that binge drinking is a risk factor for sudden death," Welty noted. "A lot of the sudden deaths that occur end up being coded as CVD deaths."

The study team is also gathering statistics on television watching time, genetic background, stress, education, and other factors that could influence CVD rates. At the 4-year point in the study, researchers will reexamine those from the first study and compile new data for comparison.

"For the next generation, we feel it is very important that the Indian people have this information so the next generation may not have to suffer as much from diabetes or heart disease," Welty said.

High Correlation Between Diabetes and Heart Disease Among American Indians

Barbara Howard, Ph.D.
Medlantic Research Institute
Washington, D.C.

After investigators in the Strong Heart Study discovered an alarmingly high incidence of diabetes among American Indians, the next question they had to ask themselves was Why? Why are American Indians one of the largest groups in the United States with a high rate of diabetes? Also, how does diabetes contribute to heart disease? What risk factors exist among diabetics, and among diabetics with heart disease?

As chairperson for the steering committee of the Strong Heart Study, Barbara Howard helped explore these issues using data from the phase 1 exam. She outlined some of the findings of the study as they relate to impaired glucose tolerance (IGT—a level of high blood sugar that falls between diabetes and nondiabetes), diabetes, and heart disease in American Indian populations. "We wanted to examine whether the prevalence of CVD differs in individuals with IGT and diabetes as compared to nondiabetics," she explained.

Howard broke her findings down into several issues. The first was, "How much diabetes and IGT exist in the three American Indian groups?"

- In Arizona, diabetes rates approached 65 to 70 percent for some age groups. Other areas reported rates of 30 to 40 percent.

  "In Arizona, among the Pima, Maricopa, and Papago communities, fasting glucose among diabetics is actually higher than in diabetics in the other two areas," Howard reported. "That means that there's not only more diabetes in Arizona but the degree of control is somewhat worse."

- IGT existed somewhat equally in all areas at a rate of 15 to 20 percent.

191

A second question addressed by the study was, "How does diabetes contribute to heart disease?"

In their initial findings, researchers discovered that heart disease was higher among men than women, and higher in South Dakota than in Arizona and Oklahoma.

Howard cited other results related to this discovery:

- **High levels of diabetes.** "Diabetes had a tremendous effect on the amount of heart disease, with the amount of heart disease being a lot higher in the individuals with diabetes," she reported.

- **Impaired glucose tolerance.** "Except for a group of men studied in South Dakota, there does not appear to be more heart disease among those with IGT," Howard noted.

- **Arizona, diabetes, and CVD.** "If you look at the number of cases, virtually all the cases of heart disease are among the diabetics."

In the third portion of the study, Howard and the other researchers looked at risk factors and asked, "What risk factors for heart disease exist in diabetics and to what degree?"

- **LDL cholesterol.** High low-density-lipoprotein cholesterol did not appear to be a factor in the diabetic patients studied. "In fact, if anything, there might be a suggestion of lower cholesterol among the diabetics." Howard said.

- **HDL cholesterol.** The study found lower levels of high-density-lipoprotein cholesterol in diabetes, which Howard termed "very significant in terms of potential effects of heart disease."

- **Triglycerides.** In subjects with IGT, triglycerides were somewhat elevated. In patients with diabetes, triglycerides were almost double compared to the nondiabetic patients.

- **High blood pressure.** "Individuals with diabetes and IGT have a clear tendency toward higher blood pressure."

- **Obesity.** "We certainly know that obesity is a risk factor for diabetes and heart disease. In both women and men, among those with IGT and diabetes, you see higher body mass indexes. They are more obese."

- **Body fat percentage.** "For men and women, it's supposed to be under 20 to 30 percent. In both groups, we found more body fat than one would expect."

- **Waist-hip ratio.** "It isn't just how much fat a person has, but where it is. If it is distributed centrally, we think it may have more of an impact on health. Again, we found a tendency in the diabetics in this group to have more of this central body fat, both in women and men."

- **Fibrinogen.** "This is a reflection of the tendency for blood to clot, and in American Indian men and women, fibrinogen levels are significantly higher among those with diabetes."

- **Insulin.** "There are a number of suggestions now that insulin itself may contribute to heart disease. Among men and women in the study, insulin levels are quite a bit higher in individuals with diabetes and IGT."

- **Smoking.** "In terms of explaining the diabetes-induced heart disease, smoking doesn't appear to be related. Diabetics, both men and women, smoked less than nondiabetics."

From these specific findings, Howard offered the following conclusions regarding the relationship between diabetes and heart disease in American Indians: "The prevalence of diabetes is higher in American Indians in Arizona," she said. "In all three communities studied, CHD is higher among those with diabetes. However, women had less heart disease than men. Finally, IGT doesn't appear to be associated with heart disease, except among American Indian men in South Dakota."

Differences in Diet Found in Communities with Higher Heart Disease Rates

Ellie Zephier, M.P.H., R.D.
Nutrition Coordinator, Strong Heart Study
Oklahoma City, Oklahoma

In a dietary study related to the Strong Heart Study, Ellie Zephier and other researchers looked at dietary differences in the three study groups of American Indians from Arizona, Oklahoma, and North and South Dakota.

Just as researchers found variations in heart disease among these three communities, the Strong Heart Study discovered numerous variations in diet among the three communities and detected clear patterns in calorie intake, fat content, fiber intake, and other related dietary issues.

Zephier summarized the findings of the study and an earlier diet study conducted on the Pima Indians in Arizona:

• The highest rate of heart disease was among the Sioux tribes in North and South Dakota.

• Coffee was the most commonly consumed product in South Dakota and Oklahoma.

• Among the Dakota group, the most commonly consumed items were fruit juice, soft drinks, milk, white bread, sugary drink mixes, and fried potatoes.

• Among the Oklahoma group, the most common items were soft drinks, fruit, fruit juice, vegetables, sugary drink mixes, and milk.

• Higher caloric intake was found among the Arizona and Oklahoma groups. The Sioux in the Dakotas ate about 500 calories fewer than other groups.

• Higher fat intake was found among the Arizona group, with the Pima Indians having the highest fat consumption based on a 24-hour recall survey.

- Levels of cholesterol are higher among the Dakota group, but cholesterol intake is actually lower than among the other two groups.

- Higher fiber intake was found among the Arizona group, with the Pima Indians appearing to eat more fiber than the other groups.

- Higher vitamin C and calcium intake was found among the Arizona group. The Pima Indians ranked about the same on sodium but had higher intakes of vitamin C and calcium.

- The Oklahoma group overall consumed a wider variety of foods than the others and also consumed more fruits and vegetables, both fresh and canned. But the Oklahoma group also ate more beef, bacon, hot dogs, potatoes, and fats.

- The Dakota group consumed more milk, white bread, fried potatoes, cereal, eggs, beans, and chicken.

In order to influence the poor dietary habits among these groups, Zephier suggested several possible interventions:

- Discourage frying food.
- Encourage the use of more beans.
- Encourage more frequent use of rice and macaroni.
- Discourage the use of eggs; encourage cereal consumption.
- Encourage the use of less fatty meats.
- Encourage the use of more decaffeinated coffee.

"Other interventions could be cooking classes and exercise classes," Zephier said. "And we need intensive nutrition education from elementary school on up."

Obesity and Heart Disease a Double Problem in Minorities

Xavier Pi-Sunyer, M.D.
Director of Obesity Research Center
Columbia University
Chief of Endocrinology, Department of Medicine
St. Luke's Roosevelt Hospital
New York, New York

While researchers know that obesity and heart disease are related, according to Xavier Pi-Sunyer it is very difficult to define the exact relationship using existing data.

"We know the metabolic adverse consequences of obesity," Pi-Sunyer said. "But we have very little data on the synergism between obesity and CVD, obesity and hypertension, obesity and diabetes."

This means that obesity and heart disease must be looked at separately, for the most part, as a "double problem" for minorities. But it doesn't mean that investigators can't continue to look for a relationship, Pi-Sunyer said. He outlined some of what is known about obesity and the risk of developing these diseases in minority groups.

- Prevalence of obesity, hypertension, diabetes, and heart disease within the same groups, with all seeming to be higher among minorities, particularly hypertension and diabetes.

- Increasing morbidity and mortality from hypertension in black populations.

- Enormously increased risk of diabetes with obesity, and high prevalence of diabetes among blacks.

- Threefold diabetes prevalence among Hispanics, and increased prevalence of diabetes among obese Hispanics.

- Twofold greater risk for hypercholesterolemia in obese patients.

- Increased mortality related to increased weight by three major studies.

"All [of the several studies] have suggested increased diabetes and increased CVD in relation to increasing central body fat."

For many reasons, central body fat seems to be a key factor in determining whether obesity will lead to the development of other diseases. Pi-Sunyer outlined some of those reasons:

- Central fat is much more lipolytically active.

- Central fat enhances the amount of fat in the liver, which doesn't seem to degrade insulin properly, causing hyperinsulinemia.

- Higher fatty acids coursing through the liver cause it to produce more glucose and raise blood insulin levels.

- Higher insulin causes sodium retention, which may lead to hypertension.

"These effects of central fat can lead to CVD, diabetes, and hypertension," he said.

In recent studies, researchers have shown the relationship between central fat and diabetes. Pi-Sunyer cited two such studies:

- Mexican Americans with central fat had much higher insulin, a higher fasting glucose, and a higher 2-hour postprandial glucose.

- In a Swedish study, participants who were quite obese showed no increased risk for other diseases if their fat was all below the waist. Patients with weight around the middle showed a six-fold risk of developing diabetes and a similar high risk for CVD and stroke.

Is Exercise the Answer?

When trying to find strategies to address obesity, researchers run into trouble when recommending exercise, dieting, and other techniques. "Many of these minority populations don't have the resources or facilities in which to exercise," Pi-Sunyer noted. "It's also hard to get people interested in modifying their behavior. We know that in America, 3 out of every 5 calories is from fat or sugar. Many of these groups are not aware of this or know that it may be harmful for their health."

To address the problem more effectively, Pi-Sunyer suggested the following strategies:

- Trying to increase energy expenditure in daily activities.
- Exercising in a group-social interaction is important.
- More frequent and more effective nutrition education.

Native Hawaiians Use Traditional Diet to Improve Worst Minority Health Status

Noa Emmett Aluli, M.D.
President, Na Pu'uwai Kaunakakai
Molokai, Hawaii

In his family practice and as president of a community-based health organization, Noa Emmett Aluli has seen Native Hawaiians ranked worst in the United States in terms of health status of minority groups.

"Most Native Hawaiians are unaware of the extent of their health problems," Aluli noted. "When compared to all races in the United States, there is evidence that Native Hawaiians suffer higher overall mortality rates for the major ailments."

Although the situation has started to improve Native Hawaiians are ranked at higher rates for most diseases compared to other minority groups. Aluli summarized the key problems as follows:

- **Death rates** are 34 percent higher than the general population.
- **Heart disease** is 44 percent higher.
- **Cancer** is 39 percent higher.

And the situation has been even worse for full-blooded Hawaiians:

- **Heart disease** is 177 percent higher.
- **Cancer** is 126 percent higher.
- **Diabetes** is 588 percent higher.

Other problems are higher cardiovascular risk levels including obesity. In fact, a study of Native Hawaiians found that 65.5 percent of males and 62.8 percent of females were overweight.

After a study of this problem, researchers found that diet was a major contributor. "One study reported that 91 percent of the people participating in the study consumed diets with greater than 30 percent of calories from fat," Aluli noted. "Contemporary Native Hawaiians consume diets which are high in saturated fat, cholesterol, sugar, and salt. Foods commonly found in the dietary recall are french fries,

198

processed sausage, ham, pork, beef, mayonnaise, butter, ice cream, eggs, pastries, cakes, pies, candies, and soda."

Traditional Diet Yields Results

In order to test the theory that a "Western" diet was causing health problems, several recent dietary programs to lower the health risks have been created that utilize traditional Hawaiian foods such as taro, fish, sweet potatoes, yams, breadfruit, green vegetables and a few fruits, seaweed, fish, some pork, fowl, salt, coconut, sugar cane, and small amounts of kukui nuts (a native Hawaiian nut used for medicine, food, and extracting lamp oil).

"It's estimated that the total fat content of the traditional Hawaiian diet ranges between 12 to 15 percent," Aluli said.

The results of these studies have been dramatic, according to Aluli. "After a 21-day traditional diet, we had significant lowering of blood cholesterol and triglycerides. The diet demonstrated total lipid lowering effects. In the Waianae Diet Program, there was also a 5.8 percent reduction in weight and an average loss of 13.4 pounds. We think the traditional diet programs will result in major changes for our worst-health status of any minority population in the United States."

Obesity Increased Among Acculturated Mexican Americans

Eunice Romero-Gwynn, Ph.D., M.P.H.
Community Nutrition Specialist
Department of Nutrition
University of California at Davis
Davis, California

Among the Latin American groups that have immigrated to the United States and given up much of their traditional diets, Mexican Americans have probably suffered the greatest problem with obesity, according to Eunice Romero-Gwynn.

"Mexican Americans, both men and women, present the greatest prevalence of obesity," she said.

Romero-Gwynn has studied food patterns of people of Mexican descent living in California to determine changes that may have taken place with acculturation. She stated that the diet of the groups she studied has become significantly higher in sources of fats and sugars. With acculturation, there has been also a decline in the consumption of traditional foods and adoption of more American types of foods. Some of the specific changes she found are:

- Increased consumption of flour tortillas (not original from Mexico), which are higher in fat than corn tortillas.

- Decreased use of lard, but significantly increased consumption of several sources of fats including margarine or butter, vegetable oil, mayonnaise, salad dressing, and sour cream.

- The increased consumption of vegetables in salads may be due to nutrition education programs that emphasize consumption of vegetables "in the American way," instead of supporting traditional ways of consuming vegetables.

- Increased consumption of sliced, white bread prepared in sandwiches (with mayonnaise and cold meats) and in toast (with margarine or butter and sugar-rich jelly).

- Increased consumption of sugar-rich drinks and beverages. These drinks have replaced the traditional low-sugar beverages—*aguas frescas de frutas* (water flavored with fresh fruit)—common in Mexico and most other Latin American countries.

- Significantly increased consumption of ready-to-eat breakfast cereals, which are often very high in sugars. These have replaced the traditional oats-and-milk hot cereals, which are lower in sugar and much lower in price.

- Decreased consumption of chilies and many traditional dishes prepared with vegetables. As a result, the diet may be lower in fiber, beta carotene, and other specific nutrients provided by vegetables. An example of a change that results in a lower diversity of vegetables is the preference for steamed white rice instead of for the traditional rice or pasta prepared with vegetables. In addition, soups and vegetable-based meat dishes have almost disappeared from the diet of second-generation Mexican Americans.

Romero-Gwynn found that there was an inverse correlation between the abandonment of traditional foods and the prevalence of obesity among the families studied.

She suggested that health and nutrition education programs emphasize the following:

- Consuming corn tortillas instead of flour tortillas.

- Reducing all types of fats, not just those rich in cholesterol (Most people think that cholesterol-free fats such as canola oils are good foods.)

- Using nonfat or low-fat mayonnaise as a spread on sandwiches and in salads.

- Preparing dips using nonfat plain yogurt and/or nonfat or low-fat cottage cheese as alternatives to mayonnaise and sour cream.

- Supporting traditional drinks, such as *aguas frescas de frutas* in place of the newly adopted high-sugar drinks.

- Emphasizing low-sugar breakfast cereals as well as the traditional milk-based atoles (a milk-based hot beverage usually consumed at breakfast or evening meal).

Romero-Gwynn believes that the retention of traditional practices and the improvement of new practices adopted in the United States may be significant contributors to decreasing the large trend toward obesity among low-income immigrants from Latin America.

"Identify healthy practices among any immigrant group and support them," she said. "When you are uncertain about a belief or practice, don't judge it. Observe, consult, and categorize it later."

Improved Data Leads to New Discoveries about Minority Health Status

Diane Makuc, Dr.P.H.
Chief, Analytical Coordination Branch
National Center for Health Statistics
Centers for Disease Control and Prevention
Hyattsville, Maryland

For many years, investigators have had difficulty getting a clear picture of the Nation's minority health status. Much of the problem has been the minority health statistics data base, or lack thereof.

However, as time goes on, the existing data base is continually improving. Information-gathering agencies like the National Center for Health Statistics (NCHS) are working to improve and expand national minority health statistics.

"Data from NCHS have been critical in identifying the significant gaps in health status among population groups," Diane Makuc said. "As a matter of fact, much of the data that was presented this morning I was happy to see came from the NCHS."

Makuc referred to several information resources from the NCHS currently in use by health care researchers and educators.

- *Health United States:* This annual publication includes a "substantial amount of minority data," according to Makuc.

- *Prevention Profile:* This publication is designed to monitor the Nation's progress toward the health objectives of Healthy People 2000, many of which have specific targets for minority populations.

Data systems that provide information on cardiovascular and pulmonary diseases for minority populations include:

- National Health Interview Survey.
- National Health and Nutrition Examination Surveys.
- Followup study of the First National Health and Nutrition Examination Survey.
- Provider surveys, including the National Hospital Discharge Survey and the Ambulatory Medical Care Survey.

202

Quoting from several of these surveys, Makuc discussed how the data have improved in recent years and what has been learned about minority death rates and health status as a result.

- In most States, Hispanic deaths are now classified in five separate subgroups. In 1987, only 18 States reported Hispanic-origin information on death certificates.

- Age-specific resident population estimates are now available for Asian, American Indian, and Hispanic populations, 1987-89.

- Heart disease death rates among persons 45 to 64 years of age were highest among black adults. 80 percent higher than the rate for white adults in 1989.

- Hispanic and Asian adults had 30 to 60 percent lower heart disease death rates than whites.

- Stroke death rates for black adults 45 to 64 years of age were 2.5 to 3 times higher than the rate for other groups.

- Pulmonary disease death rates among Hispanics and Asians 45 to 64 years of age were less than 50 percent of the rate for other groups.

- Stroke mortality for persons 65 years of age and over is about 40 percent lower for Hispanic, Asian, and American Indian persons than for whites.

- Since 1970, declines in heart disease mortality range from 27 percent for black men to 41 percent for white men.

- Asthma death rates for young blacks 5 to 34 years of age were almost four times that of young whites in 1989.

- Cigarette smoking was most prevalent among American Indian men, at a rate of 42 percent, followed by black men at 34 percent in 1989-90.

- Diabetes was twice as prevalent among Mexican Americans as among non-Hispanic whites, and 1.6 times as prevalent among blacks as among non-Hispanic whites in 1976-80.

- Between 1979 and 1987, asthma hospitalizations among children from birth to 4 years increased at an average annual rate of 4 percent for white children and 7 percent for black children.

- Relative to the number of discharges with acute myocardial infarction, whites were twice as likely to receive coronary artery bypass surgery as blacks in 1979-84.

Although some minority data have come under fire for inaccuracy, Makuc believes that the overall reliability of the resources is good. She outlined a few of the key controversies over minority health data.

- **Value of race and ethnicity data.** "Some researchers have questioned whether data should be reported by race because they say racial differences are entirely due to socioeconomic status," she said. "Several studies have shown, however, that even after controlling for socioeconomic status, substantial racial differences in health status remain."

- **Quality of race and ethnicity data on vital records and health surveys.** "This has been questioned. However, self-reported race has been shown to be a highly reliable item."

- **Potential for bias due to differences in classification of race.** "Based on data from a prospective study linking records from the census bureau to that of death certificates, overall agreement between these two sources was 99 percent."

"However, persons categorized as American Indian or Asian and Pacific Islander on the current population survey were sometimes characterized as 'white' on the death certificate," said Makuc. "Death rates for American Indians may be underestimated by about 22 percent, and death rates for Asians may be underestimated by about 12 percent."

The NCHS has been actively involved in improving minority health statistics, Makuc said, including:

- Expanding Asian statistics on health interview surveys to nine categories of Asians and Pacific Islanders.

- Oversampling blacks in surveys.

- Revising the standard birth and death certificates to include Hispanic subgroup identifications and education level.

- A resolution by the Public Health Service to improve minority health statistics by collecting and analyzing data to better understand the causes of racial disparities, improving the measurement of race and ethnicity, improving the analysis and dissemination of existing data, and addressing data gaps to improve data collection.

Lack of True Surveillance Interferes with CVD Intervention in Minority Groups

Robert Mayberry, Ph.D.
Senior Epidemiologist for Minority Health
Centers for Disease Control and Prevention
Atlanta, Georgia

For a population successfully to study, analyze, and intervene in a widespread disease such as CVD, Robert Mayberry said that the population must first have a public health surveillance system designed for "the continuous systematic collection, analysis, interpretation, and reporting of relevant health data necessary for effective planning of evaluation programs and practices, which aim to control and prevent disease, injuries, and death among the defined population."

From this somewhat involved definition of surveillance, Mayberry picked two components that he considers absolutely essential to this process: relevant health data and defined population.

In his opinion, when it comes to CVD in minority groups, the United States is lacking in both areas. "By definition, as well as by process, there really is no surveillance system for CVD in the United States," he said.

If Mayberry were able to design a national surveillance system for CVD, he would structure it so that it met most of the following guidelines:

- **Recognition, diagnoses, and reporting.** "It begins with the recognition of a disease, followed by diagnosis, which is followed by either active or passive reporting of the diagnoses to some level of coordinated center."

- **Government interaction.** "This is an interactive process between local people, State health departments, all the way up to the Federal Government. The data can be received at any of these levels and in any form."

- **Data management.** "Then there is a series of data management activities followed by the analyses and the reporting process itself."

Unfortunately, the Nation is limited in its ability to develop such a system, according to Mayberry, and the reason for this limitation is the lack of relevant health data. However, Mayberry cited several sources of information which can be of use in this process:

- Vital statistics.
- National Hospital Discharge Survey.
- Medicare data.
- National Health Interview Survey.
- Behavioral Risk Factor Surveillance System.

While these resources offer much information on minority health status, Mayberry pointed out that it may be "somewhat limited beyond some broad categories."

"If you look at medical records, people are abstract in giving information," he said. "Ethnicity—race—in the medical records is usually about 85 percent complete, whereas ethnicity data are roughly 15 percent complete."

Mayberry cited several studies that have helped in improving the data on minority health—the Framingham Study, the Finland Study, the Corpus Christi Health Project—but emphasized the lack of a national surveillance system to coordinate this effort.

Another stumbling block to progress, Mayberry said, is the lack of scientific definitions in terms of race and ethnicity. "Anthropologists have basically discounted race as a variable. They have called it an invalid consideration in these days and times," he said. "The bottom line, I believe, is that ethnicity is a social-cultural construct and in time may actually replace race as a way to classify people in regard to differences that might lead to susceptibility to disease."

Before the United States can develop a surveillance system of its own, Mayberry believes that the issue of ethnic definitions has to be addressed and that the system must allow more diversity and flexibility. He cited other issues that should also be looked at:

- Need for socioeconomic data on minorities.
- Need to overcome fears of the cost. "We have some information that indicates that a passive surveillance system, in a small state like Vermont, costs roughly $34,000 a year. So I don't think the cost is prohibitive."

Burden of CVD in Minority Women Grows Heavier as Population Ages

Irma Mebane-Sims, Ph.D.
Epidemiologist, Lipid Metabolism-Atherogenesis Branch
Division of Heart and Vascular Diseases
National Heart, Lung, and Blood Institute
National Institutes of Health
Bethesda, Maryland

The American population is aging and Americans survive well beyond 65. The health problems related to aging thus assume great importance.

One of those problems is the burden of CVD as a major cause of illness and death in minority women, especially for women past the age of menopause when the rates of CVD rise dramatically."

For many minority women in the United States, living longer means having to deal with health care problems.

"In the year 1900, there were slightly under 4 million women over the age of 50," she said. "By the time the year 2020 rolls around, there will be somewhere in the neighborhood of 50 million women over 50." According to Mebane-Sims, this means that more minority women will live long enough to develop the diseases that create the heaviest morbidity and mortality burden on the over-65 female population, namely, heart disease and cancer.

"If you look at a group of 2,000 postmenopausal women, here's what will happen to that group in a year's time: 20 will develop heart disease, 11 will develop bone loss, 6 will develop breast cancer, and 3 will develop endometrial cancer."

Mebane-Sims outlined several other trends in older minority women, including:

- In the total female population, one in three deaths in women over the age of 65 is caused by heart disease. Cancer is the number two cause of death in this group.

- In 1988, cancer (all types combined) ranked as the number one cause of death for women 45 to 64. However, in women 65 to 74, 75 to 84, and 85 and older, heart disease was the number one killer. Thus, overall for women middle-age and older, heart disease is the number one cause of death.

- Among Hispanic women, the same pattern exists.

- Although ischemic events make up the majority of heart disease deaths in women, heart attacks appear to account for less than half of these ischemic events.

- Of the 31 million hospital discharges recorded in 1988, 18.5 million occurred among women, and 16.5 million of those occurred among women 45 years of age or older.

- The leading causes of hospital stays among women 45 years and older are related to circulatory system diagnoses.

- One-third of all hospitalizations occur in women 65 and older; 60 percent of the hospitalizations for circulatory conditions happen in this age group. In 1988, approximately 15 percent of women in the United States were 65 and older.

- Average length of hospital stay is 6.1 days for women. Overall, however, increasing age results in longer stays, and circulatory conditions require longer hospitalization.

- Cerebrovascular and congestive heart failure accounts for 50 percent of the heart disease occurring in women 65 years and older.

- Smoking is relatively low among older women but increasing among younger age groups. Future cohorts of elderly women will carry the additional burdens of health risks associated with smoking.

These trends underscore the emerging importance and consequences of health issues in an aging America. Mebane-Sims also noted additional limitations of the national data currently available.

The data are too general and tend to present the information in a dichotomous fashion (men vs. women, blacks vs. whites) rather than present simultaneous information about gender, race, and age. Given the increasing importance of age and differences in the types and rates of disease/mortality by gender, race, and age, such detailed national data are important and need to be made available.

"As our minority groups get older, we have less information available in terms of the changes of risk-factor status," she said.

"One of the problems is that we have a changing dynamic within the American population. The cohorts of women who will be going through menopause in the coming years will be dramatically different, with quite a bit of exposure to oral contraceptives, alcohol use, and cigarette smoking. They will be bringing different risk factors into their elder years that will be important in estimating and intervening in their risk for cardiovascular events."

Linking Psychological Stress to CVD in Black Adults

Emmeline Edwards, Ph.D.
Associate Professor of Pharmacology and Toxicology
School of Pharmacy, University of Maryland at Baltimore
Baltimore, Maryland

When looking at risk factors that contribute to heart disease in minorities—family history, age, obesity, hypertension— Emmeline Edwards believes that one other, less talked-about risk factor must be included: psychosocial stressors.

Edwards defined psychosocial stress as follows: "An internal, subjective state that involves the perception of threat to one's well-being. The stressors would be the stimuli that would provoke the psychological stress."

Edwards, a research scientist investigating the neurobiology of stress, became involved in the subject of psychosocial stress through her work with the National Black Women's Health Project. Through her study of the existing data on psychosocial stressors, Edwards identified four factors that place psychological stress on black women:

- **Socioeconomic disadvantages.** Black women are often engaged in jobs that require lower skills and that provide decreased freedom, decreased prestige, and increased job dissatisfaction.

- **Chronic exposure to sustained, disturbing emotions.** With social disadvantages comes the increased ability to experience some level of neuroses.

- **Overload.** With lower skilled jobs, black women are required to perform repetitive tasks, such as assembly line work, and work large amounts of overtime.

- **Repressed hostility.** Black women are more likely to be placed in work situations in which they have to repress their feelings of dissatisfaction.

Scientific evidence suggests a link between psychological stress and heart disease. Edwards cited an early study which reported suppressed anger was generally related to higher blood pressure among blacks and whites. Another study reported positive correlation among diastolic blood pressure, anxiety, and suppressed hostility. Systolic blood pressure was reported to be correlated with expressed anger.

One positive finding of these studies was that stress levels seemed to go down among black women who received social support. "Unfortunately, among black American women, a very low level of both emotional support and instrumental support was available to them, so these women have not taken advantage of this coping pattern to reduce their stressors."

In addition to low levels of social support, Edwards also found very few studies on the subject of psychological stress among black women. "I would like to implore minority researchers to get themselves involved because it is very important that the population we're studying can identify with the researchers."

Early Warning Signs of CVD Found in Young Hispanics

Richard Torres, M.D.
Medical Director
Bridgeport Community Health Center
Bridgeport, Connecticut

If the health care community plans to improve the health status of Hispanics and lessen the prevalence of CVD, the first step is a recognition that CVD risk factors begin in childhood, according to Richard Torres.

As a researcher for Hispanic health issues, Torres has conducted a number of studies on CVD risk factors in adolescents. He strongly emphasized the evidence presented in an early study that the "atherosclerotic process begins in childhood."

Torres cited several studies on hypertension, diabetes, obesity, tobacco use, family history, and high serum cholesterol among Hispanics of all ages which show evidence that risk factors begin in childhood:

- **Puerto Rican Community Prevalence Study.** Found hypertension prevalence of 45 percent and diabetes prevalence of 15 percent.

- **Puerto Ricans and Health: Findings From New York City.** Found hypertension prevalence of 52 percent among Hispanics and 50 percent among blacks.

- **Florida High School Study.** Found higher prevalence of hypertension in Hispanic and black students as compared to whites.

- **Hispanic Health and Nutrition Examination Survey (HHANES) by NCHS.** Found that hypertension, obesity, and cigarette smoking were prevalent among Puerto Ricans, Mexi-

can Americans, and Cuban Americans. HDL—or good cholesterol—was also found to be lower among these groups.

- **McNamara Study.** "McNamara, in 1971, published data that
  clearly showed that early lesions begin asymptomatically and
  represent a silent disease until the clinical symptoms appear
  later in life," Torres said.

- **NCEP Program data.** Indicated that blood cholesterol levels
  are related to the extent of early lesions in adolescents, young
  adults, and children. Also, children with high blood cholesterol
  levels were found to be three times more likely to have elevated levels in adulthood.

In addition to these data, Torres offered the findings from the
Adolescent Cardiovascular Examination Survey (ACES), which was
conducted at the Bridgeport Community Health Center. The survey
looked at over 600 adolescents, ages 10 to 19, concerning risk factors
such as serum cholesterol, tobacco use, obesity, blood pressure, diabetes mellitus, family history of CVD risk factors, and medications.
About 95 percent of the cohort was of Hispanic origin.

- Five prevalent CVD risk factors were found: ethnicity, family
  history of CVD, hypercholesterolemia, obesity, and diabetes.
- Black adolescents were found to have higher blood pressure.
- One-third of adolescents reported a family history of CVD risk
  factors.
- One-fourth of those reported a family history of diabetes.
- One in six suffered from obesity.
- One in twenty had hypercholesterolemia.
- Belief systems taught by parents and relatives were found to
  be a factor in degree of risk.

To address these problems, Torres called for better screening and
better education for Hispanic adolescents. "Screening for cardiovascular risk factors and patient education on a primary care and commu-
nity-wide level needs to be performed as one means of addressing the
poor health status of Hispanic adults."

Part Three

Heart Disorders in Children

Chapter 20

If Your Child Has a Congenital Heart Defect

Introduction

The word *congenital* means inborn or existing at birth. The terms *congenital heart defect* and *congenital heart disease* are often used to mean the same thing, but the word *defect* is more accurate. The heart ailment is a defect or abnormality, not a disease. A defect results when the heart or blood vessels near the heart don't develop normally before birth.

How Congenital Heart Defects Develop

Congenital heart defects are rather uncommon. In most cases we don't know what causes them. Don't feel it's your fault for having a child with this problem.

[Things that can cause congenital heart defects include viral infections (such as German measles—rubella—in the mother during pregnancy), heredity, and alcohol and drug ingestion.]

Other factors that affect the heart's development are being studied. The truth is that we still don't know what causes most congenital heart defects.

Excerpts from American Heart Association Pub. No. 50-1109 (CP). Used by Permission. Editor's comments are bracketed.

Common Heart Defects

Patent Ductus Arteriosus (PDA)

Every baby is born with a *ductus arteriosus*. This is an open passageway between the two major blood vessels (the pulmonary artery and the aorta). [For information on how the heart works, see Chapter 1.]

Normally the passageway (ductus arteriosus) between these two arteries closes within a few hours after birth. If it doesn't, some blood that should have gone through the aorta and on to nourish the body goes back to the lungs. Failure of the ductus to close is quite common in premature infants but fairly rare in full-term babies.

If the ductus arteriosus is large, a child may tire quickly, grow slowly, catch pneumonia easily and breathe rapidly.

Septal Defects

Sometimes a baby is born with a hole in the septum. (The septum is the wall that separates the left and right sides of the heart.) This defect may be between the two upper chambers or *atria* (atrial septal defect) or between the two lower chambers or *ventricles* (ventricular septal defect). Sometimes, both upper and lower chambers are involved. These defects are sometimes called a "hole in the heart."

Atrial Septal Defect (ASD). When there's a large defect between the atria, a large amount of oxygen-rich (red) blood from the heart's left side leaks back to the right side.

Many children with this defect have few, if any, symptoms. Closing the atrial defect by open-heart surgery in childhood can prevent serious problems later in life. [T]he long-term outlook is excellent.

Ventricular Septal Defect (VSD). When there's a large opening between the ventricles, a large amount of oxygen-rich (red) blood from the heart's left side is forced through the defect to the right side. Then it's pumped back to the lungs, even though it's already been refreshed with oxygen. The heart, which has to pump an extra amount of blood, is over-worked and may enlarge.

Symptoms may not occur until several weeks after birth. Some babies with a large ventricular septal defect don't grow normally and may become undernourished. High pressure may occur in blood vessels in the lungs because there's more blood there. Over time this pressure may cause permanent damage to the walls of the vessels.

Repairing a ventricular septal defect with surgery usually restores the blood circulation to normal. The long-term outlook is good. After surgery a child must be examined regularly by a pediatric cardiologist.

Atrioventricular Canal Defect (Endocardial Cushion Defect, Atrioventricular Septal Defect). *Atrioventricular (AV) canal defect* is a large hole in the center of the heart. It exists where the wall between the upper chambers joins the wall between the lower chambers. This septal defect involves both upper and lower chambers. Also, the tricuspid and mitral valves that normally separate the heart's upper and lower chambers aren't formed as individual valves. Instead, a single large valve forms that crosses the defect.

Most infants with an atrioventricular canal don't grow normally. They also may become undernourished. Because of the large amount of blood flowing to the lungs, high blood pressure may occur there and damage the blood vessels.

In some infants, the common valve between the upper and lower chambers doesn't close properly. This lets blood leak backward from the heart's lower chambers to the upper ones. This leak, called *regurgitation or insufficiency*, can occur on the right side, left side, or both sides of the heart. With a valve leak, the heart pumps an extra amount of blood. It becomes overworked and enlarges.

In an infant with severe symptoms or high blood pressure in the lungs, surgery must usually be done in infancy. During the operation, the surgeon closes the large hole with one or two patches. Later the patch will become a permanent part of the heart as the heart's lining grows over it. The surgeon also divides the single valve between the heart's upper and lower chambers and makes two separate valves. These will be made as close to normal valves as possible.

Surgical repair of an atrioventricular canal usually restores the blood circulation to normal. However, the reconstructed valve may not work normally. The valve structures can leak or narrow. Rarely, the defect may be too complex to repair in infancy. In this case, the surgeon may place a band around the pulmonary artery to narrow it and reduce the blood flow and high pressure in the lungs. This procedure is called *pulmonary artery banding*. When a child is older, the band is

217

removed and corrective surgery is done. More medical or surgical treatment is sometimes needed.

Defects Causing Obstruction in the Heart or Blood Vessels

An obstruction to blood flow is a narrowing that may partly or completely block the flow of blood. Any one of the heart's four valves may be narrowed (*stenotic*) or completely blocked (*atretic*). The blockage may be above or below the valve. A block also can occur in vessels that return blood to the heart (veins) or that carry blood from the heart (arteries). The three defects that are the most common forms of obstruction to blood flow are: *Pulmonary stenosis, aortic stenosis and coarctation of the aorta.*

Pulmonary Stenosis. Narrowing of the pulmonary valve (*valvar pulmonary stenosis*) causes the right ventricle to pump harder to get blood past the blockage. If the stenosis is severe, especially in babies, some *cyanosis* (blueness) may occur. Older children usually have no symptoms.

Treatment is needed when the pressure in the right ventricle is high (even though there may be no symptoms). In most children the obstruction can be relieved during cardiac catheterization by *balloon valvuloplasty*. In this procedure, a special catheter containing a balloon is placed across the pulmonary valve. The balloon is inflated and the valve is stretched open. In other patients surgery may be needed. During surgery the valve can usually be opened so that it works well again.

The outlook after balloon valvuloplasty or surgery is favorable. Still, follow-up is needed to find out if the heart works normally.

Aortic Stenosis. Aortic stenosis occurs when the aortic valve didn't form properly. A normal valve has three parts (leaflets or cusps), but a stenotic valve may have only one cusp (unicuspid) or two cusps (bicuspid), which are thick and stiff.

Sometimes stenosis is severe and symptoms occur in infancy. Otherwise, most children with aortic stenosis have no symptoms. In some children, chest pain, unusual tiring, dizziness or fainting may occur. The need for surgery depends on how severe the stenosis is. In children, the surgeon may be able to enlarge the valve opening. Although surgery may improve the stenosis, the valve remains deformed. Eventually, replacing the valve with an artificial one may be needed.

A new procedure called *balloon valvuloplasty* has been used in some children who have aortic stenosis. During cardiac catheterization, a special catheter containing a balloon is placed across the constricted or narrowed valve. Then the balloon is inflated, and the valve is stretched open. The long-term results of this procedure are still being studied.

Children with aortic stenosis need lifelong medical follow-up. Even mild stenosis may worsen over time. Also, surgical relief of a blockage is sometimes incomplete. After surgery the valve keeps working in a mildly abnormal way. Some patients may have to limit how much they can do of some kinds of exercise. Check with your pediatric cardiologist about these exercise limits.

Coarctation of the Aorta. In this condition, the aorta (the main artery that carries blood from the heart to the body) is pinched or constricted. Usually no symptoms exist at birth, but they can develop as early as the first week after birth.

A baby may develop congestive heart failure or high blood pressure that requires early surgery. Otherwise, surgery usually can be delayed. A child with a severe coarctation should have surgery in early childhood. This prevents problems such as developing high blood pressure as an adult.

A surgeon doesn't have to open the heart to repair the coarctation. It can be fixed in several ways. One way is for the surgeon to remove the narrowed segment of aorta. Another option is to sew a patch over the narrowed section using part of a blood vessel to the arm or a graft of synthetic material.

The outlook after surgery is favorable, but long-term follow-up is required. Rarely, coarctation of the aorta may recur. Then another procedure may be needed. Some of these cases can be treated by a new procedure called *balloon angioplasty*. [For more information about balloon angioplasty see Chapter 36.]

Cyanotic Defects

In these defects, blood pumped to the body has less than the normal amount of oxygen. This causes a condition called *cyanosis*, which is a blue discoloration of the skin. If cyanosis is mild it may look like a "ruddy complexion." If it's severe, there's a dark blue discoloration. The degree of cyanosis may vary with age, activity or both.

Tetralogy of Fallot. The tetralogy of Fallot has four components. The first major one is a *ventricular septal defect*. The second is a *stenosis* (narrowing) at, or just beneath, the pulmonary valve. The last two components of tetralogy of Fallot are: the right ventricle is more muscular than normal: and the aorta lies directly over the ventricular septal defect. This results in blueness (cyanosis), which may appear soon after birth, in infancy or later in childhood. These "blue babies" may have sudden episodes of severe cyanosis with rapid breathing. They may even become unconscious. During exercise, older children may become short of breath and have fainting spells. These symptoms happen because there's not enough blood flowing to the lungs to supply the child's body with oxygen.

Some infants with severe tetralogy of Fallot may need an operation which will give temporary relief by increasing blood flow to the lungs with a shunt. This procedure is done by making a connection between the aorta and the pulmonary artery. Thus, some blood from the aorta flows into the lungs to get more oxygen. This reduces the cyanosis and allows the child to grow and develop until the repair can be done when the child is older.

Most children with tetralogy of Fallot have open-heart surgery before school age. The operation involves closing the ventricular septal defect and removing the obstructing muscle. If the pulmonary valve is narrow, it's opened; and if it's small, a graft or patch may be needed to finish the repair. After surgery the long-term outlook varies a great deal. Usually it's quite good, but it depends largely on how severe the defects were before surgery—especially the amount of pulmonary narrowing.

Transposition of the Great Arteries. Normally the pulmonary artery carries venous (bluish) blood from the right ventricle to the lungs to get oxygen. Then the aorta carries the oxygen-rich (red) blood from the left ventricle to the body. In transposition of the great arteries, the vessels are reversed.

Infants born with transposition survive only if they have one or more connections that let oxygen-rich (red) blood reach the body. These connections may be in the form of a hole between the two atria (*atrial septal defect*), the two ventricles (*ventricular septal defect*), or a vessel connecting the pulmonary artery with the aorta (*patent ductus arteriosus*). Most babies with transposition of the great arteries are extremely blue soon after birth because these connections are not adequate.

To improve the body's oxygen supply, a special procedure called *balloon atrial septostomy* is used during heart catheterization. It enlarges the atrial opening and helps the baby by reducing the cyanosis.

Two general types of surgery may be used to help correct the transposition. One common surgical procedure creates a tunnel inside the atria. It redirects oxygen-rich (red) blood to the right ventricle and aorta, and redirects venous (bluish) blood to the left ventricle and pulmonary artery. This operation is called a venous switch or intra-atrial baffle procedure. It has other names, too, including the Mustard procedure or the Senning procedure. It's usually done in infancy. Many factors, including the degree of cyanosis, determine how early in life a child may need surgery.

In another surgical procedure, the major arteries are switched. The aorta is connected to the left ventricle, which pumps oxygen-rich (red) blood to the body. The pulmonary artery is connected to the right ventricle, which pumps venous (bluish) blood to the lungs. This arterial switch procedure may be done in the first few weeks after birth or, depending on various factors, slightly later. If there's a large ventricular septal defect or other defects related to the transposition, the repair gets more complicated. Then other surgical procedures may be needed.

After surgery, the long-term outlook varies quite a bit. It depends largely on how severe the defects were before surgery.

Tricuspid Atresia. In this condition, there's no tricuspid valve so no blood can flow from the right atrium to the right ventricle. As a result, the right ventricle is small and not fully developed. The child's survival depends on there being an opening in the wall between the atria (*atrial septal defect*) and usually an opening in the wall between the two ventricles (*ventricular septal defect*).

Often in these children it's necessary to do a surgical shunting procedure to increase blood flow to the lungs. This reduces the cyanosis. Some children with tricuspid atresia have too much blood flowing to the lungs. They may need a procedure (*pulmonary artery banding*) to decrease blood flow to the lungs.

Other children with tricuspid atresia may have a more functional repair (Fontan procedure). In this, a connection is created between the right atrium and pulmonary artery. The atrial defect is also closed. This eliminates the cyanosis but, without a right ventricle that works normally, the heart can't work totally as it should.

Pulmonary Atresia. In pulmonary atresia, no pulmonary valve exists. Consequently, blood can't flow from the right ventricle into the pulmonary artery and on to the lungs. The right ventricle functions as a blind pouch that may stay small and not well developed. The tricuspid valve is often poorly developed, too.

Early treatment often includes using a drug to keep the PDA [patent ductus arteriosus—the opening between the pulmonary artery and aorta that exists at birth] from closing. A surgeon can create a shunt between the aorta and the pulmonary artery that may help increase blood flow to the lungs. A more complete repair depends on the size of the pulmonary artery and right ventricle. If the pulmonary artery and right ventricle are very small, it may not be possible to correct the defect with surgery. In some cases, where the pulmonary artery and right ventricle are more normal in size, open-heart surgery may produce a good improvement in how the heart works.

If the right ventricle stays too small to be a good pumping chamber, then the surgeon can connect the right atrium directly to the pulmonary artery. The atrial defect also can be closed to relieve the cyanosis. This is called a Fontan procedure.

Truncus Arteriosus. This is a complex malformation where only one artery arises from the heart and forms the aorta and pulmonary artery. Surgery for this condition usually is required early in life. It includes closing a large *ventricular septal defect* within the heart, detaching the pulmonary arteries from the large common artery, and connecting the pulmonary arteries to the right ventricle with a tube graft.

Children with truncus arteriosus need lifelong follow-up. It's important that their heart is checked regularly to see how well it's working.

Total Anomalous Pulmonary Venous Connection. In *total anomalous pulmonary venous connection* the pulmonary veins that bring oxygen-rich (red) blood from the lungs back to the heart aren't connected to the left atrium. Instead, the pulmonary veins drain through abnormal connections to the right atrium.

Symptoms may develop soon after birth. This defect must be surgically repaired in early infancy. In surgery, the pulmonary veins are reconnected to the left atrium and the atrial septal defect is closed. When surgical repair is done in early infancy, the long-term outlook is very good.

Other Complex Abnormalities

Rarely, children may have other very complicated heart defects. [Examples include a missing ventricle or a hypoplastic heart—one in which either the right or left side is incompletely formed]. In some instances, a child may have several heart defects—a complex cardiac abnormality.

[Many of the above described types of heart defects can be treated surgically. Sometimes the surgical procedures can restore normal blood circulation. Depending on the type of defect and its severity, however, surgery may be performed with a different goal. In addition, some children will need more than one operation. Ask your pediatric cardiologist to explain all planned procedures and to tell you what types of results to expect.

Depending on the type of surgery, different levels of follow-up care will be required. Some children will require life-long care. Be sure to ask your pediatric cardiologist to explain the lifetime implications your child's heart defect and the surgical procedures employed to correct or ameliorate the condition.

Preparing Your Child for Surgery

You may find it difficult to prepare a young child for a hospital stay. The American Heart Association offers the following guidelines:

- Find out what the hospital's rules are concerning visitors, toys, and clothing. Discuss ways to help your child feel more comfortable about the hospital setting. The hospital may have a social worker or nurse who can offer assistance.

223

- If a tour is permissible, take advantage of the opportunity to visit pertinent areas of the hospital with your child before the surgery.

- Give your child accurate, age-appropriate information about the surgery. Be honest, but be sensitive about how much detail to offer.

- Maintain a positive attitude. Focus on the surgery's benefits.

- Let your child know that emotions such as fear, anger, and depression are normal.

- Be available to provide emotional support. Let your child know that you will be close by during the operation.

Follow-up Care

Many types of heart defects require long-term follow-up care. Your pediatric cardiologist and surgeon will make appropriate recommendations based on your child's needs. In addition, standard pediatric care, including immunizations, will be important.

One complication you may need to guard against is bacterial endocarditis (BE). BE is a infection in the heart affecting the heart lining, a valve, or blood vessel. It develops as a result of bacteria entering the bloodstream, typically during dental procedures or during certain surgical operations such a tonsillectomy. The American Heart Association recommends that children with certain heart defects take antibiotics before undergoing any type of procedure that may place them at risk for developing BE. For further information about specific preventative treatments, contact your local American Heart Association or call 1-800-AHA-USA1.]

Chapter 21

Feeding Infants with Congenital Heart Disease: A Guide for Parents

Your Baby's Growth

[Babies with congenital heart defects frequently do not grow as quickly as healthy babies.]

Some factors related to congenital heart defects that can interfere with growth include: poor appetite, increased caloric needs, decreased food intake because of rapid breathing, frequent respiratory infections (bronchitis, pneumonia), poor absorption of nutrients from the digestive tract, or decreased oxygen in the blood (hypoxia). A baby's slow growth also may be due to hereditary or genetic conditions or pre-birth conditions. The most frequent reason for poor growth is that the baby isn't taking in enough calories or nutrients. But even if your baby seems to drink enough formula or breast milk, he or she may still gain weight very slowly.

How Much is Enough?

A baby with a heart defect often can't drink [as much milk as a normal baby] and needs more calories to gain weight. Each ounce of regular formula provides 20 calories. A baby who isn't gaining weight may need as much as 70 calories per pound (or 150 calories per kilo-

---

Excerpts from American Heart Association Pub. No. 50-1037 (CP). Used by Permission. Editor's comments are bracketed.

gram) of body weight daily for growth. Your doctor, dietitian or nurse can recommend a method to increase the number of calories in the formula or breast milk when fed by bottle.

What Kind of Nipple Is Best?

If your baby has difficulty sucking from a regular nipple, try using a soft one. Another option is to use one designed for a premature infant; it will have a hole large enough to allow the formula to flow easily. When you tip the bottle upside down, the formula should come out at a rate of several drops per second. If the hole in the nipple is too small, your baby will have to suck too hard and can swallow air. Too much air in the stomach results in spitting up the formula. You can enlarge a too-small hole with a red-hot needle or a round toothpick. Then boil the nipple for five minutes.

Starting on Solid Food

A baby with a heart defect often breathes too fast. That interferes with the ability to suck. In this case your pediatrician may suggest adding cereal to your baby's diet in the first few months. After cereals, your pediatrician will usually advise you to add strained fruits. Introducing solid foods can change your baby's nutritional intake, so discuss this with your pediatrician.

When Your Baby Can't Eat Enough

When babies are too sick or weak to take in enough food to meet their nutritional needs, they may be fed by a tube. It'll be inserted through the nose or mouth into the stomach. In rare instances, if your baby doesn't tolerate this type of formula feedings, it's possible to feed fluids containing sugar and proteins directly into the bloodstream. If your baby must be fed by either of these methods, it's still important for you to hold your baby and give him or her the pleasure that comes from sucking and caressing.

Heart Medicine and Feeding

You can give your baby medicines before or after feedings. If your child vomits, do not repeat that dose of medicine. All babies occasionally spit up milk, but usually the amount is very small. Do not mix the medicines in the bottle of formula. If your baby doesn't finish the bottle or vomits some of it, you won't know how much medicine your baby received.

If your baby is receiving digoxin and diuretics, it's important to make sure your baby gets enough potassium. [Check with your pediatrician about potassium supplements, foods rich in potassium, and the possibility of using] special diuretics that prevent potassium loss.

If your baby vomits more than twice a day or has diarrhea (loose frequent bowel movements), the formula may need to be changed. If your baby becomes ill, refuses to eat or vomits often (more than 2—3 feedings in 24 hours), he or she may require changes in medication. Contact your pediatrician for advice.

Chapter 22

Abnormalities of Heart Rhythm: A Guide for Parents

Introduction

Most infants and children have occasional changes, or irregularities, in the way their hearts beat. Sometimes you or your child's doctor will want to find out more about such an irregularity by visiting a doctor who specializes in children's heart problems and by conducting some special tests. Often parents will learn that the irregularity is the type found in normal children, and that no treatment is necessary.

In the older child or teenager who is resting, the heart beats about 70 times each minute. It beats about 140 times each minute in a newborn. The number of times the heart beats each minute is called the *heart rate*. Usually the time from one beat to the next is approximately the same, thus the heart *rhythm* is said to be regular. Heart rate changes often. For example, exercise makes the heart go faster and during sleep the heart rate will slow down. Usually, the rhythm is regular during all heart rates. If the heart is not beating regularly it is said to have an *arrhythmia*. The most common irregularity of the heart rate occurs during normal breathing. When a child breathes in, the heart rate normally speeds up for just a few seconds, slowing again after breathing out. This variation with breathing is called *sinus arrhythmia* and is entirely normal.

Excerpts from American Heart Association Pub. No. 50-058-A (CP). Used by Permission. Editor's comments are bracketed.

229

[If you would like more information about normal heart function, see Chapter 1.]

How the Cardiologist Diagnoses Disturbance of Heart Rhythm (Arrhythmia)

Arrhythmias may occur at any age. Often you and your child will not be aware of the disturbance. Your doctor may detect the abnormality during a physical examination. Usually, however, to properly identify an arrhythmia, it is necessary to record the heart's activity on an electrocardiogram (ECG or EKG). Other tests also may be required. [If you would like to learn more about the tests used to detect and diagnose arrhythmias see Chapter 6.]

Abnormalities of Heart Rhythm

Premature Supraventricular Contraction

[One of the most common types of arrhythmia called] *premature supraventricular contraction* (also known as premature atrial contraction, PAC) often occurs in newborns. When we are aware of our heart "skipping a beat" it is usually a result of this type of arrhythmia. In reality the heart does not skip a beat. What happens is that some area in the heart other than the sinus node generates an electrical signal that causes the heart to beat early, before the next regular beat. This is followed by a short pause causing the next beat to be more forceful, and the individual is aware of this more powerful beat.

Premature beats are very common in normal children and teenagers who all probably have had them at some time. They may occur spontaneously or may be caused by drugs, such as caffeine, or by anxiety or nervousness. Premature beats also may be caused by disease or injury to the heart. *Many times no cause can be found.* Usually, no special treatment is necessary. The premature beats may disappear, and even if they continue, treatment usually is not necessary and the child will remain well with no restrictions.

Ventricular Tachycardia

Ventricular tachycardia is a fast heart rate in which the beating originates in the lower chambers or ventricles. It is a serious condition that may threaten the life of a child. Fortunately, it is not common. Although the heart may not beat as fast with ventricular tachycardia as it does with supraventricular tachycardia, function of the heart is often poorer. This problem can be caused by serious disease or injury to the heart and usually requires prompt treatment. Ventricular tachycardia occasionally may occur in a child with an otherwise normal heart, and, in that case, may be less serious. This situation may not require treatment. Treatment of ventricular tachycardia includes heart medicines and treatment of the cause, if this is possible. The type of treatment and how long treatment is necessary depends upon what is causing the problem.

Bradycardia

Heart rate that is too slow is called *bradycardia*. The definition of what is too slow depends upon the age and the individual. For example, a newborn usually will not have a heart rate of less than 100 beats a minute. On the other hand, an athletically trained teenager may have a normal at rest heart rate of 50 beats a minute. In these situations, nothing is abnormal and no treatment is needed.

Sick Sinus Syndrome

Sometimes the sinus node does not work properly. This may occur after a child has open heart surgery. When sinus node function is significantly disturbed, the condition is called *sick sinus syndrome*. If the sinus node fails to cause the heart to beat, or functions too slowly, and if no other area of the heart assumes control at a fast enough rate, the child may suffer from too slow a heart rate. When this happens there may not be enough blood flow to vital organs and fainting or excessive fatigue may occur.

[Other common types of arrhythmias are discussed on Chapter 6.]

Chapter 23

Innocent Heart Murmurs

[Although it is difficult not to worry when you hear that your child has a heart murmur, there may be no cause for concern. If the doctor tells you that the murmur is an "innocent" heart murmur, it means that the sound is considered normal. Although your doctor may want to perform some tests to verify the diagnosis, once the tests are completed they will probably not have to be repeated.]

Innocent murmurs are sounds made by the blood circulating through the chambers and valves of the heart or through blood vessels near the heart. They are sometimes called a "functional murmur," "physiologic murmur" or "vibratory murmur." The doctor can hear these murmurs by listening to your child's heart through a stethoscope

[According to the American Heart Association, many children may have innocent heart murmurs at some stage during of their development. The sounds may come and go or get softer and louder; they may change with emotional swings. There is a good chance that they will disappear altogether by the time your child reaches adulthood.]

Excerpts from American Heart Association Pub. No. 51-1005 (CP). Used by Permission. Editor's comments are bracketed.

Chapter 24

You, Your Child, and Rheumatic Fever

[Rheumatic fever] is an inflammation that may affect many parts of the body. It can also affect the heart. [Streptococcal infections, the kind that cause strep throat and scarlet fever, cause rheumatic fever.]

[Rheumatic fever does not always cause permanent heart damage, but when it does the result is called rheumatic heart disease. Rheumatic heart disease refers to the resulting] inflammation and scarring of the heart valves.

[O]nce a child has had rheumatic fever, he or she becomes so susceptible to another attack that the child should take medication (usually penicillin or sulfa) continuously. These drugs prevent strep throat and so protect against a recurrence of rheumatic fever.

You should help your child avoid a strep throat by making sure he or she follows the doctor's orders to take penicillin or sulfa. These drugs, injected once a month or taken daily by mouth, are very effective in preventing rheumatic fever recurrences.

[Children] with rheumatic heart disease [need to take antibiotics] before undergoing any dental or surgical procedure likely to allow bacteria to enter the bloodstream. These antibiotics are *in addition* to those taken to prevent recurrent attacks of rheumatic fever.

[One of the difficulties parents face when children get sick with a sore throat is determining whether or not it is the result of a strep-

Excerpts from American Heart Association Pub. No. 50-1014 (CP). Used by Permission. Editor's comments are bracketed.

tococcal infection. Sore throats from other causes do not result in rheumatic fever.

The American Heart Association reports that these symptoms are associated with streptococcal infections:

- A sore throat that appears abruptly
- A complaint that it hurts to swallow
- An elevated temperature

Symptoms alone, however, cannot diagnose streptococcal infections. Your pediatrician may want to order some tests to aid in making an accurate diagnosis.]

Chapter 25

Simpler Treatment Helps Children with Kawasaki Syndrome

A new treatment regimen may reduce the mortality risk for children with acute Kawasaki syndrome, according to Dr. Jane W. Newburger, associate professor of pediatrics at Harvard Medical School in Boston, Massachusetts. The results of a 3-year multicenter study conducted by Dr. Newburger and 19 coinvestigators suggest that a variation in the established therapy for Kawasaki syndrome reduces patient risk for developing coronary artery aneurysms—balloon-like swellings of blood vessels.

Kawasaki syndrome, also known as mucocutaneous lymph node syndrome, was first identified by Dr. Tomisaku Kawasaki in 1967. Although the etiology of Kawasaki syndrome remains unknown, epidemiologic features suggest that this systemic disorder is triggered by an infectious agent. Patients, primarily infants and children, usually develop rashes; swelling of the hands and feet; enlarged lymph nodes in the neck; "strawberry" tongues; high fevers that last 5 days or more; and dry, cracked lips.

Conventional treatment for Kawasaki syndrome has been high-dose aspirin in combination with a 4-day course of gamma-globulin, the protein component of blood that contains most of the body's disease-fighting antibodies. Dr. Newburger and her colleagues have shown that a large, single-dose infusion of intravenous gamma-globulin (IVGG) is more effective than and as safe as the conventional 4-day treatment.

NCRR Reporter, March 1992.

"We were motivated initially by a desire to decrease costs and improve patient comfort," says Dr. Newburger. "We discovered, however, that the single-dose infusion not only costs less and is more comfortable for the patient, but also works better."

The therapeutic effectiveness of IVGG plus aspirin compared with regimens of aspirin alone was first demonstrated in an earlier multicenter study conducted by Dr. Newburger and her colleagues. Their clinical evaluation showed that four consecutive daily infusions of IVGG combined with high doses of aspirin lowered the incidence of coronary artery disease, a severe complication of acute Kawasaki syndrome.

The worldwide incidence of Kawasaki syndrome has increased alarmingly during the last 20 years, notes coinvestigator Dr. Masato Takahashi, professor of pediatrics at the University of Southern California School of Medicine in Los Angeles. The rise has been so dramatic that Kawasaki syndrome has surpassed acute rheumatic fever as the leading cause of acquired heart disease in children. Although Asian children, particularly those of Japanese and Korean descent, appear to have a predilection for the disorder, cases have been documented in children from all ethnic groups, adds Dr. Takahashi.

Kawasaki syndrome in its acute stage is characterized by vasculitis, or inflammation of the blood vessels. Dr. Takahashi explains that large aneurysms of the coronary arteries may cause serious complications. "Giant aneurysms may occasionally rupture and cause massive hemorrhages, but more often we notice occlusion of the aneurysmal artery by a clot or narrowing of arterial segments by scar tissue adjacent to the aneurysm. In either case the patient may develop myocardial infarction [heart attack]." Dr. Takahashi notes that 1 to 2 percent of untreated patients with Kawasaki syndrome die from myocardial infarction as a complication of giant aneurysms, which by definition have internal diameters of 8 millimeters or more.

Drs. Newburger and Takahashi, working with other specialists in Kawasaki disease at seven medical centers, studied 549 children who had acute Kawasaki syndrome. All patients were treated with IVGG and high-dose aspirin; 276 received the conventional 4-day regimen of IVGG infusions, and 273 received high-dose single infusions of IVGG. The researchers reported that children receiving the single-infusion regimen had a shorter period of fever and more rapid resolution of inflammation.

To check for coronary artery abnormalities, patients in both treatment groups underwent two-dimensional echocardiography, a noninvasive diagnostic method that uses ultrasound to outline the shapes of organs and tissues. Echocardiograms were performed when the patients were first enrolled in the study and then at 2- and 7-week followup visits. According to Dr. Newburger, "The children receiving the standard 4-day infusions of gamma-globulin were almost twice as likely to have coronary artery abnormalities such as dilatations or aneurysms than were the patients who received single infusions of gamma-globulin."

The majority of smaller aneurysms in Kawasaki syndrome patients regress spontaneously, explains Dr. Takahashi. "Giant aneurysms present the most risk to patients," he says. "Among the patients who had no coronary abnormalities prior to treatment, no giant aneurysms developed in the single-infusion group, but three children who received 4-day infusions did develop giant aneurysms."

Researchers have yet to uncover the reason gamma-globulin and aspirin are effective in treating Kawasaki syndrome. "Additional basic research into the etiology of Kawasaki syndrome is needed before a more specific therapy can be designed," Dr. Newburger says. She suggests that future studies could explore the usefulness of either an increased dose or repeated infusions of gamma-globulin for selected high-risk patients.

During the acute phase the patients received aspirin—in addition to IVGG—in doses that for an average 1-year-old child are approximately equivalent to 12 1/2 tablets of baby aspirin, or more than 3 adult aspirin tablets per day, according to Dr. Takahashi. After the 14th day of illness the aspirin doses were drastically reduced.

"Children with acute Kawasaki syndrome are given these large aspirin doses every day through the 14th day of illness, which may cause complications for children who are sensitive to aspirin," he says. "Use of high-dose aspirin is a carryover from the days when we did not have a more effective anti-inflammatory agent in the form of IVGG."

Dr. Takahashi and other investigators are currently engaged in a prospective study comparing the effects of high-dose versus low-dose aspirin in combination with single-infusion gamma globulin. "Children with Kawasaki syndrome have a high platelet count, and platelets tend to adhere to each other quite easily and initiate blood coagulation," he notes. Platelets are small particles in the blood that play a key role in blood coagulation. "We think that the aspirin is necessary to prevent thrombosis, or blood clotting, by inhibiting platelet function. However, prevention of these complications does not require a large dose of aspirin; a very small dose is sufficient."

Drs. Newburger and Takahashi say that continued research may lead to an even more effective, less toxic treatment for Kawasaki syndrome. They expect that future studies will consider whether repeated treatment of high-risk patients will reduce mortality and whether better treatment can be developed for patients who show adverse reactions to high doses of aspirin.

—by Jeanne Baker

Additional reading:

1. Newburger, J. W., Takahashi, M., Beiser, A. S., et al., A single intravenous infusion of gamma-globulin as compared with four infusions in the treatment of acute Kawasaki syndrome. *New England Journal of Medicine* 324:1633-1639, 1991.

2. Shackelford, P. G. and Strauss, A.W., Kawasaki syndrome. *New England Journal of Medicine* 324:1664-1666, 1991.

3. Barron, K. S., Murphy, D. J., Sr., Silverman, E. D., et al., Treatment of Kawasaki syndrome: A comparison of two dosage regimens of intravenously administered immune globulin. *Journal of Pediatrics* 117:638-644, 1990.

4. Newburger, J. W., Takahashi, M., Burns, J. C., et al., The treatment of Kawasaki syndrome with intravenous gamma-globulin. *New England Journal of Medicine* 315:341-347, 1986.

5. Furusho, K., Kamiya T., Nakano, H., et al., High-dose intravenous gamma-globulin for Kawasaki disease. *Lancet* 2:1055-1058, 1984.

The research described in this article was supported by the General Clinical Research Centers Program of the National Center for Research Resources and by the National Heart, Lung, and Blood Institute.

Chapter 26

Cholesterol in Children

This booklet will help you understand:

- How blood cholesterol in children is related to heart disease later in life.
- Which children should get their cholesterol tested and what to expect afterwards.
- How the whole family can eat in a low-saturated fat, low-cholesterol way.
- How to help your child follow a prescribed diet to lower cholesterol.

This booklet describes changes you and your family can make in your eating patterns to help lower blood cholesterol levels and prevent heart disease. Please note that these changes apply to children ages 2 to 19. Medical authorities agree that infants under age 2 years should not be placed on cholesterol-lowering diets.

This guide is part of a series. Other booklets in the series are for 7 to 10 year olds, 11 to 14 year olds, and 15 to 18 year olds. [For ordering information contact the National Cholesterol Education Program, NHLBI Information Center, P.O. Box 30105, Bethesda, MD 20824-0105.]

Taken from NIH Pub. No. 92-3099.

Cholesterol Is a Family Affair

Do you know your blood cholesterol level? Is it high?

Your child's blood cholesterol level can be related to your level. If you have high blood cholesterol or heart disease, there is a greater chance that your child has high blood cholesterol. Children whose blood cholesterol levels are high, in general, tend to have higher levels as adults and be at greater risk for heart disease. That is why controlling blood cholesterol levels is a family affair.

All healthy Americans, 2 years of age or older, should eat in a way that is low in saturated fat and cholesterol. We now know that eating this way lowers blood cholesterol levels and reduces the risk of heart disease.

Heart disease is still the number one killer of both men and women in the United States. More than 6 million Americans have symptoms of heart disease. High blood pressure, smoking, and obesity, as well as high blood cholesterol increase your risk of getting heart disease. The good news is that you can change these risk factors and reduce your family's risk of heart disease.

How Does Blood Cholesterol Affect Heart Disease?

Heart Disease Has Its Start Early in Life

Atherosclerosis may start very early in life, yet not produce symptoms for many years. Over the years, cholesterol and fat build up in the arteries. This narrows the arteries and can slow or block the flow of blood to the heart. This process is known as "atherosclerosis." Most heart attacks are caused by a clot forming at a narrow part of an artery which cuts off the blood and oxygen supply to the heart muscle. Most coronary heart disease is due to blockages in these same arteries.

We know that lowering blood cholesterol in adults slows the fatty buildup in the walls of the arteries and reduces the risk of heart disease and heart attack. Lowering blood cholesterol levels in children is likely also to help reduce their risk of heart disease when they become adults.

Cholesterol: Your Body Needs It And Makes Its Own

Cholesterol is a soft, waxy substance. Your body needs cholesterol to function normally. Cholesterol is present in all parts of the body, including the brain, nerves, muscle, skin, liver, intestines, and heart. It is a part of cell membranes. And it is important for the production of hormones, vitamin D, and bile acids—which help to absorb fat.

Your blood cholesterol level is affected not only by the saturated fat and cholesterol in your diet, but also by the cholesterol made in your liver. In fact, your body makes all the cholesterol it needs. The saturated fat and cholesterol in your diet only help to increase your blood cholesterol level.

Lipoproteins Carry Cholesterol in Your Blood

Cholesterol travels in your blood in packages called lipoproteins. They are often referred to as LDLs and HDLs.

- LDLs: Low density lipoproteins (LDLs) carry most of the cholesterol. If your LDL level is high, cholesterol and fat can build up in your arteries and cause atherosclerosis. This is why LDL-cholesterol is often called "bad cholesterol."

- HDLs: Cholesterol is also packaged in high density lipoproteins (HDLs). HDLs carry cholesterol back to your liver. Here it is processed or removed from your body. Removal helps prevent cholesterol from building up in your arteries. So, HDLs are often referred to as "good cholesterol."

What Affects Blood Cholesterol Levels?

Many Factors Influence Blood Cholesterol Levels

Diet. Among the factors you and your family can do something about, diet has the greatest effect on blood cholesterol levels.

- Saturated fat raises blood cholesterol levels more than anything else you eat.

- Dietary cholesterol also increases blood cholesterol levels.

Changing your family's way of eating will be a very important step to control or lower blood cholesterol.

243

Weight. In children, as in adults, obesity is related to increased total blood cholesterol levels. Losing weight has been shown to lower these levels. Children who are obese are more likely than other children to become obese adults. Obesity, by itself, also increases the risk of heart disease.

Genetic factors. Genes, i.e., heredity, play a major role in determining blood cholesterol levels and how well your child will be able to lower the level by diet. Because of their genes, a very small number of people have a high blood cholesterol level even if they eat a cholesterol-lowering diet.

Smoking. Cigarette smoking is related to lower HDL-cholesterol levels, and also increases the risk of heart disease.

Physical activity. Regular exercise throughout life is associated with a lower risk of heart disease. We also know that regular exercise may help control weight and increase HDL-cholesterol. Aerobic exercise helps strengthen the heart and improve the circulatory system as well.

Sex and age. In the United States, the average total cholesterol level in children is about 160 mg/dL. At birth, total cholesterol levels are about 70 mg/dL and rise to between 100 to 150 mg/dL during the first few weeks of life. At 2 years of age, these levels increase to about 160 mg/dL in boys and to 165 mg/dL in girls. They stay at about these levels until puberty. Between 12 and 18 years, total cholesterol in boys declines slightly to about 150 mg/dL. Levels in girls also decline slightly. At age 20, blood cholesterol levels in both men and women start to rise.

Alcohol. You may have heard that modest amounts of alcohol can improve HDL-cholesterol levels. However, it is not known whether this protects against heart disease. Because drinking alcohol can have serious harmful effects, it is not recommended as a way to prevent heart disease.

Shared Habits and Genes

Families share similar habits including eating, exercise, smoking, and drinking. Families also share similar genes. The shared habits and genes influence cholesterol levels in families. Clearly, as a family you can do something about your shared habits:

- Eat foods lower in saturated fat and cholesterol. This will help to lower blood cholesterol levels and maintain a healthy weight. In fact, most people are able to control or lower their blood cholesterol levels by eating this way.

- Exercise regularly.

- If you smoke, STOP. As your child's role model, help him or her avoid taking up the habit.

- Be aware that friends, fads, and advertising also influence eating, exercise, smoking, and other habits.

Does Your Child Need a Cholesterol Test?

As a Parent, You Need To Know Your Cholesterol Level

If your blood cholesterol was ever "high" (240 mg/dL or greater), your child's blood cholesterol level will need to be checked. [The following groups apply to persons 20 years of age or older.]

- 240 mg/dL or greater: High
- 200-239 mg/dL: Borderline-high
- Less than 200 mg/dL: Desirable

Any cholesterol level above 200 mg/dL, even in the "borderline-high" group, increases your risk for heart disease. Levels less than 200 mg/dL put you at lower risk.

Most Children Do Not Need To Have Their Cholesterol Levels Checked

Most children do not need to have their blood cholesterol tested. The National Cholesterol Education Program and the American Academy of Pediatrics agree that children, 2 years of age or older, and teenagers should have their blood cholesterol levels measured if they have *one* of the following:

1. At least one parent who has ever had high blood cholesterol (240 mg/dL or greater).

2. A parent or grandparent who got heart disease before 55 years of age.

3. Parents whose medical history is not known, especially in children with other risk factors for heart disease [such as chgarette smoking, high blood pressure, obesity, diabetes, or physical inactivity].

Getting your child's total cholesterol level measured is easy and can be part of a regular visit. The doctor will take a small sample of blood from the finger or arm. Your child can usually eat and drink before this test. The [following list] can help you understand your child's total blood cholesterol test. Even if you do not know your blood cholesterol level or your family history for heart disease, your doctor may measure your child's cholesterol level. If your child's cholesterol is high, heart disease may run in your family. So, be sure to ask your doctor to measure your cholesterol level too. Your spouse and any other children in the family should also have their levels checked. All family members who have an elevated cholesterol level need to take steps to lower it—it is a family affair.

Some children with high blood cholesterol grow up to be adults with normal levels. That's why not all children need to have their cholesterol tested. But children with a family history of high cholesterol or early heart disease who have high cholesterol levels are at increased risk of heart disease as an adult. That's why these children need to be tested. If their blood cholesterol is high, they can begin taking steps to lower their levels.

Total Blood Cholesterol Levels in Children and Teenagers from High Risk Families

- Less than 170 mg/dL: Acceptable
- 170-199 mg/dL: Borderline
- 200 mg/dL or greater: High

NOTE: These groups apply only to children ages 2 to 19 years who have a parent with high blood cholesterol or a family history of early heart disease.

What Is a Cholesterol Profile?

The "cholesterol profile" is a detailed set of blood measurements. It includes measurements of LDL-cholesterol, HDL-cholesterol, and triglyceride levels. This is done because LDL and HDL provide more accurate information on the risk of getting heart disease.

Your doctor should check your child's cholesterol profile if:

- Your child's total cholesterol is "high" (200 mg/dL or greater).
- Your child's total cholesterol level is "borderline" (170 mg/dL or greater) after two measurements are averaged, or
- A parent or grandparent had heart disease before age 55.

In order to do a cholesterol profile, your doctor will take a blood sample from your child's arm. Your child must not eat or drink anything, except water, for 12 hours before the test.

Check below for the acceptable, borderline, and high LDL-cholesterol levels for children and adolescents:

- 130 mg/dL or greater: High
- 110-129 mg/dL: Borderline
- Less than 110 md/dL: Acceptable

NOTE: These groups apply only to children ages 2 to 19 years who have a parent with high blood cholesterol or a family history of early heart disease.

Next Steps Based on Your Child's Cholesterol Level

Acceptable. Children with an acceptable total or LDL-cholesterol level should adopt the same eating pattern as all healthy Americans, namely one lower in saturated fat and cholesterol. This will help keep their cholesterol level low.

Borderline and High. If your child's total cholesterol level is either high or borderline, your doctor will likely do a cholesterol profile. This will show your child's LDL-cholesterol level. If the LDL level is high or borderline, your child will require a Step-One Diet. This diet is basically the same eating pattern suggested for all healthy children. However, children given the Step-One Diet will have to follow the eating pattern more closely. The doctor will check their cholesterol levels more often to see how they are responding to the diet.

A few children who are not able to lower their cholesterol level enough may need the Step-Two Diet. This diet is lower in saturated fat and cholesterol to help produce the biggest change. Information about the Step-One and Step-Two Diets [is given below].

Aim for Acceptable Blood Cholesterol Levels

Your child's blood cholesterol level should begin to fall within a few weeks after starting the Step-One Diet. Ideally the goal should be:

1. Acceptable total cholesterol—less than 170 mg/dL, or

2. Acceptable LDL-cholesterol—less than 110 mg/dL.

After starting the Step-One Diet, your doctor will most likely check your child's cholesterol level on a regular basis. If the goal is not met after a certain period of time on the Step-One Diet, your doctor will likely have your child try the Step-Two Diet. If the goal is still not met after 6 months to 1 year on the diet, some children with extremely high levels may need to be given drugs along with the diet.

Make Heart-Healthy Eating a Family Routine

What your family eats has a large impact, not only on their blood cholesterol levels, but on their general health as well. All children and teenagers need to eat a nutritious diet. They need to eat a variety of foods that provide enough calories and nutrients—carbohydrates, protein, fat, vitamins, and minerals. This helps them grow and develop properly. It is also important as they become more physically active. A nutritious and "heart-healthy" diet is also low in saturated fat, total fat, and dietary cholesterol. As you know, this type of diet is important to lower blood cholesterol and maintain it at acceptable levels.

Did you know that what parents eat influences what their children eat? Do you make a habit of eating fatty fried foods or rich, high-fat desserts? Children learn these eating patterns early in life. They learn to enjoy the taste of high-fat foods. They can also learn to enjoy the taste of fruits, vegetables, and grains if you show them how.

Changing established eating habits can often be difficult for you and your children, especially teenagers. It is much easier to start by making changes at home that everyone in your family over 2 years old can follow. Buy and prepare foods low in saturated fat, total fat, and dietary cholesterol for the whole family.

Help Your Child Eat Right And Exercise

Telling children and teenagers to eat right and exercise is good; showing them is better. Here are some tips to help your children develop healthful habits.

Be a model. Set a good example. Adults, particularly parents, are a major influence on children's behavior. Children are also influenced by television, radio, magazines, newspapers, ads, friends, brothers and sisters, and others who may not conform to your ways. So, eat a heart-healthy diet and your children will be more likely to do the same. Exercising with your child also sets a good example.

Know the dietary guidelines to lower blood cholesterol. Knowing how diet, blood cholesterol and heart disease are related will help you guide your family to lower their blood cholesterol levels. Knowing the basics on choosing foods low in saturated fat, total fat, and cholesterol is important to your success.

Know the food groups. Know the food groups and the low-saturated fat, low-cholesterol choices within each group. This will help you buy and provide such foods and snacks at home.

Stock the kitchen. Stock the kitchen with low-saturated fat, low-cholesterol foods from each of the food groups. Prepare these foods in large quantities to be frozen for quick use later. Foods such as casseroles, soups, and breads can be frozen in individual servings for a quick meal. The whole family will then have low-saturated fat, low-cholesterol meals on hand. Teach children how to choose healthy snacks.

Teach basic food preparation skills. Teach children how to clean vegetables, make salads, and safely use the stove, oven, microwave, and toaster. Children who have basic cooking skills appreciate food more and are more inclined to try new foods.

249

Let children help. Let children help with or even do the grocery shopping. The supermarket is an ideal place to teach children about foods. Teach them how to read food labels. Involve children in meal planning and preparation. Encourage them to prepare snacks, bag lunches, and breakfast. This will help them become responsible and fulfill a need for independence.

Plan family meals. Eating meals together as a family can really help foster heart-healthy eating habits in children. The more you create a "family setting" where everyone shares the same nutritious meals, the more children will accept healthful eating as a way of life. Try to maintain regular family meals every day—breakfast, lunch or dinner, or all three. This way, the whole family can learn about healthful eating and build good eating habits.

Encourage physical activity. Make time for physical activity. Encourage children to get some exercise throughout the day and especially on the weekends. Take trips that involve activities like hiking, swimming, and skiing. Join in the fun. Ride bikes, run, skate, or walk to places close by. Give your child a splash or dance party. Use your backyard or park for basketball, baseball, football, badminton, or volleyball.

Know the Dietary Guidelines for Lowering Blood Cholesterol Levels

In order to help your family eat in a way that is lower in saturated fat and cholesterol, you need to know some dietary guidelines. They are consistent with the "Dietary Guidelines for Americans" and include choosing a variety of foods that provide the following nutrients:

- Less than 10 percent of calories from saturated fat,
- An average of no more than 30 percent of calories from fat,
- Less than 300 milligrams of dietary cholesterol a day,
- Enough calories to support growth, and to reach or maintain a healthy weight.

The whole family (except infants under 2 years who need more calories from fat) should follow these guidelines. This may look complicated, but you will soon see that it is really easy if you take some general steps [outlined in the sections below].

These guidelines are basically the same as the Step-One Diet. The Step Two Diet, however, is different because it is lower in saturated fat and cholesterol as shown below:

- Less than 7 percent of calories from saturated fat,
- Less than 200 milligrams of dietary cholesterol a day.

If you want to check whether you are following the above guidelines, [you will need to do some simple mathematical calculations]. Briefly, each gram of fat (of any type) provides 9 calories per gram. So, if your child eats 1,800 calories per day, 10 percent of those calories from saturated fat is equal to 20 grams of saturated fat allowed per day. This information is provided because food labels list fat information in grams, not percent of calories.

Remember, the Step-One and Step-Two Diets are recommended for children with elevated blood cholesterol levels. If your doctor prescribes one of these diets, help your child to follow it closely. Registered dietitians or qualified nutritionists can provide additional information to help children and their families adjust to this way of eating and still include some favorite foods.

Eating Patterns Help Your Child Follow the Guidelines

Following the dietary guidelines to lowering blood cholesterol levels can be easy if you think of them in terms of food. Foods make up your eating patterns. So, knowing the foods to choose is the first step. Choosing these foods from each of the food groups every day will help assure that your family is following the guidelines recommended for all healthy Americans. And, eating a variety of foods will help assure your child is getting all of the nutrients needed for growth. Don't worry about whether your child eats specific numbers of servings from each group every day as long as your child's cholesterol level is in the acceptable range....

Once your child is put on the Step-One or Step-Two Diet, allow him or her time to grow into the pattern. Be flexible, yet encourage your child to eat enough of the right kinds of foods. Remember, these diets can also be enjoyed by the whole family.

Calories. Children and teenagers need calories to grow and develop. The suggested eating patterns are not low in calories, although they are low in saturated fat, total fat, and cholesterol. Some calories are replaced by calories from carbohydrates to maintain normal growth. Do not restrict your child's calorie level while on a low-fat diet. This can cause growth problems. Children with high blood cholesterol who follow the Step-One or Step-Two Diet should be followed closely by their doctor.

Obesity. Most children who are obese and still growing taller should not lose weight. Instead, they should eat in a way that keeps their weight the same while they continue to grow taller. Obese teenagers who are at their adult height should be encouraged to follow a weight-loss diet under a doctor's care to achieve desirable weight. It's also good to develop lifelong habits of regular exercise to help in weight control.

Protein and Vegetarianism. Protein is vital to growth and development. An eating pattern low in saturated fat, total fat, and dietary cholesterol does not mean cutting out all animal products or becoming a vegetarian. It means you replace fatty cuts of meat with lean meat, fish, and poultry, and whole-milk dairy products with low-fat or nonfat dairy products.

Vegetarian diets, if well planned, are not low-protein diets and may offer nutrition and health benefits which include lower blood cholesterol levels. But, not enough calories and other nutrients from strict vegetarian diets have caused poor growth and vitamin and mineral deficiencies. Vegetarian diets for children and teenagers require careful thought. Meeting with a registered dietitian can be helpful.

Protein and Building Muscle. Some teenagers, especially boys, believe that protein builds muscle. Most Americans eat more protein than they need. So, eating even more won't necessarily build muscle. Some foods high in protein, such as fatty cuts of meat and whole milk products, are also high in fat and saturated fats. If your teenager insists on eating more protein, choose those high-protein foods that are lower in total fat and saturated fat. Skim milk, for example, has as much protein as whole milk. Carbohydrate foods from the breads, cereals, pasta, rice, dry peas and beans group are important for athletes of all ages and also provide protein.

Teenage girls. Teenage girls may often avoid milk and other dairy products to control body weight. Weight-conscious teenagers should be taught that fat provides calories, and encouraged to avoid fad diets and select foods from all the food groups. Choosing a wide variety of low-fat foods, including low-fat dairy products, and increasing physical activity will help with weight control.

Read Food Labels. Many foods have labels that tell you how much saturated fat and cholesterol they have. Did you know that even low-fat foods can be high in cholesterol? And some products may not contain cholesterol but are still high in fat and saturated fat. Make a habit of reading food labels to help you select foods low in both saturated fat and cholesterol.

Shop for Foods That Are Low in Saturated Fat and Cholesterol

Stocking your kitchen with a variety of foods that are low in saturated fat, total fat, and cholesterol will help you and your family eat in a heart-healthy way. These heart-healthy choices are described by food group....

Food Groups

Meat, poultry, fish, and shellfish are important sources of protein and other nutrients in your child's diet. They also provide saturated fat and cholesterol. Lean cuts of beef, such as top round, are lower in saturated fat and cholesterol than fattier cuts such as regular ground beef. Chicken without skin has less saturated fat and less total fat than chicken with skin. And even though two chicken hot dogs have a lot less saturated fat than beef hot dogs they have more saturated fat than even chicken with the skin. Fish such as haddock has less saturated fat and cholesterol than either chicken or beef. And, foods with less fat contain fewer calories as well.

To help lower your child's blood cholesterol level, choose leaner meats as well as chicken, turkey, fish, and shellfish more often. Remember, all of these foods contain some saturated fat and cholesterol. So, the number of servings and serving size your child eats are also important. For variety, consider dry beans or legumes as a main dish instead of meat. They are high in protein and very low in fat. Or, stretch small amounts of meat with pasta, rice, or vegetables for hearty dishes.

253

Meat. Lean cuts of beef (round, sirlion, chuck, lion), veal (all trimmed cuts), pork (tenderloin, fresh leg, shoulder—arm or picnic), and lamb (arm, let, loin) are available. These cuts of meat can be tender and tasty if prepared the right way. Some people think that only the well-marbled cuts of meat (meat with white fat running through it) taste good. However, tasty cuts do not have to be high in fat.

Beef, veal, and lamb cuts are "graded" based on the amount of marbling in the meat. "Prime" is the top grade and has the most fat. "Choice" has less fat and "select" least of all. "Select" grades of meat can also be tender if braised or stewed. Before preparing any meat, be sure to trim the fat off.

Remember, your child's diet can include meat, especially the lean cuts. For teenage girls, who are more likely to get iron deficiency anemia, lean meat is an especially important source of iron.

High-fat processed meats (like bologna, salami, beef or pork hot dogs, and sausage) should be eaten less often. Sixty to eighty percent of their calories come from fat—much of which is saturated. The good news is that a few lower-fat beef hot dogs have recently been developed. Organ meats (like liver, sweetbreads, and kidneys) are relatively low in fat, but are high in cholesterol. They too should be eaten less often—once a month is okay on the Step-One Diet—and even less often on the Step-Two Diet.

Poultry. In general, poultry has less saturated fat than meat, especially when the skin is removed. Chicken and turkey are excellent choices for your family's new eating pattern. When choosing poultry, keep these tips in mind:

- Eat chicken and turkey without skin to reduce the saturated fat.
- Bake roast or broil do not fry.
- In choosing processed poultry products like chicken hot dogs, bear in mind that they contain more fat and cholesterol than fresh chicken. However, some are lower in fat than similar beef or pork products.

Fish and Shellfish. Most fish, such as haddock or halibut, is lower in saturated fat and cholesterol than meat and poultry. Fish also provides protein and other nutrients, so it is a good choice.

Shellfish varies in cholesterol content. Some, like shrimp and crayfish, are relatively high, and some, like clams and lobster, are low. All shellfish has less fat than meat, poultry, and most fish. So, shellfish can certainly be eaten occasionally.

Some fish, like tuna, salmon, and mackerel—the high-fat fish—are rich in "omega-3" fatty acids, a polyunsaturated fatty acid. Some people believe that these omega-3 fatty acids, commonly called "fish oils," lower blood cholesterol levels. This does not appear to be the case. However, eating fish is a good choice since it is low in saturated fat. Taking fish oil supplements for treating high blood cholesterol is not recommended. It may lead to undesirable side effects over time.

Dairy Products

Whole milk dairy products are major sources of saturated fat and cholesterol. However, dairy products are also a great source of calcium. Children and adolescents need calcium for the proper growth and development of strong bones. Girls, especially, need to eat foods high in calcium. By choosing low-fat, skim, and nonfat dairy products more often than high-fat dairy products you not only cut back on saturated fat and cholesterol but in most cases you get more calcium per serving. Dairy products are often added to foods, like casseroles, pizza, cookies, and sauces. So, even if your children do not eat much cheese or drink much milk, they may be getting quite a lot of high-fat dairy products without knowing it.

Milk. Milk provides many nutrients, especially calcium, that are essential for growth and development. Choose more often either 1 percent or skim milk instead of whole milk (3.3 percent) or 2 percent milk. The lower fat types provide as much or more calcium and other nutrients as whole milk. Yet they have much less saturated fat and cholesterol and fewer calories. Children over age 2 can drink 1 percent or skim milk and still get the nutrients they need.

Cheese. When people cut back on meat, they often eat more cheese. Most cheeses, particularly those prepared with whole milk or cream, are actually higher in saturated fat than meat or poultry. Cholesterol, however, is about the same in the high-fat cheeses, meat, and poultry...

Determining which cheeses are high or low in saturated fat and cholesterol can be confusing. Cheeses are often labeled as part-skim milk, low-fat, imitation, processed, natural, hard, or soft. As a rule, imitation cheeses (made with vegetable oil), part-skim milk cheese, and cheeses advertised as "low-fat" are usually lower in saturated fat and cholesterol than are natural and processed cheeses (which are made with whole milk). However, even part-skim milk cheese and low-fat cheeses are not necessarily lower in fat than many meats. Remember it this way:

- Natural, processed, and hard cheeses, like cheddar, Swiss or American, are highest in saturated fat.
- Low-fat and imitation cheeses may have less saturated fat.
- Many meats have less saturated fat than many of these cheeses.

Therefore, when you can, replace natural, processed and hard cheeses with low-fat and imitation cheeses. Read the label.

When your child has the urge for cheese, try the following:

- String cheese
- Part-skim mozzarella
- Low-fat cottage cheese
- Farmer cheese

If your child is on the Step-One Diet, choose low-fat cheeses that have no more than 6 grams of fat in 1 ounce. If your child is on the Step-Two Diet, choose low-fat cheeses that havve no more than 2 grams of fat in 1 ounce.

Ice Cream. Children love ice cream. But, ice cream is made from whole milk and cream. It contains a large amount of saturated fat and cholesterol. Try frozen desserts, like ice milk and low-fat frozen yogurt, which are lower in saturated fat. Also try sorbet and popsicles, which contain no fat.

Make your own ice cream substitutes:

- Tangy yogurt cubes. Combine 6 ounces of undiluted frozen fruit juice concentrate with 8 ounces plain low-fat yogurt and freeze in ice cube trays or paper cups.

- Homemade popsicles. Freeze orange and other juices on a stick.

• Floats. Combine ice milk with carbonated fruit juice.

Eggs

Egg yolks are high in cholesterol: each contains about 213 mg. So, they should be eaten in moderation. On the Step-One Diet your child can eat 3 to 4 yolks a week. This includes those in processed foods and many baked goods. On the Step-Two Diet your child should eat even less. Egg whites which contain no cholesterol can be eaten freely.

In recipes, whole eggs can be replaced with egg whites. For most cake or cookie recipes, you can substitute egg whites for one to two eggs; in some, up to three to four. Since egg substitutes are made mainly of egg white, they also may be used to replace eggs (all or some) in dishes such as scrambled eggs, omelets, and some baked items.

Fats and Oils

Foods included in this group will be high in either saturated, polyunsaturated, or monounsaturated fatty acids. Lard, fatback, and butter are high in saturated fat. Solid shortenings and some commercial salad dressings contain moderate amounts of saturated fats. So, limit how much you use of these foods, especially in your cooking.

Instead of butter, use margarine since it is higher in polyunsaturated fatty acids. Choose those liquid vegetable oils that are highest in unsaturated fats, like canola (rapeseed oil), safflower, sunflower, corn, olive, sesame, and soybean oils in cooking and salad dressings. When you shop, read food labels. Choose margarines and oils that have more polyunsaturated fat than saturated fat.

Some vegetable oils, like coconut, palm, and palm kernel oil, are saturated These vegetable fats, often called "tropical oils," can be found in commercially baked goods such as cookies and crackers, nondairy substitutes such as whipped toppings and coffee creamers, cake mixes, and even frozen dinners. They also can be found in some snack foods, like chips, candy bars, and buttered popcorn. Many companies have removed tropical oils from their products in order to help reduce their saturated fat content.

Also, vegetable oils can become saturated by hydrogenation—a process that makes them solid. They are called hydrogenated vegetable oils.

257

When choosing foods that contain tropical oils or hydrogenated vegetable oils, read the label before you buy. Choose those products lowest in saturated fat.

Since avocados, olives, nuts, and seeds are high in fat, they are often grouped with fats and oils. Although the fat in nuts and seeds is mostly unsaturated fat, they are very high in calories. They can fit into the eating plan if used in small amounts and not too often. Peanut butter can be a good choice for children's sandwiches, and nuts and seeds can be an after school treat.

Fruits and Vegetables

Fruits and vegetables contain no cholesterol, are very low in saturated fat, and are low in calories, except for avocados and olives (see Fats and Oils). Cutting back on high-fat foods cuts out some calories. Eating more fruits and vegetables is a good way for the whole family to replace those calories. Fruits can be a tasty snack or dessert. Even vegetables can be disguised as snacks and interesting side dishes. When chopped into small pieces, vegetables can be added to most favorite recipes without the child even noticing. By eating more of these foods your child can get more vitamins, minerals, and fiber and less saturated fat and cholesterol.

Breads, Cereals, Pasta, Rice, and Dry Peas and Beans

Breads, cereals, pasta, rice, and dry peas and beans are all high in complex carbohydrates and low in saturated fat. Replace foods high in saturated fat with those high in complex carbohydrates.

Your child might like some of the following suggestions:

- Try pasta with tomato sauce, or spaghetti with oil and herbs for supper as the main dish. Add low-fat cheese or small amounts of meat or fish and vegetables for extra punch.

- Combine rice with vegetables or smaller portions of meat, chicken, or fish.

- Use dry peas and beans (like split peas, lentils, kidney beans, and navy beans) as main dishes, casseroles, soups, or other one-dish meals without high-fat sauces. Chili without lots of meat is a good low-fat, one-dish meal.

Cereals, both cooked and dry, are usually low in saturated fat. Some that contain coconut or coconut oil, like many types of granola, are not. In fact, most granolas are high in fat. Compare the cereal labels. Choose those lower in fat, particularly saturated fat.

Most breads and rolls also are low in fat. Choose the whole-grain types for more fiber. Some commercially baked goods, [such as croissants, muffins, biscuits, butter rolls, and doughnuts] are often made with large amounts of saturated fats.

Read the labels on baked goods to figure out their fat content. Instead of buying the high-fat types, you can make your own muffins and quick breads using unsaturated vegetable oils and egg whites or substitutes. In most recipes, you can replace one whole egg with two egg whites.

Foods from this group can be great snacks for children at any age. Instead of snacks high in saturated fat, encourage your child to try low-fat crackers (like graham crackers); ready-to-eat cereal; and whole-grain bread with low-fat cheese, peanut butter, or lean meat. Even pizza can be lower in fat and saturated fat when made with low-fat cheese on an English muffin or low-fat crackers. Remember to leave off the pepperoni, sausage, and extra cheese toppings.

Sweets and Snacks

Sweets and snacks often are high in saturated fat, cholesterol, and calories. Commercial cakes, pies, cookies, cheese crackers, and some types of chips are examples of such foods. Once again, the key is to read labels carefully. Choose those that contain primarily unsaturated fats and are low in total fat and calories.

Candy made mostly of sugar (for example, hard candy, gum drops, candy corn) has very little or no fat. It can be a snack now and then. Other candies, especially chocolate, should be limited because they are high in saturated fat.

If your child likes to eat pies, cakes, or cookies, try some tasty alternatives to the high-saturated fat and high-cholesterol types. Fig bars, ginger snaps, graham crackers, homemade cake and cookies made with vegetable oils and egg whites or substitutes, or angel food cake are all options. New baked goods have been developed which contain no cholesterol and very little fat. Some items, like frozen dairy desserts and puddings, are even made with fat substitutes. Even though these new products may be low in saturated fat and cholesterol, they are not always low in calories. Pay attention to serving sizes, especially for children who are overweight.

Remember, most desserts can be made at home. Substitute unsaturated oil or margarine for butter and lard, skim milk for whole milk, and egg whites or substitutes for egg yolks. This reduces their saturated fat and cholesterol, although total fat remains high. If your child has a weight problem, they should be eaten only once in a while. For snacks, try instead a piece of fruit, some vegetable sticks, unbuttered popcorn, or breadsticks.

Changing Eating Patterns Takes Time

All of the changes suggested above don't have to happen at once. Take it day by day. Aim for the target of change: less saturated fat, total fat, and cholesterol in your child's diet each day. This is especially important if your child has a high blood cholesterol level.

The first step is to look at your child's current eating pattern and begin to plan alternatives. Write down a typical day's menu for your child. Is your child eating too many high-fat foods? Is your child eating from all the food groups?

Don't try to cut out all the high-saturated fat and high-cholesterol foods at one time. Instead, try to substitute one or two more appropriate foods each day. If your child rarely eats foods high in saturated fat, these foods once in a while won't raise your child's blood cholesterol level. If you expect a high-saturated fat, high-cholesterol day, have your child eat a low-saturated fat, low-cholesterol diet the day before and the day after.

Changing eating patterns takes time. Start with easy-to-do changes followed by harder ones. For example, instead of limiting pizza, try pizza with vegetables and low-fat cheese. Make "lasting" changes rather than rapid changes that will last only a short time. Soon enough your child will be eating in a way that is lower in saturated fat and cholesterol.

Heart-Healthy Meals and Snacks

Breakfast

Children as they get older, especially girls, may often skip breakfast. It is important to begin the day with a good breakfast. Breakfast is an easy meal to introduce good-tasting heart-healthy foods.

- Serve toast (whole-grain types), English muffins, bagels, and hot or cold cereal with skim milk. These are quick and easy to prepare.

- Serve unsweetened or barely sweetened cereals as often as you can. Adding fruit to unsweetened cereal makes it special, and at the same time, increases nutrients and fiber without adding fat.

- For special events or weekend treats, try pancakes, muffins, or French toast made with egg whites or egg substitutes and skim milk. Add some sweet syrup or fruit sauce, neither of which contains fat, to make it more appealing to children.

- For a more hearty breakfast, add some low-fat meat such as sliced poultry or lean ham to a bagel or an English muffin.

Lunch

Choosing lunch at school gives children the chance to make the right food choices for themselves. Packing a lunch offers them the chance to plan their own heart-healthy meals. Whether your child buys a school lunch or takes a packed lunch, discuss some tips for eating right. Try some of these:

- Sliced turkey, lean roast beef, chicken, or tuna fish are good choices for lower-fat sandwiches. Even add a bit of sliced processed low-fat cheese.

- Peanut butter and jelly is also okay, especially on whole grain bread. For more nutritional punch, create peanut butter and mashed bananas with raisins or carrots.

- Whole-wheat, rye, pumpernickel, or bran breads add more fiber to a sandwich and taste good too.

- Try some of last night's pasta salad or cold baked chicken with herbs for a switch from sandwiches for lunch.

- Pack some snacks such as apples, bananas, grapes, raisins, nuts, or seeds. Also, put in prepackaged juices or other types of unsweetened beverages.

Some lunches provided at school may be high in saturated fat and cholesterol. Check the menu in advance. If low-fat choices are not available on a certain day, you and your child can pack a lunch. However, if your child's school never offers heart-healthy choices, try to arrange that it does so. Work with your PTA or school system to promote a school lunch program which offers heart-healthy choices.

Dinner

Dinner may pose a problem for busy parents who have little time to shop and cook. Many rely on high-fat convenience foods like creamy, canned soups and boxed macaroni and cheese dinners. Replace these with foods lower in saturated fat and cholesterol that are quick and easy to prepare:

- Chicken breasts, fish fillets, and lean hamburgers take little time to prepare. Broil, bake, or microwave, rather than fry.

- Vegetables can be steamed or microwaved in minutes.

- Vegetable stew can be made with rice or pasta and shavings of lean meat instead of a lot of chunks. Meat contributes protein, vitamins, and minerals like iron. Children should not avoid eating meat. It is a good idea to "stretch" meat by using it in a combination dish, like stew.

- Many ethnic dishes can also be low in fat and quick and easy to prepare. Try Chinese stir fries of rice, peppers, mushrooms, and water chestnuts with thin strips of beef or chicken. Pizza can be made with low-fat cheese and vegetable toppings rather than sausage or pepperoni.

- Some TV dinners and other convenience meals can be low in saturated fat and cholesterol. Look for dinners that provide foods from different food groups including vegetables, fruits, and breads. Choose less often those that contain battered, fried, or deep fried items. Read the labels and compare. Choose the one lowest in total fat and saturated fat.

Snacking Is Okay

Snacking is not a bad word. What your child eats matters more than when it is eaten. Children are growing quickly and need calories. Young children's appetites and stomachs may be small, so they may tend to eat smaller amounts at one time. They may not be able to eat enough calories at a meal to meet their energy needs. So, snacks may need to be part of their eating pattern.

Preteens and teenagers also may need extra nutrition and calories to get them through their growth spurts or athletic programs. Snacks can help meet their energy needs without being high in saturated fat and cholesterol. Instead, they can be rich in carbohydrates and fiber.

Plan for snacks. We all tend to eat what's handy. So, stock your kitchen with nutritious, low-saturated fat, low-cholesterol snack foods from all of the food groups. See below for some suggestions.

Let the snack foods you serve at home be the "good eating guide" when your child is away from home. Some of these snacks are now also found in vending machines. Your child just needs to choose them.

Like anything else, snacking can be overdone. If snacking leads to eating too much, it can lead to weight gain. Or, if snacks come mainly from the "Sweets and Snacks" group, your child may not get enough of the nutrients provided by other foods.

Low-Saturated Fat, Low-Cholesterol Snacks

- Snack mix of cereal, dried fruit, and small amounts of nuts and seeds
- Cold cereal, dry or with low-fat milk
- Peanut butter and jelly sandwich
- Fruit juice and vegetable juice
- Peanuts in a shell or other dry roasted nuts
- Toast with jam or jelly
- Fruit leather
- Low-fat cheese pizza on English muffin
- Celery stalk filled with peanut butter
- Vegetable soup and low-fat crackers
- Candy (nonchocolate fat-free types)

- Skim milk with graham crackers
- Raisins and other dried fruit
- Frozen grapes or bananas
- Flavored low-fat yogurt
- Low-fat cookies

Recipies and Healthy Fast Foods

There is no reason to stop using your favorite recipes and cookbook. You can change tried and true recipes to low-saturated fat, low-cholesterol recipes. The tips for substitutes in the [list] below will help you get started.

- In place of 1 tablespoon butter, use 1 tablespoon margarine or 3/4 tablespoon oil.
- In place of 1 cup shortening, use 2/3 cup vegetable oil
- In place of 1 whole egg, use 2 egg whites
- In place of 1 cup sour cream, use 1 cup yogurt (plus 1 tablespoon cornstarch for some recipies)
- In place of 1 cup whole milk, use 1 cup skim milk

Experiment! find the recipes that work best with these changes.

Convenience Foods and Fast Foods Can Be Heart Healthy

Stopping now and then at a fast food restaurant with friends or family does no harm. However, these days children may be eating fast and convenience foods three or more times a week. By serving heart-healthy meals and snacks at home, you can plan for fast-food meals once in a while. Also, some fast and convenience foods are now lower in saturated fat and cholesterol than they used to be. See the [Figure 26.1] for a comparison of some of children's fast food favorites.

Here are some ways to avoid eating too much saturated fat and cholesterol while enjoying convenience. Try some of these tips:

- Order a small plain hamburger. It is lower in fat than fried or battered fish and chicken or anything with cheese.

- Try lean roast beef and grilled or broiled chicken sandwiches or pita pockets filled with small pieces of meat and vegetables.

Fast Food Favorites: A Comparison

Product	Saturated Fat (grams)	Dietary Cholesterol (milligrams)	Total Fat (grams)	Total Calories
Cheese pizza, 1 slice	2	9	3	140
Pepperoni pizza, 1 slice	2	14	7	181
Bean burrito	3	3	7	224
Beef and cheese burrito	5	85	12	317
Hamburger	4	36	12	275
Cheeseburger	6	50	15	320
French fries, regular	4	0	12	235
French fries, large	6	0	19	355
Grilled chicken breast sandwich	1	60	9	310
Chicken nuggets, 6 pieces	6	62	17	290
Beef hot dog, on bun	6	27	15	265
Vanilla low-fat frozen yogurt cone	0	2	1	105
Vanilla soft serve ice milk cone	4	28	6	164
Vanilla shake	5	32	8	314
Vanilla ice cream, 1 cup (10% fat)	9	59	14	269
Cola, 12 oz.	0	0	0	151

Source: USDA Handbook 8-21; individual manufacturers for items not available from USDA.

Figure 26.1

- Select the small serving; order the regular hamburger instead of the jumbo.

- Order a plain baked potato instead of French fries.

- Create a salad at the salad bar. Limit toppings of cheese, fried noodles, bacon bits, and salads made with mayonnaise. Also, limit salad dressings that add saturated fat and cholesterol.

- Try ethnic cuisine—many such as Chinese and mid-Eastern are becoming fast food.

- Choose pizza with vegetable toppings such as mushrooms, onions, or peppers. Avoid extra cheese, pepperoni, or sausage.

- Create convenience foods at home by freezing low-fat casseroles, soups, and leftovers in single serving sizes.

[Figure 26.2] shows how some of these small changes can add up to big savings in saturated fat, total fat, cholesterol, and calories.

Sample Menus: Step-One and Step-Two Diets

The differences between the eating pattern suggested for all healthy Americans, the Step-One Diet, and Step-Two Diet appear to be small. BUT they are very important for lowering your child's blood cholesterol level. All of the small changes add up to improve your child's blood cholesterol level.

Take a look at the sample menus [at the end of this chapter]. There are three sets of menus, each set for a different age range. The samples of the suggested eating pattern, Step-One, and Step-Two Diets have the same number of calories as the sample menu of the current eating pattern. However, they have much less saturated fat, total fat, and cholesterol. And, the sample menus show that because the fat in the current eating pattern was so calorie rich, the new eating patterns actually allow your child to eat more food!

The menus show how you can change a child's current eating pattern to one that is lower in saturated fat, total fat, and cholesterol, and be consistent with the Step-One and Step-Two Diets. (The nutrient analysis for each sample menu [follows the menus].)

Sample Fast Food Meals:
How Small Changes Add Up

Meal	Saturated Fat (grams)	Dietary Cholesterol (milligrams)	Total Fat (grams)	Total Calories
Typical meal #1 Chicken nuggets Large French fries Vanilla shake	17	94	45	959
Lower-fat choice #1 Grilled chicken breast sandwich ½ small French fries 12 oz. cola Low-fat frozen yogurt cone	3	62	16	684
Typical meal #2 Cheeseburger Large French fries 12 oz. cola Vanilla ice milk cone	16	78	40	990
Lower-fat choice #2 Hamburger ½ small French fries 12 oz. cola Low-fat frozen yogurt cone	6	38	19	649

Figure 26.2

Look across the menus and compare the highlighted items.

- Some items show simple changes in the type of food offered which lowers the saturated fat and cholesterol content of the menu. For example, across the sample menus for breakfast, you will see a change from whole milk to 1% milk to skim milk. Likewise, the dinners in sample menu 2 show a change from fried chicken to skinless broiled chicken, and change the butter on the vegetables to regular or tub margarine.

- Other changes in the actual foods offered can also help to reduce saturated fat and cholesterol. For example, the lunches in sample menu 2 show replacing a cheeseburger with a hamburger for Step-One, and with a tuna sandwich made with water-pack tuna for Step-Two.

- Sample menu 3 suggests choosing a roast beef sandwich instead of a beef hot dog with chili for lunch, and chicken cacciatore (made with skinless chicken and pasta) instead of lasagna (made with regular ground beef and whole milk mozzarella) for dinner.

You may notice that the Step-Two Diet calls for adding more margarine as tub margarine, which is highly unsaturated. By using only skim milk, low-fat cheese, and the leanest meat on the Step-Two Diet, you have removed many hidden sources of saturated fat. Since the Step-Two Diet has the same amount of total fat and calories as the other eating patterns it's okay to replace these saturated fats with more tub margarine.

As you can see, learning to eat the heart-healthy way means choosing more foods low in saturated fat and cholesterol. It's important to remember that you can have variety within any given day.

You Can Lead Your Child To Food, But You Can't Make Him Eat

The most carefully planned heart healthy meal is no good if your child does not eat it. Younger children may just be picky eaters going through a stage. Older children may have "reasons" for being picky. Children can be encouraged to eat foods lower in saturated fat and cholesterol but should not be made to eat them. You need to be creative and give them choices:

- Let your child help fix the meal. Helping makes eating more fun.

- Make the meal attractive. For younger children, make a face on top of casserole or cut foods with a cookie cutter to make fun shapes.

- If your child doesn't like a certain lower fat food, serve it with something your child does like. Disguise an unliked food in other foods. For example, add the food to casseroles or soups, or bake it into muffins or quick breads.

- Above all, be a good role model yourself—let your eating patterns be the example for others.

Choosing to eat in a heart-healthy way is a family affair. It becomes even more important if someone in the family has high blood cholesterol. If your child has high blood cholesterol, talk to them about it. They may not understand why they need to eat this way and may be afraid of sudden changes. Encourage children to eat for the health of their heart, yet don't make too big a deal about it. If your child is growing well, he or she is probably getting enough to eat. So don't worry about it. If your child gets stuck on one food or refuses to make any changes, discuss the problem with your doctor or a dietitian.

HELP!

If you want more help in planning low-saturated fat, low-cholesterol eating patterns, visit a registered dietitian or other qualified nutritionist. They can help you design an eating pattern suited to your own child's needs and likes. Dietitians may be found at local hospitals, and state and district chapters of the American Dietetic Association (ADA). The ADA keeps a list of registered dietitians. By calling the Division of Practice (312-899-0040), you can request names of dietitians in your area. Others can be found in public health departments, health maintenance organizations, cooperative extension services, and colleges. You can also call the ADA's consumer nutrition hotline at 800-366-1655.

Dietitians can help you by giving further advice on shopping and preparing foods, eating away from home, and changing your child's eating habits to help maintain the new eating pattern. Their skill will help you and your child set short-term targets for change. This will help your child reach the blood cholesterol goal without greatly changing your family's eating patterns and lifestyle.

The National Cholesterol Education Program has produced booklets for children of different age groups: ages 7 to 10, 11 to 14, and 15 to 18. These booklets are designed to help children understand blood cholesterol levels and the need to eat in a way that is low in saturated fat, total fat, and cholesterol. To order these booklets and others for adults with high blood cholesterol, contact:

National Cholesterol Education Program
NHLBI Information Center
P.O. Box 30105
Bethesda, Maryland 20824-0105

Sample Menus 1

With School Lunch for Children 7 to 10 Years

Current Eating Pattern	Suggested Eating Pattern or Step-One Diet	Step-Two Diet
Breakfast ¹/₂ cup orange juice 1 packet oatmeal with maple and brown sugar 1 cup whole milk	**Breakfast** ¹/₂ cup orange juice 1 packet oatmeal with maple and brown sugar 1 cup 1% milk	**Breakfast** ¹/₂ cup orange juice 1 packet oatmeal with maple and brown sugar 2 tsp. tub margarine 1 cup skim milk

School Lunch
oven fried chicken with skin
¹/₂ cup mashed potatoes
¹/₂ cup green beans with butter
¹/₂ canned pear
1 cup whole milk
	School Lunch
	oven fried chicken with skin
	¹/₂ cup mashed potatoes
	¹/₂ cup green beans with butter
	¹/₂ canned pear
	1 cup 2% milk
		Bag Lunch
		ham sandwich:
		  2 slices bread
		  2 oz. lean ham
		  2 tsp. mayonnaise, lettuce, tomato, pickle
		1 medium banana
		1 cup skim milk

Snack
ham sandwich:
  2 slices bread
  1 oz. ham luncheon meat
  lettuce, tomato, pickle
  ¹/₂ tbsp. mayonnaise
1 medium cola
	Snack
	turkey sandwich:
	  2 slices bread
	  1-¹/₂ oz. turkey luncheon meat
	  1 oz. low-fat cheese
	  lettuce, tomato, pickle
	  1 tsp. mayonnaise
	1 medium cola
		Snack
		turkey sandwich:
		  2 slices bread
		  1-¹/₂ oz. turkey luncheon meat
		  1 oz. low-fat cheese
		  lettuce, tomato, pickle
		  1 tsp. margarine or tub margarine
		1 medium cola

Dinner 1 serving tuna macaroni casserole ¹/₂ cup carrots and peas 1 small roll ¹/₂ cup applesauce water or noncaloric beverage	**Dinner** 1 serving tuna macaroni casserole ¹/₂ cup carrots and peas 1 small roll 1 tsp. margarine ¹/₂ cup applesauce water or noncaloric beverage	**Dinner** 1 serving tuna macaroni casserole ¹/₂ cup carrots and peas 2 tsp. margarine ¹/₂ cup applesauce water or noncaloric beverage
Snack 1" x 2" chocolate brownie 1 cup whole milk	**Snack** 4 medium commercial oatmeal cookies 1 cup 1% milk	**Snack** 4 medium homemade oatmeal cookies, made with tub margarine 1 cup skim milk

Sample Menus 2

With Fast Food Lunch for 11 to 14 Year-Old Girls

Current Eating Pattern	Suggested Eating Pattern or Step-One Diet	Step-Two Diet
Breakfast	Breakfast	Breakfast
1 cup orange juice	1 cup orange juice	1 cup orange juice
1 cup presweetened cereal	3/4 cup corn flakes	3/4 cup corn flakes
1 cup whole milk	1 cup 1% milk	1/2 English muffin
		1 tsp. margarine
Fast Food Lunch	Fast Food Lunch	1 cup skim milk
1 cheeseburger	1 hamburger, quarter pound	
1 regular order French fries	lettuce, tomato, onions	Bag Lunch
3 packets catsup	1 regular order French fries	tuna sandwich:
1 small cola	1 packet catsup	2 slices bread
	1/2 box animal crackers	3 oz. water pack tuna
Snack	1 medium cola	tomato, celery, relish
2 medium ginger snaps		4 tsp. mayonnaise
water or noncaloric beverage	Snack	3/4 oz. bag pretzels
	4 multi-grain, low-fat crackers	4 homemade oatmeal cookies
Dinner	3/4 oz. low-fat cheese	1 medium cola
1 breaded and fried chicken breast	water or noncaloric beverage	
with skin		Snack
1 boiled potato with butter	Dinner	4 multi-grain, low-fat crackers
1/2 cup broccoli with butter	3 oz. broiled chicken breast,	3/4 oz. low-fat cheese
1 small roll	no skin	water or noncaloric beverage
1 tsp. margarine	1 boiled potato with margarine	
1 cup iced tea	4 broccoli spears with margarine	Dinner
	4 tomato slices	3 oz. broiled chicken breast,
Snack	1 slice bread	no skin
3/4 oz. American cheese	1/2 cup strawberries	1 boiled potato with tub margarine
4 crackers	1 container nonfat yogurt	4 broccoli spears with tub margarine
1/2 cup fruit drink	water or noncaloric beverage	4 tomato slices
		1 slice bread
	Snack	2 tsp. margarine
	1 commercial cupcake	1/2 cup strawberries
	1 cup 1% milk	1 container nonfat yogurt
		water or noncaloric beverage
		Snack
		1 homemade cupcake
		1 cup skim milk

Sample Menus 3

With Fast Food Lunch for 15 to 19 Year-Old Boys

Current Eating Pattern	Suggested Eating Pattern or Step-One Diet	Step-Two Diet
Breakfast 1 cup orange juice ½ cup granola cereal 1 cup whole milk	**Breakfast** 1 cup orange juice ¾ cup presweetened corn flakes 1 bagel 1 tsp. margarine 1 cup 1% milk	**Breakfast** 1 cup orange juice ¾ cup presweetened corn flakes 1 bagel 2 tsp. margarine 1 cup skim milk
Fast Food Lunch 1 beef hot dog on bun with chili 1 oz. potato chips 1 medium cola	**Sandwich Shop** roast beef sandwich 2 cups tossed salad 2 tbsp. Thousand Island dressing 1 oz. bag corn chips 1 medium cola	**Sandwich Shop** roast beef sandwich 2 cups tossed salad 3 tbsp. Thousand Island dressing 1 medium cola

Snack
2 oz. chocolate candy bar
1 medium cola
	Snack
	ham and cheese sandwich:
	  2 slices bread
	  1 oz. low-fat ham
	  1 oz. low-fat cheese
	2 tsp. mayonnaise, lettuce, tomato, pickle
	4 commercial oatmeal cookies
	1 cup orange juice
		Snack
		turkey and cheese sandwich:
		  2 slices bread
		  1 oz. turkey breast
		  1 oz. low-fat cheese
		  lettuce, tomato, pickle
		  2 tsp. mayonnaise
		¾ oz. bag pretzels
		5 gingersnaps
		1 cup orange juice

Dinner 1 serving beef lasagna (4"x3") 2 cups tossed salad 3 tbsp. Thousand Island dressing 1 slice French bread 2 brownies (1"x2") 1 cup whole milk	**Dinner** 3 oz. chicken cacciatore ½ cup green beans 1 cup white rice 1 tsp. margarine 1 slice bread 15 grapes 1 cup nonfat yogurt with fruit flavor water or noncaloric beverage	**Dinner** 3 oz. chicken cacciatore ½ cup green beans with tub margarine 1 cup rice with tub margarine 1 slice bread 1-½ tsp. margarine 15 grapes 1 cup nonfat yogurt with fruit flavor water or noncaloric beverage
Snack 1 cup frozen yogurt 1 medium cola	**Snack** 6 homemade peanut butter cookies 1 cup 1% milk	**Snack** ⅛ of 9" homemade apple pie 1 cup skim milk

273

Age	Nutrients	Current Eating Pattern	Suggested Eating Pattern or Step-One Diet	Step-Two Diet
7 to 10 Year-Old Children	Calories	2,008	2,005	1,966
	Total fat (% of calories)	35	29	29
	Saturated fat (% of calories)	15	11	7
	Cholesterol (milligrams)	261	188	126
11 to 14 Year-Old Girls	Calories	2,219	2,240	2,248
	Total fat (% of calories)	35	29	27
	Saturated fat (% of calories)	15	10	6
	Cholesterol (milligrams)	264	188	159
15 to 19 Year-Old Boys	Calories	2,998	3,026	2,993
	Total fat (% of calories)	36	30	29
	Saturated fat (% of calories)	15	9	7
	Cholesterol (milligrams)	258	224	157

Title: *Nutrient Analysis*

Part Four

Cardiovascular Pharmacological Interventions

Chapter 27

Clot-Busting Drugs to Turn Off Heart Attacks

Every year, about 1.5 million Americans suffer a heart attack. Of that number, one-third die within one year, 100,000 before they can be hospitalized. Typically, a blood clot develops in one of the arteries to the heart, preventing oxygen-rich blood from that part of the heart muscle. The greater the blockage and the longer it continues, the more of the heart muscle that is lost. Substantial loss of heart muscle can lead to heart failure and death.

But over the past several years, researchers have developed drugs called thrombolytic agents that can help dissolve the clots. Blood can then again flow through the artery, preventing further damage to the heart. Last fall, FDA approved alteplase (trade name Activase), one of a new class of thrombolytic agents known as tissue plasminogen activators (TPA). In addition, FDA approved the expanded use of another thrombolytic agent, streptokinase (trade names Kabikinase and Streptase). These approvals mean that heart attack victims have greater reason for hope than ever before that they will successfully recover from their attacks.

Alteplase is a genetically engineered copy of a protein produced naturally by the body. In 1979, scientists in Belgium first purified TPA and showed that it could dissolve clots in laboratory animals. But the amount produced in the body, or from most human cells in culture, is so minute that large-scale production would be impractical. So, in

---

FDA Consumer, February 1988; February 1990.

1981, Genentech Inc., of South San Francisco, Calif., began using recombinant DNA technology to produce enough alteplase to be tested in heart attack victims.

Genetically engineered alteplase is made by introducing the human gene that holds the instructions for producing the protein into cells originally derived from the ovaries of Chinese hamsters. The inserted gene programs the cells to consistently produce large quantities of alteplase.

Clinical trials of alteplase began in 1984. In all, Genentech's alteplase has been tested in more than 4,000 patients. It has been shown in controlled clinical trials to dissolve clots in 71 percent of heart attack patients when injected within six hours after symptoms occur. In separate trials, the drug significantly improved heart function when given within four hours.

One of the largest studies, sponsored by the National Heart, Lung, and Blood Institute, was known as the Thrombolysis in Myocardial Infarction Trial. This study included alteplase and streptokinase. Streptokinase—made by Behringwerke AG, a German firm represented in the United States by Hoechst-Roussel Pharmaceuticals Inc. of Somerville, N.J., and KabiVitrum AB of Stockholm, Sweden, which has offices in Alameda, Calif.—has been licensed for use in treating heart attacks since 1982. Until last fall, however, the use of streptokinase, which is derived from *Streptococci* bacteria, was limited because it could be administered only by inserting a catheter directly into the coronary artery. This procedure could only be done in hospitals that have special coronary care units.

But recent data from clinical trials, including one involving more than 11,000 patients, have shown that streptokinase given intravenously—by a needle inserted into a vein—reduces the death rate among recipients by 20 percent to 25 percent when given within six hours after a heart attack. "The most dramatic result—a 47 percent reduction in mortality," said FDA Commissioner Frank E. Young, M.D., Ph.D., "was observed when streptokinase was administered within one hour of the onset of symptoms." In separate studies, it was shown to improve heart function.

Alteplase and streptokinase can be used to treat the vast majority of heart attack victims, but should not be given to patients at high risk of hemorrhaging. This includes patients with internal bleeding; a recent stroke, surgery or major injury; long-standing, uncontrolled high blood pressure; or a bleeding disorder. Both drugs also should be used with caution in people over 75, in pregnant women, and where bleeding is a significant hazard.

Bleeding within the brain was one of several issues that concerned the Cardiovascular and Renal Drugs Advisory Committee—an advisory committee made up of nongovernment experts—on May 29, 1987. This committee advised FDA to obtain more data on safety and effectiveness before approving alteplase.

Data submitted later showed that the bleeding problem occurred more frequently at higher doses, but at the recommended dose of 100 milligrams it occurred only in 0.4 percent of patients. Bleeding occurred at about the same rate with streptokinase when given at recommended dosages.

The committee also recommended FDA find out whether a change in manufacturing procedures at Genentech made any difference in alteplase's safety and effectiveness. Data submitted by the manufacturer showed that it did not. In addition, the committee questioned whether alteplase's ability to dissolve clots actually, as theorized, limited heart damage. Subsequent data showed that it did.

Robert E. Windom, M.D., assistant secretary for health, observed that although changes in diet, anti-smoking campaigns, and other factors have helped reduce deaths from heart disease, coronary heart disease "remains America's number one killer, responsible for about 768,000 deaths each year—or about a third of all deaths," he said. "At some point in their lives," Dr. Windom added, "one out of every four or five people will feel the pain and constriction of a heart attack—pressure or pain in their chest or pain in their left arm." When that happens, he advised, "Don't waste time hoping against hope that the pain will go away . . . get help quickly."

—by Catherine Carey

Catherine Carey is a member of FDA's public affairs staff.

Third Clot Dissolver Approved for Heart Attacks (2/90)

FDA has approved a third intravenous blood-clot-dissolving (thrombolytic) drug for preventing permanent damage to the heart muscle following a heart attack. Known generically as anistreplase, the product is being marketed by both Beecham Laboratories and Upjohn Co. under the trade name Eminase.

Anistreplase is administered as a single injection lasting two to five minutes. The other two thrombolytics—alteplase (or TPA) and streptokinase—are administered over a period of one to three hours. The labeling for all three products advises that they should be administered as soon as possible after heart attack symptoms begin.

In clinical studies, anistreplase opened blocked arteries of 72 percent of heart attack victims who received it within six hours of onset of symptoms. Improved heart function was documented in a study of patients given the drug within four hours of onset of symptoms. Studies also showed that the number of deaths occurring after 30 days was reduced by 47 percent and after one year by 38 percent.

Chapter 28

Antiarrhythmic Drugs

Researchers at Duke University Medical Center in Durham, North Carolina, have developed methods to test the efficacy of antiarrhythmic drugs in the prevention of unexpected increases in heart rate known as paroxysmal supraventricular arrhythmias.

In a recent trial involving 23 patients with recurrent supraventricular arrhythmias, Dr. Edward L. C. Pritchett, professor of cardiology and clinical pharmacology and program director of the General Clinical Research Center at Duke, and his colleagues found that propafenone reduced the rate of arrhythmia recurrence to approximately one-fifth the rate seen during treatment with placebo (a harmless inactive treatment). Patients used portable electrocardiogram (ECG) recorders to document arrhythmic attacks and transmitted the recordings to the investigators by telephone.

According to Dr. Pritchett, the research is significant not only because it demonstrates the efficacy of propafenone but also because it provides a reliable method to test the efficacy of antiarrhythmic drugs in general. "Now we have a procedure that can be used reliably to assess the ability of an antiarrhythmic drug to suppress a patient's arrhythmia," he says. "This was the third study we have conducted using the same methodology. The other two have led to the only Food and Drug Administration (FDA) approvals since 1968 of drugs to treat these disorders. Those drugs are verapamil, which was approved in 1986, and flecainide, which was approved in 1991."

NCRR Reporter, January/February 1993.

An arrhythmia is a defect in the heart's electrical conduction system that causes it to beat irregularly and, as a result, to pump blood ineffectively. The two types of arrhythmia studied by Dr. Pritchett's group are paroxysmal atrial fibrillation—in which the many individual muscle fibers of the heart's small chamber, the atrium, suddenly begin to beat rapidly and chaotically—and paroxysmal supraventricular tachycardia, which is characterized by a rapid, regular rhythm.

"The heart rate will go from a resting rate of 60 to 80 beats a minute to an average rate of about 200 beats a minute," explains Dr. Pritchett. "It may continue to be that high for periods of a few minutes to several hours. During that time patients are aware of palpitations in their chest. They may also get light-headed, develop chest pain, feel anxiety, and become short of breath."

These disorders affect people of all ages, according to Dr. Pritchett. He estimates that about 1.5 million people in the United States suffer from these two types of arrhythmia. About one-third of patients with arrhythmias also suffer from another form of heart disease.

The sporadic nature of these disorders has made it difficult to prove that drugs are effective against them, says Dr. Pritchett. "The average patient who has one of these arrhythmias will have about one attack every 3 weeks. Some patients will only have one attack every few months.

"Until the telephone monitoring system became available, it was very difficult to actually document that a patient had an arrhythmia. You cannot put somebody in the hospital and wait for 3 weeks to see whether he has an attack."

Dr. Pritchett explains that the portable ECG monitor, developed by the Maryland-based company Survival Technology, is an instrument about the size of a cigarette pack. It has two outside wires that are attached to bracelets, like expansion bracelets for a wristwatch. If the patient puts the bracelets on and presses a button on the monitor, it will record his ECG for 30 seconds. If the patient then punches another button on the monitor, it will play his ECG back as a whining tone that can be carried over a telephone. In the research center an instrument can turn the tone back into the wave form of an ECG.

"It's a completely portable, battery-operated system," Dr. Pritchett says. "When patients feel their hearts beating abnormally, they can attach the monitor to themselves and take a recording for us.

It obviates the need for the patient to go to an emergency room or a physician's office when he has an attack. The monitor has a memory, so the patient can call in and play back the ECG when it's convenient."

According to Dr. Pritchett, the devices are very simple to operate. "You don't have to be technically proficient. They're a lot easier to run than a VCR, for example. It does require a motivated patient, but the technical skills required are not difficult to master."

The propafenone study began with a "dose-finding phase," in which researchers tested patients' responses to different doses of the drug. Thirty-two patients entered the study, but nine dropped out because of adverse effects, according to Dr. Pritchett.

In the randomized phase of the study, the remaining 23 patients received either propafenone or a placebo daily until they had a recurrence of arrhythmia (measured on the portable monitor) or for 60 days, whichever came first. Neither the patients nor the physicians administering the medication knew who was receiving the drug and who was receiving the placebo.

Then the treatments were switched: patients who had received propafenone got placebo, and those who had received placebo were started on propafenone. Patients continued the second treatment either for another 60 days or until their arrhythmia recurred.

The researchers used statistical techniques to compare the time to the first recurrence of arrhythmia while patients received placebo with the time to recurrence while they were receiving propafenone. They estimated that the recurrence rate of arrhythmia during treatment with propafenone was approximately one-fifth of the recurrence rate during treatment with placebo.

Dr. Pritchett says more studies involving larger numbers of patients may be required before there is sufficient evidence of propafenone's effectiveness in patients with atrial fibrillation and supraventricular tachycardia to warrant FDA approval of the drug to treat these disorders. Propafenone is already approved for the treatment of some other types of arrhythmia.

For him and his colleagues, Dr. Pritchett says, the greatest satisfaction is in having developed a method to test the efficacy of antiarrhythmic drugs that enables the FDA to reasonably consider whether the drugs work. "That has been one of our goals since I came to Duke 18 years ago," he notes.

The group initially researched fundamental questions about arrhythmias in humans, he says. "But on a very practical level it turns out that what we have done has had a major impact on the way antiarrhythmic drugs are tested."

—by Eleanor L. Mayfield

Additional reading:

1. Pritchett, E. L., McCarthy, E. A., and Wilkinson, W. E., Propafenone treatment of symptomatic paroxysmal supraventricular arrhythmias. *Annals of Internal Medicine* 114:539-544, 1991.

2. Pritchett, E. L. and Lee, K. L., Designing clinical trials for paroxysmal atrial tachycardia and other paroxysmal arrhythmias. *Journal of Clinical Epidemiology* 41:851-858, 1988.

3. Antman, E., Beamer, A. D., Cantillon, C., et al., Long-term oral propafenone therapy for suppression of refractory symptomatic atrial fibrillation and atrial flutter. *Journal of the American College of Cardiology* 12:1005-1011, 1988.

4. Pritchett, E. L., Smith, M. S., McCarthy, E. A., et al., Observations on the spontaneous occurrence of paroxysmal supraventricular tachycardia. *Circulation* 70:1-6, 1984.

5. Pritchett, E. L., Hammill, S. C., Reiter, M. J., et al., Life-table methods for evaluating antiarrhythmic drug efficacy in patients with paroxysmal atrial tachycardia. *American Journal of Cardiology* 52:1007-1012, 1983.

Dr. Pritchett acknowledges the research contributions of registered nurse Elizabeth McCarthy and Drs. William Wilkinson, Walter Clair, and Richard Page. The research described in this article was supported by the General Clinical Research Centers Program of the National Center for Research Resources; the National Heart Lung, and Blood Institute; and Knoll Pharmaceuticals, Inc.

Chapter 29

Low-Dose Estrogen May Reduce Postmenopausal Cardiac Risks

Low-dose estrogen prescribed for women at menopause to prevent osteoporosis and relieve discomfort has the additional benefit of improving the balance of cholesterol-carrying lipoproteins in the blood. As a result it may help protect older women against their increased risk of heart disease, according to researchers at Harvard Medical School and Brigham and Women's Hospital in Boston, Massachusetts.

"As far as we can determine, this is the first time that a placebo-controlled trial of estrogen doses this low [0.625 mg per day] has been conducted in postmenopausal women," says Dr. Frank M. Sacks, assistant professor of medicine at Harvard Medical School and a clinical investigator at Brigham and Women's Hospital.

Gynecologist Dr. Brian W. Walsh, director of the menopause clinic at Brigham and Women's Hospital, conducted the study with Dr. Sacks and gynecologist Dr. Isaac Schiff in 31 healthy postmenopausal women who had normal levels of blood lipid, or fat. Before and after estrogen therapy the Boston scientists measured the women's blood levels of three classes of lipoproteins: very-low-density lipoproteins (VLDL), which are fat-laden proteins carrying cholesterol and triglyceride; low-density lipoproteins (LDL), which are VLDL that have shed triglyceride and transport cholesterol to body cells; and high-density lipoproteins (HDL), the so-called "protective" lipoproteins that return excess cholesterol to the liver where it can be metabolized and then

Research Resources Reporter, July/August 1992.

excreted with the bile. VLDL and LDL primarily contain fat and cholesterol; HDL consists mainly of protein.

The 31 women, whose average age was 56, were nonsmoking nonobese women who were not heavy drinkers and had no known risk factors for heart disease. None had taken estrogen for at least 5 weeks before their entry into the study. The investigators measured the women's fasting lipoprotein levels before treatment and during the 10th to 12th week of each treatment sequence.

They received, in random order, 3-month sequences of a placebo—a harmless inactive treatment—and two dose levels (0.625 and 1.25 mg per day) of estrogen tablets. During the last 2 weeks of each sequence the scientists determined the women's blood lipoprotein levels. After each of the three regimens the hormone progesterone was administered for 10 days to induce withdrawal bleeding, similar to the normal flushing of proliferative uterine tissue that occurs at the end of a menstrual period.

The Boston investigators found that the low and the high estrogen doses decreased the average LDL cholesterol by 15 and 19 percent, respectively, and increased the "protective" HDL-cholesterol level by 16 and 18 percent. "The fact that the lower estrogen dose appears as effective as the higher dose in improving cholesterol levels seems to me the most important aspect of our findings," says Dr. Walsh. "It's particularly important because adverse effects are more common with the higher dose."

In low- and high-dose estrogen-treated women VLDL-triglyceride levels rose by 24 percent and 42 percent, respectively. Although elevations in triglycerides, which are fats, may not be desirable, Dr. Sacks says they should pose no problem for most women, "except those women who have very high triglyceride levels to start with. About 1 in 500 women might fit this category and should be monitored very closely," he cautions. "Their risk of pancreatitis [inflammation of the pancreas] could be serious."

In a subsequent study of nine postmenopausal women the researchers examined how estrogen treatment effectively lowers LDL as it raises VLDL and triglycerides. Human estrogen (estradiol) was given in tablet form. To measure the effect on lipoprotein metabolism the scientists gave the women a 14-hour infusion of a nonradioactive variant, or isotope, of the amino acid leucine after an overnight fast at the end of each estrogen treatment period. The labeled leucine was incorporated into apolipoprotein B, which is the main protein component of VLDL and LDL. Because VLDL is converted to LDL the researchers could monitor the production and catabolism of the two lipoproteins through the common apolipoprotein B component.

Based on these studies the Boston investigators concluded that orally administered estrogen increases the production of VLDL by the liver and its secretion into the blood. However, most of the additional VLDL is apparently cleared directly from the blood without being converted to LDL. At the same time, the catabolism, or breakdown, of LDL is stimulated so that the net result is a lower LDL blood concentration and a higher VLDL concentration.

Dr. Sacks notes that throughout their lives women have a lower incidence than men of cardiovascular disease, although the differences begin to narrow when women reach the sixth decade of life. The diminished estrogen production in menopause and its effects on lipoprotein metabolism apparently push women toward the male risk level at that stage. Nevertheless, only 15 to 20 percent of postmenopausal women in the United States receive estrogen replacement therapy, according to an estimate by Dr. Walsh. He believes that these findings may encourage more women to take low-dose estrogen.

A randomized, prospective clinical study would be needed for conclusive proof of the benefits of postmenopausal estrogen therapy, the Harvard clinicians say. "It will be an extremely important but difficult study to do, particularly the randomization," Dr. Sacks says. "Women tend to want either the estrogen or the placebo. A large population of women will be needed to answer all the questions."

Earlier studies suggested that long-term estrogen administration may pose an increased risk of breast cancer and cancer of the endometrium, the inner lining of the uterus. Whether a breast cancer risk will persist with low-dose estrogen is unclear, the scientists say. Certainly the risk is believed to be less than with the higher dose studied. But breast cancer is not rare in the United States, as Dr. Sacks points out. According to the American Cancer Society, approximately one of every nine women will develop breast cancer in her lifetime. It is estimated that 180,000 new cases will be diagnosed in 1992, so even a small increased risk could have an important impact. While the debate continues about the breast cancer risk, the scientists say that the risk of endometrial cancer has been substantially diminished since progesterone treatment was added to estrogen therapy for postmenopausal women.

The present study may further focus attention on women's health issues, the Boston clinicians believe, as did a 10-year followup report on the Nurses' Health Study published by other Harvard scientists in late 1991. The authors of that nonrandomized study, which included 48,470 postmenopausal women, found a lower incidence of heart disease in women receiving estrogen supplementation than in women who received no estrogen.

"A large-scale, prospective, randomized study of low-dose estrogen will be difficult, but the difficulties will not be insurmountable," Dr. Sacks says. "And for scientific proof, such a trial is essential." A change in cholesterol is not the only ultimate endpoint; there are important questions relating to heart disease and cancer that may be resolved by such a study, according to the investigators.

—by Jane Collins

Additional reading:

1. Walsh, B. W., Schiff, I., Rosner, B., et al., Effects of postmenopausal estrogen replacement on the concentrations and metabolism of plasma lipoproteins. *New England Journal of Medicine* 325:1196-1204, 1991.

2. Stampfer, M. J., Colditz, G. A., Willett, W. C., et al., Postmenopausal estrogen therapy and cardiovascular disease: Ten-year follow-up from the Nurses' Health Study. *New England Journal of Medicine* 325:756-762, 1991.

3. Barrett-Connor, E. and Bush, T. L., Estrogen and coronary heart disease in women. *Journal of the American Medical Association* 265:1861-1867, 1991.

4. Henderson, B. E., Paganini-Hill, A., and Ross, R. K., Decreased mortality in users of estrogen replacement therapy. *Archives of Internal Medicine* 151:75-78, 1991.

5. Sacks, F. M. and Walsh, B. W., The effects of reproductive hormones on serum lipoproteins: Unresolved issues in biology and clinical practice. *Annals of the New York Academy of Science* 592:272-285, 1990.

The research described in this article was supported by the General Clinical Research Centers Program of the National Center for Research Resources; the National Heart, Lung, and Blood Institute; Bristol-Myers/Mead Johnson Laboratories; and the American Heart Association.

Chapter 30

FDA Drug Actions

Manufacturer Withdraws Heart Drug (12/91)

The manufacturer of the anti-arrhythmic medication Enkaid (anconoid hydrochloride) will withdraw the drug from the market effective Dec. 16, because of continuing uncertainty about the drug's effectiveness.

Bristol-Myers Squib Co., of Evansville, Ind., announced the withdrawal of Enkaid, used to treat irregular heartbeat, on Sept. 16. The company warned, however, that patients should not stop taking the drug unless advised to do so by their physicians.

"In some cases, physicians may judge that patients with life-threatening ventricular arrhythmias who are already successfully managed on Enkaid should not be changed to another medication," said E.J. Fox, M.D., vice president of the firm's Bristol Laboratories division. For these patients, the Enkaid Continuing Patient Access Program will provide the medication free of charge to eligible patients who were being treated with Enkaid for life-threatening ventricular arrhythmias as of Sept. 16, 1991.

Questions about whether Enkaid can decrease the risk of sudden cardiac death among patients who have survived heart attacks and have non-life-threatening arrhythmias were first raised during a study by the National Institutes of Health (NIH). Patients given

---

FDA Consumer, December 1991, July-August 1993, October 1993.

Enkaid, as well as those taking two other drugs in the study, had a higher death rate from heart attacks than patients receiving a placebo.

NIH removed Enkaid and Tambocor (flecainide), manufactured by 3M Riker, St. Paul, Minn., from the study in April 1989, and Bristol announced that Enkaid should be prescribed only for patients with life-threatening ventricular arrhythmias.

NIH stopped the trial completely last August after seeing the same negative results with the final drug under study, Ethmozine (moricizine), manufactured by Du Pont Pharmaceuticals, Wilmington, Del.

At press time neither of the other two firms had taken any actions concerning their drugs.

FDA approved Enkaid for marketing in December 1986.

Deaths with Highest Dose Of New Heart Drug (7-8/93)

Doctors should stop prescribing the highest dosage level of the new heart drug Manoplax, FDA recommended in April.

The agency made the recommendation after learning that patients taking 100 milligrams of Manoplax (flosequinan) a day had a significantly increased risk of dying.

Boots Pharmaceuticals, manufacturer of Manoplax, sent "Dear Doctor" letters last April 23 and May 24 recommending that patients receiving a 100-milligram daily dose of flosequinan should have their dose lowered to either 75 mg or 50 mg daily.

FDA advised that patients on Manoplax should not alter their use of the drug without consulting their physicians. The agency notified doctors and pharmacists about the problem immediately after making the recommendation.

Manoplax was approved by FDA in December 1992 for managing congestive heart failure in patients who do not respond to or cannot tolerate other medications. Boots Pharmaceuticals was evaluating the effects of the higher dose on survival of patients with severe congestive heart failure when the problem was found. The manufacturer and FDA are further evaluating clinical study data to see if certain groups of patients taking 75 mg daily may also have a higher mortality risk.

Heart Drug Withdrawn (10/93)

Boots Pharmaceuticals withdrew its new heart drug Manoplax (flosequinan) from the market in July after data from a clinical trial indicated that patients taking the drug had an increased risk of hospitalization or death. Data from the trial also showed that the drug's beneficial effects on symptoms of heart failure do not appear to last beyond the first three months of therapy.

FDA advises that patients taking Manoplax should consult their doctors immediately, but should not stop or change their use of the drug before getting medical advice. Patients who discontinue Manoplax may need to adjust the dosage of other medications they are taking for heart failure.

Both the company and FDA had notified doctors as early as last April to stop using the 100-milligram dose of Manoplax because preliminary results from the clinical trial showed that patients taking this dosage had a significantly increased risk of dying. Lower doses (75 and 50 milligrams) did not seem to pose a problem. The warning severely curtailed the use of the drug in the United States; at the time it was withdrawn, only about 2,000 patients were still taking it.

When approved in late December 1992, Manoplax was the first in a new class of vasodilators, medications that decrease the pressure in the blood vessels against which the heart must push. The drug, released for marketing in late March 1993, was approved for managing congestive heart failure in patients who do not respond to or cannot tolerate other medications.

Boots Pharmaceuticals will continue to make the drug available under investigational procedures to patients already receiving it who are unable to tolerate withdrawal. For more information, call (1-800) 356-2225.

Chapter 31

Aspirin:
A New Look At an Old Drug

In purses and backpacks, in briefcases and medicine chests the world over, millions of people keep close at hand a drug that has both a long past and a fascinating future. Its past reaches at least to the fifth century B.C., when Hippocrates used a bitter powder obtained from willow bark to ease aches and pains and reduce fever. Its future is being shaped today in laboratories and clinics where scientists are exploring some intriguing new uses for an interesting old drug.

The substance in willow bark that made ancient Greeks feel better, salicin, is the pharmacological ancestor of a family of drugs called salicylates, the best known of which is the world's most widely used drug—aspirin.

Americans consume an estimated 80 billion aspirin tablets a year. The *Physicians' Desk Reference* lists more than 50 over-the-counter drugs in which aspirin is the principal active ingredient. Yet, despite aspirin's having been in routine use for nearly a century, both scientific journals and the popular media are full of reports and speculation about new uses for this old remedy. The National Library of Medicine's main computerized catalog includes more than 2,700 scientific articles about aspirin. And those are only the English language publications that have appeared in the last five years.

Yet aspirin's beginnings were rather unspectacular. Nearly 100 years ago, a German industrial chemist, Felix Hoffmann, set about to find a drug to ease his father's arthritis without causing the severe

FDA Pub. No. 95-3212.

stomach irritation associated with sodium salicylate, the standard anti-arthritis drug of the time. In the forms then available, the large doses of salicylates used to treat arthritis—6 to 8 grams a day—commonly irritated the stomach lining, and many patients, like Hoffmann's father, simply could not tolerate them.

Figuring that acidity made salicylates hard on the stomach, Hoffmann started looking for a less acidic formulation. His search led him to synthesize acetylsalicylic acid (ASA), a compound that appeared to share the therapeutic properties of other salicylates and might cause less stomach irritation. ASA reduced fever, relieved moderate pain, and, at substantially higher doses, alleviated rheumatic and arthritic conditions. Hoffmann was confidant that ASA would prove more effective than salicylates then in use.

His superiors, however, did not share his enthusiasm. They doubted that ASA would ever become a valuable, commercially successful drug because at large doses salicylates commonly produced shortness of breath and an alarmingly rapid heart rate. It was taken for granted—incorrectly as it turns out—that ASA would weaken the heart and that physicians would be reluctant to prescribe it in preference to sodium salicylate, a drug they at least knew. Hoffmann's employer, Friedrich Bayer & Company, gave ASA the now-familiar name aspirin, but in 1897 Bayer didn't think aspirin had much of a future. It could not have foreseen that almost a century after its development aspirin would be the focus of extensive laboratory research and some of the largest clinical trials ever carried out in conditions ranging from cardiovascular disease and cancer to migraine headache and high blood pressure in pregnancy.

How Does It Work?

The mushrooming interest in aspirin has come about largely because of fairly recent advances in understanding how it works. What is it about this drug that, at small doses, interferes with blood clotting, at somewhat higher doses reduces fever and eases minor aches and pains, and at comparatively large doses combats pain and inflammation in rheumatoid arthritis and several other related diseases?

The answer is not yet fully known, but most authorities agree that aspirin achieves some of its effects by inhibiting the production of prostaglandins. Prostaglandins are hormone-like substances that influence the elasticity of blood vessels, control uterine contractions, direct the functioning of blood platelets that help stop bleeding, and regulate numerous other activities in the body.

In the 1970s, a British pharmacologist, John Vane, Ph.D., noted that many forms of tissue injury were followed by the release of prostaglandins. In laboratory studies, he found that two groups of prostaglandins caused redness and fever, common signs of inflammation. Vane and his co-workers also showed that, by blocking the synthesis of prostaglandins, aspirin prevented blood platelets from aggregating, one of the initial steps in the formation of blood clots.

This explanation of how aspirin and other nonsteroidal anti-inflammatory drugs (NSAIDs) produce their intriguing array of effects prompted laboratory and clinical scientists to form and test new ideas about aspirin's possible value in treating or preventing conditions in which prostaglandins play a role. Interest quickly focused on learning whether aspirin might prevent the blood clots responsible for heart attacks.

A heart attack or myocardial infarction (MI) results from the blockage of blood flow not *through* the heart, but *to* heart muscle. Without an adequate blood supply, the affected area of muscle dies and the heart's pumping action is either impaired or stopped altogether.

The most common sequence of events leading to an MI begins with the gradual build-up of plaque (atherosclerosis) in the coronary arteries. Circulation through these narrowed arteries is restricted, often causing the chest pain known as angina pectoris.

An acute heart attack is believed to happen when a tear in plaque inside a narrowed coronary artery causes platelets to aggregate, forming a clot that blocks the flow of blood. About 1,250,000 persons suffer heart attacks each year in the United States, and some 500,000 of them die. Those who survive a first heart attack are at greatly increased risk of having another.

Could Aspirin Help?

To learn whether aspirin could be helpful in preventing or treating cardiovascular disease, scientists have carried out numerous large randomized controlled clinical trials. In these studies, similar groups of hundreds or thousands of people are randomly assigned to receive either aspirin or a placebo, an inactive, look-alike tablet. The participants—and in double-blind trials the investigators, as well—do not know who is taking aspirin and who is swallowing a placebo.

Over the last two decades, aspirin studies have been conducted in three kinds of individuals: persons with a history of coronary artery or cerebral vascular disease, patients in the immediate, acute phases of a heart attack, and healthy men with no indication of current or previous cardiovascular illness.

The results of studies of people with a history of coronary artery disease and those in the immediate phases of a heart attack have proven to be of tremendous importance in the prevention and treatment of cardiovascular disease. The studies showed that aspirin substantially reduces the risk of death and/or non-fatal heart attacks in patients with a previous MI or unstable angina pectoris, which often occurs before a heart attack.

On the basis of such studies, these uses for aspirin (unstable angina, acute MI, and survivors of an MI) are described in the professional labeling of aspirin products, information provided to physicians and other health professionals. Aspirin labeling intended for the general public does not discuss its use in arthritis or cardiovascular disease because treatment of these serious conditions—even with a common over-the-counter drug—has to be medically supervised. The consumer labeling contains a general warning about excessive or inappropriate use of aspirin, and specifically warns against using aspirin to treat children and teenagers who have chickenpox or the flu because of the risk of Reye syndrome, a rare but sometimes fatal condition.

Aspirin for Healthy People?

Once aspirin's benefits for patients with cardiovascular disease were established, scientists sought to learn whether regular aspirin use would prevent a first heart attack in healthy individuals. The findings regarding that critical question have thus far been equivocal. The major American study designed to find out if aspirin can prevent cardiovascular deaths in healthy individuals was a randomized, placebo-controlled trial involving just over 22,000 male physicians between 40 and 84 with no prior history of heart disease. Half took one 325-milligram aspirin tablet every other day, and half took a placebo.

The trial was halted early, after about four-and-a-half years, and the findings quickly made public in 1988 when investigators found that the group taking aspirin had a substantial reduction in the rate of fatal and non-fatal heart attacks compared with the placebo group. There was, however, no significant difference between the aspirin and placebo groups in number of strokes (aspirin-treated patients did slightly worse) or in overall deaths from cardiovascular disease.

A similar study in British male physicians with no previous heart disease found no significant effect nor even a favorable trend for aspirin on cardiovascular disease rates. The British study of 5,100 physicians, while considerably smaller than the American study, reported three-quarters as many vascular "events." FDA scientists believe the results of the two studies are inconsistent.

The U.S. Preventive Services Task Force, a panel of medical-scientific authorities in health promotion and disease prevention, is one of many groups looking at new information on the role of aspirin in cardiovascular disease. In its *Guide to Clinical Preventive Services*, issued in 1989, the task force recommended that low-dose aspirin therapy "should be considered for men aged 40 and over who are at significantly increased risk for myocardial infarction and who lack contraindications" to aspirin use. A revised *Guide*, scheduled for publication in the fall of 1994, is expected to include a slightly revised recommendation concerning aspirin and cardiovascular disease but no major change in advice to physicians about aspirin's possible role in preventing heart attacks.

Better understanding of aspirin's myriad effects in the body has led to clinical trials and other studies to assess a variety of possible uses: preventing the severity of migraine headaches, improving circulation to the gums thereby arresting periodontal disease, preventing certain types of cataracts, lowering the risk of recurrence of colorectal cancer, and controlling the dangerously high blood pressure (called preeclampsia) that occurs in 5 to 15 percent of pregnancies.

None of these uses for aspirin has been shown conclusively to be safe and effective, and there is concern that people may be misusing aspirin on the basis of unproven notions about its effectiveness. Last October, FDA proposed a new labeling statement for aspirin products advising consumers to consult a doctor before taking aspirin for new and long-term uses. The proposed statement would read, "IMPORTANT: See your doctor before taking this product for your heart or for other new uses of aspirin because serious side effects could occur with self treatment."

299

The Other Side of the Coin

While examining new possibilities for aspirin in disease treatment and prevention, scientists do not lose sight of the fact that even at low doses aspirin is not harmless. A small subset of the population is hypersensitive to aspirin and cannot tolerate even small amounts of the drug. Gastrointestinal distress—nausea, heartburn, pain—is a well-recognized adverse effect and is related to dosage. Persons being treated for rheumatoid arthritis who take large daily doses of aspirin are especially likely to experience gastrointestinal side effects.

Aspirin's antiplatelet activity apparently accounts for hemorrhagic strokes, caused by bleeding into the brain, in a small but significant percentage of persons who use the drug regularly. For the great majority of occasional aspirin users, internal bleeding is not a problem. But aspirin may be unsuitable for people with uncontrolled high blood pressure, liver or kidney disease, peptic ulcer, or other conditions that might increase the risk of cerebral hemorrhage or other internal bleeding.

New understanding of how aspirin works and what it can do leaves no doubt that the drug has a far broader range of uses than Felix Hoffmann and his colleagues imagined. The jury is still out, however, on a number of key questions about the best and safest ways to use aspirin. And until some critical verdicts are handed down, consumers are well-advised to regard aspirin with appropriate caution.

—by Ken Flieger

Ken Flieger is a writer in Washington, D.C.

Chapter 32

Questions and Answers about Chelation Therapy

Over the past twenty years people suffering from a type of hardening of the arteries called atherosclerosis have been hearing about a "miracle cure" called chelation (pronounced "kee-lay-shun") therapy. But they may not know that the American Heart Association and other medical and scientific groups have spoken out against this form of treatment.

Chelation therapy is the administration of a man-made amino acid called EDTA into the veins. (EDTA is an abbreviation for ethylendiamine tetraacetic acid. It's marketed under several names, including Edetate Disodium, Endrate and Sodium Versenate.) EDTA is most often used in cases of heavy metal poisoning (lead or mercury), because it's able to latch onto or bind these metals, creating a compound that can be excreted in the urine.

Besides binding heavy metals, EDTA also chelates (naturally seeks out and binds) calcium, one of the components of atherosclerotic plaque. In the early 1960s, this led to speculation that EDTA could be used to remove calcium deposits from atherosclerotic plaque. The idea was that once the calcium was removed by regular treatments of EDTA, the remaining elements in the atherosclerotic plaque would break up and the plaque would clear away. The narrowed arteries would be restored to their former state.

Excerpts from American Heart Association Pub. No. 50-074-A (CP). Used by Permission.

Based upon this thinking, chelation therapy has been proposed both as a treatment for existing atherosclerosis and to prevent athero- sclerosis from forming in the future.

After carefully reviewing all of the available scientific literature on this subject, the American Heart Association has concluded that the benefits claimed for this form of therapy aren't scientifically proven. That's why the AHA doesn't recommend this type of treat- ment.

Supporters of chelation therapy rely on personal testimonies of people who have used the therapy. And there are many people who claim that because they underwent chelation therapy their lives were saved, their health was improved or their circulation was restored to their arms and legs.

The American Heart Association can't say why some people feel better after undergoing chelation therapy. And the AHA doesn't deny that some people actually may feel better after treatment. So what's the problem?

The problem is that the AHA questions whether these patients feel better because of chelation therapy. It's possible that patients feel better, not because of chelation therapy, but because of something else.

For example, chelation therapists usually require their patients to make changes in their lifestyles. These changes can include quitting smoking, losing weight, eating more fruit and vegetables, avoiding foods high in saturated fats and exercising regularly. These are healthy changes for anyone to make, and patients make them at the same time that they're undergoing chelation therapy. That's what clouds the issue, because these *lifestyle changes* have been shown to improve the quality of life and improve patients' sense of well-being. In fact, the AHA has advocated these lifestyle changes for many years.

The American Heart Association believes that these lifestyle changes (also called risk factor modifications) are probably why the condition of some patients improves. The AHA believes that patients don't feel better because of chelation therapy with EDTA, but because of better, healthier habits that they adopt.

There's another reason why some patients may feel better after undergoing treatment. That reason is psychological. Many physicians are familiar with symptoms in a diseased person disappearing for no apparent reason, due to a placebo effect. This could be a another rea- son why some patients report that they feel better after they've spent $3,000 to $5,000 for chelation therapy.

Part Five

Cardiovascular Surgical Interventions

Chapter 33

Cardiovascular Spare Parts

The human cardiovascular system is highly efficient, yet enormously complex. A thousand times each day, the muscular heart pumps five quarts of blood through the arteries, to the smaller arterioles and finally the microscopic capillaries, and then through ever larger venules and veins, back to the heart.

The journey of blood through the capillaries alone covers more than 60,000 miles! In such an intricate and interconnected system, it's easy to see how a single glitch can profoundly affect health.

Medical researchers have devised some ingenious ways to replace malfunctioning cardiovascular parts. Substitute heart valves have been in use for three decades, and replacement blood, blood vessels, and even a heart are being developed.

Many of these inventions are carefully crafted combinations of synthetic materials and biological substances, designed to hopefully equal nature, yet at the same time mimic the body closely enough so that the immune system does not reject the new part. Plus, these products must present a smooth surface for blood to flow over. Even the tiniest uneven surface can rupture a passing platelet, triggering the chemical cascade of clotting that can obstruct blood flow to a vital organ.

FDA Consumer, May 1990; September 1990; March 1991; June 1992; October 1994.

Red Blood Cell Substitutes

Blood is a complex mixture of red cells, white cells, and platelets, suspended in a watery, protein-rich plasma. Because these components must be present in specific proportions, duplicating nature's recipe is a daunting task. But the rise in blood-borne infections, such as hepatitis and AIDS, has made the idea of a blood substitute quite appealing. The next best thing, many researchers think, is a substance that can do the work of red blood cells in transporting and delivering oxygen to the body's tissues and removing wastes. The hemoglobin protein in red blood cells normally carries out this function.

A safe and effective red cell substitute must meet strict criteria. "It must be absolutely disease-free, have a long storage life, and it must do the job for an extended period of time," says Joseph Stocks, M.D., a blood banking expert at the Maine Medical Center in Portland.

Several types of chemicals can carry oxygen. In 1965, Leland Clark, Ph.D., at the University of Cincinnati, showed that some chemicals soak up so much oxygen they could supply the vital gas to an animal immersed in it. He put a mouse in a beaker filled with silicone oil. The animal's lungs quickly filled and it sank—but kept breathing! Silicone oil proved too toxic, so Clark next worked with perfluorochemicals (PFCs), organic compounds containing the element fluorine.

Clinical trials with PFCs began in 1978, and the first red cell replacement using these chemicals was approved by the Food and Drug Administration in January 1990. The product, Fluosol, is a mixture of two PFCs, a mild detergent, and lipid molecules from egg yolk. Its use is very restricted.

"Fluosol was approved as an oxygen-carrying drug in limited amounts, to be used during balloon angioplasty in the coronary arteries," explains Joseph Fratantoni, M.D., of FDA's Center for Biologics Evaluation and Research.

With balloon angioplasty, an inflated balloon is used to press plaque against artery walls, opening up the blocked vessel. Blood flow to the neighboring area is temporarily impeded during the procedure, which may cause chest pain and change in heart muscle function. But Fluosol, infused through a narrow tube in the balloon, keeps the area oxygenated.

Previous attempts to deliver blood through the balloon failed because a very small tube must be used, and the red cells are too large to squeeze through. But a Fluosol particle is only 1/900th the volume of a red blood cell, and the preparation is half as thick as blood. With the protective effect of Fluosol, it may be possible to extend the angioplasty technique to more patients.

Fluosol may have other applications. Clinical trials are under way to examine its use following administration of "clot-busting" drugs such as streptokinase and tissue-plasminogen activator. After a clot is dissolved, the rush of blood through the opened region can damage tissue. Fluosol may stem this tide by allowing a steadier trickle of fluid past as the clot breaks apart. It may also help to save heart muscle normally deprived of oxygen during a heart attack and to oxygenate donated organs awaiting transplant.

An obvious red cell substitute is the hemoglobin molecule itself, which would probably not trigger an immune reaction if freed from the red blood cells that normally contain it. (Such an immune reaction can occur if a mismatched blood transfusion, containing cells from incompatible blood types, is given.)

There would be no compatibility problem with freed hemoglobin, but it could carry disease, unless purified. Researchers at Somatogen Inc. in Broomfield, Colo., have circumvented these problems by mass-producing human hemoglobin in genetically engineered bacteria and yeast, providing a pure and abundant source of the molecule, much as human insulin is supplied to diabetics.

But use of single hemoglobin molecules outside of their red cell carriers presents several problems. The molecules are broken in two in the body, and can then squeeze through the one-cell-thick walls of the capillaries and easily enter the kidney tubules to be excreted before delivering oxygen where it's needed. In addition, without co-factors contained in the red cell, hemoglobin cannot efficiently bind oxygen delivered by the lungs, and also loses antioxidant biochemicals that normally protect surrounding cells from damage by too much oxygen.

Fortunately, clever chemists have already overcome these technological hurdles. They link individual hemoglobin molecules together, or chemically augment them. This provides the bulk the molecules need to stay in circulation. The molecule can even be further modified so that it not only binds and transports oxygen, but relinquishes it easily to oxygen-depleted tissues.

Several companies are applying these chemical manipulations to human hemoglobin derived from donated blood, starting with a "crosslinking" technique developed by Quest Blood Substitute, Inc., in Detroit. Werner Wahl, Ph.D., vice president for science and technology at Quest, explains: "When you crosslink hemoglobin molecules, you add a chemical reagent to tie two or more of them together. There are lots of kinds of chemicals you can use, but some are better than others. Exactly how you crosslink determines the characteristics of the hemoglobin."

Each company then introduces its own chemical modifications. One substitute, for example, follows crosslinking with a special pasteurization process to eliminate viral contaminants.

A compromise between a free, "naked" hemoglobin molecule and nature's red cell packaging is to enclose hemoglobin in a fatty bubble called a liposome, forming a structure called a "neohemocyte." Biologically, this makes sense. "Evolution spent an awful lot of time and energy wrapping hemoglobin in a membrane. So, maybe it isn't surprising that when you unwrap the package, there is trouble," says Fratantoni.

At the University of California at San Francisco, pharmaceutical chemist C. Anthony Hunt, Ph.D., is wrapping hemoglobin in the same type of capsules used to enclose ink in "carbonless carbon" paper and scents in "scratch 'n sniff" papers. But so far in animal studies, the immune system rapidly seeks and destroys these neohemocytes.

Brave New Blood Vessels

Delivery of blood through open vessels is crucial to cardiovascular function. Block a vessel with plaque or a clot, and blood flow backs up, robbing nearby tissues of vital oxygen. Blood can only flow through a smooth conduit. So far, none of the several methods to unclog or replace blocked arteries keeps them smooth indefinitely. Plaque that is scraped away or pressed against the artery wall recurs. A transplanted blood vessel may provoke the recipient's immune system to reject it, and taking a vessel from the patient's own body involves surgery at two sites rather than just one.

Synthetic blood vessels cause problems too. "There is a great need for a living artery equivalent that has the properties of an actual artery," says Eugene Bell, Ph.D., chief scientific officer of Organogenesis, Inc., in Cambridge, Massachusetts. "No small-caliber, synthetic vascular graft presently exists that will remain unplugged by blood clots."

That company's "living blood vessel equivalent," now being tested in animals, is a flexible yet strong tubule mimicking the triple-decker structure of real blood vessels. It is built of an inner layer of tile-like cells (called endothelium), a middle layer of smooth muscle, and an outer layer of connective tissue. The cells, which come from human cadaver arteries, are grown in the laboratory and then molded into the tubules. A very important step is the removal of molecules on the cells that are most likely to trigger an immune attack. A woven-in Dacron mesh lends strength to the tubules.

The blood vessel equivalent can be made in any length or width, and can tolerate the pressure exerted by blood hurtling through the circulatory system. The vessel replacements can be stitched to their natural counterparts so seamlessly that blood clots are not likely to form. Bell foresees eventual use of the living blood vessel equivalent in cardiac bypass surgery, and in replacing damaged arteries in the brain and legs.

Another possible blood vessel replacement is Dacron vessels coated with the patient's own endothelial cells. Because the body recognizes these cells as "self," it does not reject the replacement vessel. By adding certain growth factors, the cells are coaxed to knit a one-cell-thick endothelial lining on the interior of the Dacron tubules smooth enough to prevent clotting. In cell culture experiments conducted by Stuart Williams, Ph.D., and co-workers at Jefferson Medical College in Philadelphia, the lining began to form immediately.

Valves

Heart valves are flaps of tissue embedded in thin sheets of connective tissue. Located at strategic points in the heart, the valves keep blood flowing in one direction. About seven different types of artificial valves are approved for use by FDA. Some are similar to the first device, which resembled a ball in a cage. It was implanted in a 52-year-old man in 1961 by Albert Starr, M.D., and M.L. Edwards, M.D.

"It's hard to beat the original Starr-Edwards model," says John Watson, chief of the devices and technology branch of the National Heart, Lung, and Blood Institute. "Claude Pepper was one of the original people in Congress who helped form the institute, and he subsequently received a Starr-Edwards valve. He lived for 20 years and died from something unrelated. The fundamental design has been refined in terms of surgical technique and clinical management, but really there have been no significant breakthroughs."

But opinion varies. Says William Letsing, M.D., of FDA's Office of Device Evaluation, "The Starr-Edwards is a 1960s type valve. Many newer models, such as the St. Jude, have much better hemodynamics and a higher state of technology."

When natural heart valves do not close properly, are abnormally thick, or are damaged by rheumatic endocarditis (a complication of rheumatic fever that can also sometimes follow strep throat), replacement valves are lifesaving. After open-heart surgery became possible in the 1950s, surgeons first tried to treat valve disease by scraping away the calcium deposits causing the problem. But it was clear that replacing, rather than repairing, the valve would be more effective. Today mechanical prosthetic heart valves are built of a ceramic and a metal (such as titanium). Pig valves and cow pericardium (outer heart muscle) are also fashioned into valves that are mounted on synthetic bases called stents.

About 75,000 people receive replacement heart valves in the United States each year. Mechanical models are generally used for those under 65 because of superior long-term durability, and for children, who tend to deposit calcium on biological valves. Older patients are usually given animal models that do not last as long because they are less likely to calcify or be blocked by clots and may not require replacement. Many patients with mechanical replacement valves must take anti-clotting drugs because they otherwise would have a considerably increased risk of a dangerous clot forming.

But even a medical device as successful as heart valves can be improved. Charles Peskin, Ph.D., a mathematician at New York University, uses computer modeling to design better valves. Depicting the heart and its circulation in three dimensions, he alters the curvatures of the discs and angles of the pivot points so that the smoothest possible blood flow is achieved.

"We think of clotting purely as a chemical process, but it also depends on fluid mechanics," Peskin says."If the blood stagnates in a pool, a clot will form. We're trying to design a valve so there will be no regions of stagnation." One of Peskin's heart valve designs is being patented, but his device is still a long way from an FDA application.

The Artificial Heart

In the 1980s, four men lived for varying amounts of time with artificial hearts. But problems were rampant. The plastic, metal and Velcro of the heart attracted bacteria to areas inaccessible to many antibiotics. The device also caused blood clots, triggering strokes.

As a result, life for the "permanent" artificial heart recipient was difficult. Recipient William Schroeder, for example, suffered from strokes, seizures, fever, and depression on many of his record-setting 620 days with the Jarvik-7 device, which was then used predominantly as a short term "bridge to transplant." But even this temporary use was halted in January 1990.

The attachment of the Jarvik device to the bulky exterior equipment is thought to be a route of infection. So many scientists hope a fully implantable, electrically driven artificial heart can be developed. Other artificial hearts are under development at the University of Arizona in Phoenix, the University of Utah in Salt Lake City, Pennsylvania State University in Hershey with 3M Corp., the Cleveland Clinic Foundation with Nimbus, Inc., Temple University in Philadelphia with Abiomed, Inc., the Minneapolis Heart Institute, and the Texas Heart Institute in Houston.

Ventricular Assist Devices

A currently more fruitful area of research is the electrically powered implantable ventricular assist device, a pump used to support the patient's left ventricle, the chamber that must work most vigorously to send blood throughout the body. The 1970s and 1980s saw a variety of experimental left ventricular assists, all tethered to outside support equipment. Used as a bridge to transplant, the device is promising.

In a study reported by R. Gaykowski, L. Barker, and W. Yates at the 34th annual meeting of the American Society for Artificial Internal Organs, 92 heart patients received Jarvik-7 devices while awaiting a heart transplant. Of these 92, 63 received donor hearts, and 35 of these survived, a survival rate after transplant of 56 percent. In a similar evaluation of patients using the ventricular assist to sustain them until a donor heart became available, survival after transplant was 82 percent.

The difference in performance between the two devices may be anatomical location or technology complexity. "The technology for both devices is similar. But control of the total artificial heart is more difficult, because there are both left and right ventricles that must be integrated," says the National Heart, Lung, and Blood Institute's Watson.

One type of totally implantable ventricular assist device is a blood pump about the size of a softball, inserted beneath the heart in the muscles of the abdomen. Blood from the left ventricle is diverted to the pump, which then sends it to the aorta, the largest artery in the body. The pump senses when to boost the blood by way of an electrically driven control unit that monitors the cardiac cycle.

The control unit, about the size of a deck of cards, is also implanted in muscle. The miniature electrical engine and rechargeable battery are charged from the outside by a coil and battery pack worn by the patient. The external coil is coupled to a second coil implanted under the skin of the abdomen.

"We expect to begin implanting the device in people for clinical study in the fall of 1991. We are now in the process of fabricating the systems, selecting clinical centers, and developing protocols that will require an IDE [investigational device exemption] from the FDA," says Watson.

Many cultures have regarded the heart as the center of a person's being. In the coming century, scientists hope to beat heart disease by a prudent combination of prevention and an arsenal of cardiovascular spare parts.

—by Ricki Lewis, Ph.D.

Ricki Lewis has a Ph.D. in genetics and teaches biology at the State University of New York at Albany.

Shiley C-C Heart Valve Alert (9/90)

People with Bjork-Shiley 60° C-C (Convexo-Concave) heart valves and those in their households should be aware of the symptoms of valve failure, according to a letter Shiley Inc. sent last March to physicians and emergency room workers.

The letter was based on a report in the May 1988 *Journal of the American College of Cardiology* by Loren Hiratzka, M.D., and others— an independent panel Shiley had convened to evaluate its C-C valves. As a result of strut fractures, Shiley took its larger C-C valves off the market in October 1985 and withdrew the smaller sizes in November 1986. (See "Shiley Ends Sale of Heart Valve" in the Updates section of the February 1987 *FDA Consumer.*)

Although strut fractures are quite rare, they can occur without warning and are life-threatening. Patients may notice a change or absence of valve sound. Signs and symptoms may be similar to those of congestive heart failure, heart attack, and other cardiac conditions: shock, low blood pressure, sudden and rapidly progressive breathing difficulty due to severe fluid accumulation in the lungs, chest pain, irregular heartbeat, and impaired or loss of consciousness.

Patients and household members should know which hospitals can perform emergency valve replacement. Patients are advised to carry their implant card in wallet or purse and to wear a medical alert bracelet or similar article containing implant information.

Shiley told physicians that chest x-rays can help diagnose problems but that echocardiography or fluoroscopy may also be needed. A malfunctioning valve should be immediately replaced. However, removal of a valve in the absence of signs of malfunction is not advised because the risk posed by replacement surgery is far greater than the risk of strut fracture. According to the letter, the annual risk of fracture ranges from about 2 valves per 10,000 to about 29 per 10,000, depending on the size and date of manufacture. The risk of death from elective reoperation is likely greater than 5 out of 100.

Shiley Heart Valve Notification (3/91)

People who have a certain type of artificial heart valve manufactured by Shiley Inc. are being notified about rare, but often fatal, valve fractures under a plan that has been developed by the device's Irvine, Calif., manufacturer and accepted by FDA.

Under the plan, the nonprofit foundation Medic Alert is asking all heart specialists in the United States and Canada for the names of patients implanted with the Bjork-Shiley 60-degree convexo-concave heart valve ("C-C" valve). Hospital administrators are also being asked to search their records to locate C-C valve patients. (A plan to notify foreign governments about the U.S. program is also being developed.)

Medic Alert will then send an information kit about the C-C valve, along with a letter addressed to each patient, to the patient's doctor.

"When one of these valves fractures, the patient's life can sometimes be saved if the valve is replaced quickly," says FDA Deputy Commissioner James S. Benson. "That's why it is important for C-C valve patients to ask their doctors how to recognize early signs of valve fracture and what to do should it occur.

"We hope that the Shiley program will encourage this dialogue between implant patients and physicians, and we will be closely monitoring it to be sure people are being reached with the information they need."

Replacing an intact valve is generally not recommended, because the surgical risk far outweighs the risk of fracture.

In addition to the information kit, the Shiley plan includes an international implant registry operated by Medic Alert. Once enrolled, patients will receive an ID card and a bracelet or neck chain that indicates the wearer has a C-C valve and provides special information for emergency medical personnel.

About 82,000 people worldwide—23,000 in the United States and Canada—have a C-C valve. FDA has been notified of 313 fractures, 204 of which were fatal.

New Risk Information On One Heart Valve (6/92)

The risk of fracture for certain types of Bjork-Shiley convexo-concave (C-C) heart valves may be up to four times higher than previously estimated for some patients. Valve fracture is often fatal.

FDA has asked the manufacturer, Shiley Inc., of Irvine, Calif., to notify patients and physicians of the new estimates based on a study reported in the Feb. 1 issue of *The Lancet*.

"It is important to remember that this new risk information applies only to Shiley C-C valves, not to other makes and models," said James Benson, director of FDA's Center for Devices and Radiological Health. "Even with the C-C valves, the increased fracture risk is confined to the large size valves, and only those that are implanted in the mitral position. The risk figures have not appreciably changed for C-C valve patients who have the smaller size valves or who have their valves in the aortic position." About 6,000 patients in the United States have the larger valves (29 millimeters or greater). These patients should talk to their doctors about what the new risk numbers mean for them. This is especially true for the subgroup at greatest risk: patients with larger valves welded between Feb. 1, 1981, and June 30,1982, which were implanted in the heart's mitral position. Their fracture rate may be as high as 1 percent.

According to the study reported in *The Lancet*, patients in this group who were under the age of 50 when their valves were implanted may be at higher risk than those who were over 50.

FDA believes the risk over an eight-year period may be high enough for some of these individuals that they and their doctors may want to consider replacing intact valves. The agency recommended that physicians and patients make the decision to replace a valve on a case by case basis, depending on the new fracture figures and the patient's medical status, lifestyle, and wishes.

FDA asked Shiley to send letters to patients with all sizes of C-C heart valves informing them of the risk of fracture. FDA also asked Shiley to send letters to physicians providing detailed risk information, discussing the option of valve replacement, and enclosing a copy of the report in *The Lancet*.

Shiley withdrew its 60-degree C-C valves from the market in 1986, but some 23,000 patients in the United States and Canada had valves implanted before the withdrawal. FDA has received about 350 reports of 60-degree valve fractures among the roughly 82,000 C-C valves implanted worldwide.

In a program begun in 1990, FDA asked Shiley to notify implanted patients of the fracture problems. At that time, replacement of intact valves was not recommended because the surgical risk was thought to far outweigh the fracture risk.

Shiley Agrees to Pay Government Millions (10/94)

Shiley, Inc., a subsidiary of Pfizer, Inc., will pay the United States as much as $20 million as a result of making false statements to FDA. Shiley made the statements to get a mechanical heart valve the company knew was subject to life-threatening fracture approved by FDA and to keep it on the market. The Department of Justice and FDA announced the settlement last June 30. The valve is the Bjork-Shiley 60-degree Convexo-Concave (C-C) heart valve.

The firm agreed to pay $10.75 million in fines and reimbursement to the government for payments made for Shiley heart valves. Shiley will also pay possibly millions more for medical costs the government has incurred since January 1992, as stated in the agreement, or would otherwise incur in the future through Medicare, Medicaid, CHAMPUS, federal hospitals, or other government programs due to fracture or elective replacement of the valve. The agreement, made under the False Claims Act, settles the government's claims against Shiley. (Shiley earlier agreed in a class-action lawsuit to reimburse patients not covered by government programs for surgical replacement and damages. Other patients filed separate actions.)

The settlement should not affect decisions about whether individual patients should have their valves replaced. Patients should consult their doctors to decide their best course of action.

Shiley first marketed the C-C valve in 1979, but withdrew it from the market in 1985 and 1986 after FDA took steps to withdraw the approval. Of an estimated 31,368 implanted in the United States, 196 have fractured. On average, two of every three fractures are fatal.

The government says that Shiley:

- falsely asserted the C-C valve caused fewer blood-clotting complications than other models

- falsely asserted a series of manufacturing changes had corrected a serious design defect

- did not provide FDA with all the data it had concerning fractures during laboratory testing

- argued—to keep marketing the valve after the fracture problem became evident—that the fracture risk was outweighed by the purported blood-clotting advantage, which did not prove to be as significant as represented to FDA

- rebuilt scrap valves

- rewelded valves an excessive number of times

- polished, rather than rewelded, cracked valve struts

- falsified employee identification numbers on cards attached to bags of reworked valves, including more than 3,000 "baggie cards" with inaccurate identification numbers.

(See "Shiley Saga Leads to Improved Communication" in the January-February 1994 *FDA Consumer*.)

Chapter 34

Using Smart Lasers to Unclog Arteries

A laser microsurgery system that identifies fatty deposits and re-opens clogged arteries promises to alleviate some of the risks associated with current treatments for atherosclerosis, according to researchers at the Massachusetts Institute of Technology in Cambridge and the Cleveland Clinic Foundation in Cleveland, Ohio. Called LAS II (for Laser Angiosurgery System II), the system is unique in that a single catheter is used for both diagnosis and treatment, and computer control of the cutting lasers protects against accidental removal of healthy tissue, says Dr. Michael S. Feld, professor of physics and director of the MIT George R. Harrison Spectroscopy Laboratory. LAS II is now being used in a clinical trial to unblock the coronary arteries of 10 patients at the Cleveland Clinic.

Artery disease is the leading cause of death and disability in the United States, says Dr. Feld, and a common manifestation involves the accumulation of calcified fatty deposits known as atherosclerotic plaques, which can obstruct blood flow and thus lead to stroke or heart attack. Today one of the most widely used and inexpensive methods for unblocking arteries is balloon angioplasty, in which a narrow balloon is inserted into the clogged region and inflated, opening the passage by pushing the plaque against the vessel walls. This treatment, however, traumatizes the artery by abrading and distending it. Trauma is a recognized cause of restenosis, or recurrence of blockage,

---

NCRR Reporter, October 1991.

he says. "In developing LAS II, our overall goal was to find a less traumatic way to remove plaque and thereby avoid the high rate of restenosis associated with balloon angioplasty."

The cornerstone of the LAS II system is the concept that diagnosis guides treatment, says Dr. Feld. A catheter containing 12 optical fibers each approximately as thick as a human hair—is inserted into a clogged artery, and the rounded tip is pressed against the plaque.

The system uses laser-induced fluorescence spectroscopy to determine which parts of the tip are touching plaque and which parts are in contact with normal tissue. Higher energy ablation, or cutting, lasers are then fired over the optical fibers in contact with the plaque to remove a thin layer of it, leaving the healthy vessel intact. As the catheter gradually advances through the artery, the diagnosis/ablation sequence is repeated until the entire plaque is removed.

The LAS II system integrates four separate lines of research: catheter design, spectroscopy, ablation, and computer control. For nearly a decade Dr. Feld and his colleagues have worked toward reducing arterial trauma by improving catheter design and choosing the best lasers for diagnosis and tissue removal. (For more information on medical uses of lasers see the *Research Resources Reporter*, April 1991, January 1991, May 1988, and October 1987.)

"Our first objective in developing the system was to have nontraumatic delivery of light. To achieve that we developed the concept of multiple fibers in the catheter," says Dr. Feld. The 12 quartz fibers are arranged in the catheter such that the light they emit overlaps and covers the entire face of the optical shield, a rounded transparent structure at the tip. The optical shield is about the size of the head of a pin and has the same diameter as the catheter, 1.6 mm.

Although other laser ablation systems may use multiple fibers, the distribution of laser light is uneven, producing what Dr. Feld calls a "Swiss cheese" effect. "Other systems may remove only about 20 percent of the blockage, which means that 80 percent of the plaque is left in place, and the catheter has to push through it. This is a significant source of trauma," he says. "In contrast, LAS II removes plaque over the entire face of the shield, so the catheter is not pushed through partly clogged arteries."

The key to uniformly removing diseased tissue is the computer-controlled feedback loop, says Dr. Richard P. Rava, a principal research scientist at the George R. Harrison Spectroscopy Laboratory. Using the diagnostic laser, the computer identifies the fibers that are abutting plaque and subsequently instructs those fibers to fire varying doses of ablation laser light.

"The diagnostic laser, a small nitrogen-dye laser, emits a blue light with a wavelength of 480 nm. The diagnostic light is fired down each fiber one at a time," says Dr. Rava. As a result, the tissue at the catheter tip fluoresces, and the signals are retrieved by each fiber and analyzed by the computer.

"We tested almost all of the wavelengths of light from 250 to 550 nm for their diagnostic usefulness, and a few different regions were particularly sensitive to atherosclerosis," says Dr. Rava.

The 480 nm wavelength was chosen in part because the blue light penetrates 300-400 micrometers into the tissue, whereas the ablation light removes only 100-150 micrometers of plaque. "The device always 'sees' more than it is about to ablate, which is another safety precaution that helps to prevent accidental removal of healthy artery," adds Dr. Rava.

A second reason for choosing 480 nm, Dr. Rava says, is that this wavelength allows the spectrograph to distinguish three types of material important to atherosclerosis: structural proteins, ceroid, and hemoglobin.

"When an atherosclerotic plaque is growing, the structural protein collagen accumulates in the top layer of the tissue, which our spectroscopy can detect. As the disease progresses, the body begins to break down some of the lipids and fats into a highly fluorescent material called ceroid, which the artery can't get rid of," says Dr. Rava. "As the ceroid content rises, the plaque becomes more extensive and the artery more diseased."

Based on the proportions of ceroid and structural proteins at each fiber tip, the computer categorizes the 12 overlapping regions as "normal," "soft plaque," or "calcified plaque" and the results are displayed on a computer touch screen.

Once the diagnosis is complete, the computer initiates the ablation sequence. "The computer does a statistical analysis to determine the probability that the tissue in front of each fiber is plaque. If the probability is greater than 70 percent, and if at least three contiguous fibers all give the same information, then the computer instructs the ablation lasers to fire down those fibers," says Dr. John R. Kramer, a staff cardiologist who is overseeing the clinical aspects of the LAS II research at the Cleveland Clinic. Ablation light is never fired down only one fiber.

"In practice, the countercheck is that the surgeon and the computer operator can see the diagnostic information on the computer touch screen in front of them," he says. "If either person finds fault with the diagnosis he can release a foot pedal, which interrupts the ablation sequence."

Several factors were considered in choosing the appropriate wavelength for ablation, says Dr. Feld. The ideal wavelength, he says, would not only cleanly remove calcified and fibrous tissue but also be nonmutagenic, have a short penetration depth, and be able to be conducted through optical fibers. "Our studies showed that wavelengths shorter than about 400 nm—in the ultraviolet range—were acceptable for removing tissue. The commonly used XeCl (xenon chloride) excimer laser, which emits light at 308 nm, seemed perfect, but we were concerned with the fact that that wavelength is known to be mutagenic," he says.

The investigators therefore decided to use 355 nm ablation light from a modified Nd:YAG (neodymium yttrium aluminum garnet) laser, which is the most commonly used laser source for medical applications, says Dr. Feld. At this wavelength possible mutagenic effects of radiation are avoided.

One snag with this selection, however, was that the light pulses produced by commercially available Nd:YAG lasers are too brief to be carried over optical fibers at the desired energies. Such high-energy, short pulses could destroy the fibers. "To overcome this obstacle, we developed a technique for 'stretching' the pulses," says Dr. Feld. Using two Nd:YAG lasers, the researchers were able to manipulate and tailor the light pulses, stretching their duration from 10 ns to 200 ns, which allowed the light to be carried through the optical fibers with enough energy to remove tissue.

In the clinical trial, which began in May, LAS II is being used to remove plaques from the coronary arteries of patients who undergo bypass surgery. Coronary bypass involves grafting a blood vessel, usually from the leg, to the vessels surrounding the heart, thereby bypassing a blockage and reestablishing blood flow. LAS II will be used to treat either the bypassed blockage or another nearby plaque that might compromise the graft, says Dr. Kramer. He is now in the process of selecting patients for the procedure.

Although the catheter is designed for percutaneous (through the skin) application, usually performed by inserting the catheter through a vein in the thigh, in the clinical trial LAS II will be used during bypass surgery. "When done percutaneously, however, we envision that the LAS II procedure could one day be done in the catheterization laboratory as quickly as a balloon angioplasty," says Dr. Robert M. Cothren, a project scientist at the Cleveland Clinic who has collaborated with Dr. Feld for 8 years. Dr. Cothren will operate the computer during most of the clinical trial.

"The amount of time that the ablation lasers are actually on is very short for a relatively small lesion, but the system only fires when the catheter tip is in good contact with the lesion. Establishing and maintaining good contact may be the most time-consuming part," he says.

Medical followup will include taking an angiograph, or x-ray image, of the treated area after 6 months, says Dr. Cothren. "We chose a 6-month time frame because that is when problems often begin following balloon angioplasty."

Meanwhile, the researchers are evaluating ways to further improve their "smart" laser system. "The diagnostics will become much more sophisticated in the future," says Dr. Kramer. "Instead of retrieving only three pieces of chemical information—information about structural proteins, ceroid, and hemoglobin—we may one day gather information about as many as 100 body chemicals using infrared Raman spectroscopy, and the computer will have a lot more to analyze."

Raman spectra can detect many of the molecular substances that result from atherosclerosis, says Dr. Rava, including calcifications, cholesterol, cholesterol esters, fatty acids, collagen, and elastin. "Each compound can be detected individually and fairly easily," he says. The drawback, however, is that with current technology, retrieving a high-quality Raman signal may take as long as 20 to 30 minutes, whereas the fluorescence spectroscopy now used in the LAS II system is done with one 10-nanosecond pulse, he says. The researchers are now considering ways to reduce the time needed for Raman analysis.

"Obviously, balloon angioplasty is a much simpler and much less expensive technique than the LAS II procedure, but if we can offer the patient a better long-term solution by reducing the incidence of restenosis, then LAS II offers a real advantage," says Dr. Cothren.

—*by Victoria L. Contie*

Additional reading:

1. Albagli, D., Cothren, R., Jr., Dasari, R. R., et al., LAS II: An integrated system for spectral diagnosis, guidance, and ablation in laser angiosurgery. In *Future Directions in Interventional Cardiology, II* (Vogel, J. H. K., ed.). Chicago, Illinois: C. V. Mosby, in press.

2. Sacks, B. A., Feld, M. S., and Greenfield, A. J., Laser angiosurgery. In *Peripheral Vascular Imaging and Intervention* (Kim, D. and Orron, D., eds.). Chicago, Illinois: C. V. Mosby, in press.

3. Richards-Kortum, R., Mehta, A.,Hayes, G., et al. Spectral diagnosis of atherosclerosis using an optical fiber laser catheter. *Progress in Cardiology* 118:381-391, 1989.

The research described in this article was supported by the Biomedical Research Technology Program of the National Center for Research Resources, the Cleveland Clinic Foundation, and G. V. Medical, Inc.

Chapter 35

Coronary Artery Bypass Graft Surgery

What is Coronary Artery Bypass Graft Surgery?

Bypass surgery is an operation in which a section of vein, usually the saphena vein from the leg, is removed and sewn onto the aorta, the large artery leaving the heart. The other end of the vein is then attached to a branch of the coronary artery. In effect, this procedure detours the blood around the damaged or blocked areas of the coronary arteries so that the blood flow to the heart is increased.

[Leg veins are the most commonly used veins for bypass surgery, although other veins may also be used. The reason leg veins are preferred is that they are longer than many other veins and can be taken without having a negative impact on circulation. In addition, leg veins are usually less affected by atherosclerosis.]

What Will Bypass Surgery Accomplish?

The purpose of bypass surgery is to improve the flow of blood to the heart muscle. And a greater blood flow to the heart can mean fewer episodes of chest pain (angina) or no episodes at all. Second, it can reduce your need for medication and improve your capacity for exercise. While the operation may not prolong your life, it should improve the quality of your life.

Excerpts from American Heart Association Pub. No. 50-047-B (CP). Used by Permission. Editor's comments are bracketed.

What about Hospital Admission?

Admission to the hospital is usually scheduled for two or three days before your operation. This allows time for pre-operative testing. This time is also when you will be given instructions about clearing your lungs of mucus, different coughing techniques and deep breathing exercises.

Is It Common to Be Frightened or Nervous Before the Operation?

It's perfectly normal to be a little nervous before any operation. You can reduce your nervousness by understanding why you need the operation, by meeting members of the team of physicians who will be caring for you, and by asking questions to clear up your doubts. Sometimes a mild sedative can help you relax, too.

What Happens the Day Before Surgery?

The day before your operation, the surgical staff will visit you to discuss the details of your surgery and to answer any questions you have. The anesthesiologist will make an evaluation, and will tell you how he or she plans to maintain your vital body functions during the operation. The anesthesiologist will also ask you questions about your medical and surgical history and whether you're allergic to any medications that might be used.

On the same day, much of your body hair will be shaved off. This helps reduce the risk of infection. During your evening shower, the places on your leg and chest where incisions will be made will be scrubbed with antiseptic surgical soap for the same reason.

What Happens on the Day of the Operation?

When it's time for your operation, hospital attendants will move you into the operating room on a rolling bed. Once you're in the operating room, the anesthesiologist will administer an anesthetic drug to make you fall asleep and to prevent you from feeling pain during the operation.

How Long Do Bypass Operations Usually Last?

Coronary artery bypass graft surgery usually takes from three to six hours. The length of the operation depends on its complexity. As you'd expect, the more bypasses that must be attached, the more time the operation will take. Then, too, every operation poses its own unique set of problems. Because of this, it's impossible to pinpoint the length of time a particular operation will take.

Most hospitals have places where patients' families wait during surgery. Be sure your surgeon knows where your family will be during the operation so there won't be any communications difficulties.

What Happens Immediately After the Operation?

When the operation is over, you'll be taken to a recovery room or an intensive care unit. This is where you'll be when you wake up from the anesthesia. It's possible that when you first wake up you may have difficulty moving your arms and legs. This isn't too unusual; it's due to the anesthesia. In a short time you'll recover and coordination won't be a problem.

How Soon After the Operation May the Family Visit?

Close relatives are usually allowed in the recovery room or intensive care unit within an hour or two after the operation. The effects of the anesthesia won't have worn off yet, so if they do visit, they'll find that you're still sleeping.

Is Fever Common?

Everyone runs a fever after having bypass surgery: it's perfectly normal. Sometimes fever may cause you to perspire heavily during the night or even during the day. Taking aspirin or an aspirin substitute usually brings relief, but the fever may continue for three or four days after surgery.

What Can Be Done to Speed Recovery?

[Several actions can help speed your recovery. These include:

1. Deep breathing exercises and coughing.

2. Frequent position changes.

3. Progressive increases in activity]

Can Leaving the Hospital Cause Mixed Feelings?

It's not at all unusual to feel apprehensive or depressed about returning home. Sometimes these feelings result because patients feel scared about leaving the security of the hospital, with its expert medical team and equipment. They think that going home is risky. It's important to remember, however, that your doctor won't let you go home until he or she thinks that your condition has stabilized and continued recovery at home is possible.

[Once you return home from the hospital, you may need to make some changes in your lifestyle:

1. You may need to modify your diet. Refer to suggestions in Chapter 56 or consult with a doctor or dietitian.

2. Maintain the proper weight for your height. In addition to diet modifications, you may need to begin an exercise program. Consult with your doctor before beginning an exercise program. Suggestions on exercising can be found in Chapter 58.

3. Stop smoking.

4. Your doctor may recommend that you avoid working under stress or strict deadline pressures.]

How Long Should I Wait Before Returning to Work?

For people who have sedentary office jobs, four to six weeks is the average. People who must perform heavy work will have to wait longer. In some cases, a person may not be able to return to his or her former job. If that's your case, contact the State Vocational Rehabilitation Agency for information and help.

Chapter 36

Balloons to Bypass Bypass Surgery

Percutaneous transluminal coronary angioplasty. Quite a mouthful to say and practically impossible to remember. A more common name for the procedure, balloon angioplasty, is not only easier to pronounce, but gives us a clue as to what's involved. A half-inch-long balloon that looks like a tiny hot dog when inflated plays a crucial role in this medical technique.

Balloon angioplasty is an increasingly important alternative to coronary bypass surgery for improving blood flow to the heart. Although angioplasty probably won't ever entirely replace bypass surgery, it is being done more and more each year. Figures from the National Center for Health Statistics show that nearly seven times as many angioplasties were done in 1985 as in 1982; 82,000, up from 12,000. Although many more people have bypass surgery—170,000 in 1982 and [230,000]* in 1985, the rate of increase is much lower. And it's very likely that the number of angioplasties will continue to rise dramatically. So, what is this procedure and why is it so popular?

To pump blood, the heart muscle itself requires a large supply of oxygen-rich blood that is delivered through the coronary arteries. When one or more of these arteries becomes clogged with deposits of fat, the heart may not receive enough blood to do its job properly. Balloon angioplasty widens the artery's channel, helping to improve the blood supply to the heart, while relieving pain and lessening the chances of having a heart attack.

FDA Consumer, May 1988.

The procedure demands a high degree of skill on the part of the doctor. With the patient under local anesthesia, the physician gently threads a guiding catheter (a thin, flexible tube) toward the heart by entering and passing it through an artery in the leg. The physician carefully watches the catheter's progress on an X-ray screen. A second catheter, tipped with a deflated balloon, is introduced through the guiding catheter and advanced to the constricted area. When the tip reaches the blockage, the tiny balloon is blown up, compressing the soft, fatty deposits against the artery's inner walls. If necessary, the balloon can be inflated more than once. It's then deflated, and the catheter is slowly withdrawn from the body. In the hands of an expert (such as the physician who developed balloon angioplasty, the late Dr. Andreas Gruentzig of Emory University Hospital in Atlanta), the procedure can take as little as 20 minutes. In a day or so, the patient can go home.

Balloon-tipped catheters used in coronary angioplasty are regulated by FDA's Center for Devices and Radiological Health. The first such catheter received FDA approval in March 1980.

Balloon angioplasty seems like a miracle compared to the much more complicated bypass surgery, which involves taking a vein from another part of the body—usually the leg—and sewing it at one end to the aorta (the largest artery coming from the heart) and at the other end to the diseased coronary artery "downstream" from the blockage, thus bypassing the obstruction. This surgery requires general anesthesia, many hours on the operating table, use of a heart-lung machine, and a longer recuperative stay in the hospital.

Neither procedure would be necessary if arteries leading to the heart didn't clog up to begin with. Atherosclerosis—the buildup of fatty deposits known as plaque on the inside artery wall—is a progressive disease, usually connected with aging, though the process may begin early in life. (Fatty streaks have been found in the arteries of children, and autopsies of young men dying of other causes revealed many cases of advanced atherosclerosis.)

No one knows exactly what causes atherosclerosis. What is known is that people at greatest risk are those who smoke, have high blood pressure, or have high levels of cholesterol in the blood. Other risk factors are diabetes, a sedentary lifestyle, a family history of heart disease, and being male. (In people under 45, coronary artery disease is 10 times more prevalent in men than in women.) Coronary artery disease is the major cause of heart attacks, suffered by almost 700,000 Americans each year.

Besides the coronary arteries, other arteries in the body may be affected by atherosclerosis. When narrowed arteries in the head and neck impair blood flow to the brain, a stroke may occur. Clogged arteries in the legs and feet can cause pain and difficulty in walking. Left untreated, these obstructions interfere with circulation so severely as to cause gangrene, leading to amputation. Insufficient blood flow to the kidneys can cause high blood pressure.

A chilling fact is that many people with coronary artery disease don't know they have it. That's because the heart doesn't begin to complain until its blood supply is severely disturbed. It takes a sizable narrowing—more than 50 percent—of at least one artery before the heart sends out warning signals.

Chest pains are most often the first symptom. They occur when the heart needs more oxygen, usually on exertion, signaling that the blood supply to the heart is inadequate. This temporary lack of oxygen causes no permanent damage; medicine can relieve the pain known as angina, and permit many sufferers to live normal lives.

But in time the clogging may become so severe that medication can't control the symptoms. Pain may occur at rest as well as on exertion; the chances of complete blockage and heart attack increase. At that point, the patient may require more aggressive treatment—bypass surgery or balloon angioplasty.

Patient selection is very important. The procedure works best on people who have had angina less than a year, who are under 65, and who have only one obstruction in one artery (though angioplasty is now being done on people with multiple obstructions in all three of the main coronary arteries). The procedure is generally less successful in women than in men. As with any technical procedure, a physician who has done many balloon angioplasties is more likely to have a higher success rate.

Many people are not candidates for angioplasty because the procedure has some limitations. Over half the people with coronary artery disease can't undergo angioplasty because the blockage(s) is too severe or because the heart has been damaged by past heart attacks. Those with an obstruction in the left main artery usually don't qualify either, because angioplasty of this artery—which supplies the largest amount of heart muscle with blood—allows for no mistakes. A nick in the left main artery could cause heart attack or sudden death. Also, plaque that has become calcified (hardened by calcium) may rule some people out, since the balloon doesn't work as well when deposits are hard.

However, doctors are now using a laser device to remove even hardened blockages in leg arteries. Should it prove to be safe and effective in destroying blockages in coronary arteries, FDA could approve it for that use as well. Occlusions must also be accessible by catheter. Even with improved catheters, many blocked areas just can't be reached, especially those located at or after sharp bends in the artery or where the artery separates into two branches. Clogged areas longer than three-fifths of an inch are not suitable for dilation because of an increased risk of damaging the artery with the catheter guidewire. In all, fewer than one-third of persons with coronary artery disease are eligible for the procedure.

Another requirement for balloon angioplasty is that the patient must also be able to undergo bypass surgery. In about 3 percent to 5 percent of patients, the dilated artery immediately closes up again after the catheter is removed, and bypass surgery must be performed right away to prevent a heart attack. For this reason, a bypass surgical team should always be on standby.

Physicians who perform angioplasty must also be prepared for other emergencies, because if an artery is accidentally punctured, blood may fill the sac that contains the heart (the pericardium), causing a buildup of pressure on the heart (cardiac tamponade). Heart failure may result. A heart attack may also occur if a clot forms in the dilated area, or if an artery goes into spasm.

One problem that is frustrating to some individuals—and their cardiologists—is reblockage of arteries that have been widened by angioplasty. This happens—unpredictably—to about one-third of the patients within a year of the balloon treatment. The reasons for recurrent blockages are unknown. Often angioplasty will have to be repeated—it has been done as often as four times in the same artery—or coronary bypass surgery will have to be performed.

Balloon angioplasty does not cure coronary artery disease. It aims to relieve pain and improve blood flow to the heart, and is successful in about 85 percent to 90 percent of cases. Death following the procedure or death associated with bypass surgery after unsuccessful angioplasty occurs in about 1 percent to 2 percent of the patients, the same as for bypass surgery alone.

Since 1968, the mortality rate from cardiovascular disease has declined about 2 percent a year, according to the *Morbidity and Mortality Weekly Report* (Oct. 24, 1986), published by the U.S. Centers for Disease Control in Atlanta. It may be that changes in lifestyle—increased attention to a healthful diet, exercise, and reduction in smoking—are making a difference. Certainly playing a part are the development of drugs that dissolve blood clots in the heart and arteries, better diagnostic tests, better surgical procedures, and new techniques, such as balloon angioplasty.

—*by Evelyn Zamula*

Evelyn Zamula is a free-lance writer in Potomac, Md.

Correction: Bypass Surgery

*In the article "Balloons to Bypass Bypass Surgery" in the May 1988 *FDA Consumer*, the number of coronary bypass operations performed in the United States in 1985 was reported incorrectly. The correct number is 230,000. (from *FDA Consumer* September 1988, p. 7)

Chapter 37

Implanted Defibrillators and Pacemakers

On a Boston subway train in December 1990, John Thomas' heart stopped its normal steady beating. Instead, it began to quiver ineffectively in a type of cardiac arrest called fibrillation.

Automatically, built-in protection came to the rescue. A medical device implanted in Thomas' abdomen delivered an electric shock to his malfunctioning heart, jolting it back to regular rhythm.

"I lost consciousness for just a few seconds," says Thomas, 36, a social worker in Boston. "Nobody on the subway knew. I wasn't even sure what had happened." That same day, his doctor confirmed the device had indeed responded.

The device is a cardioverter defibrillator, one of the newest heart-rhythm regulators in pacemaker-defibrillator evolution. ("Cardioverter" indicates the capability to deliver low-energy shocks.) Thomas needs the device to treat primary ventricular fibrillation, a condition in which the lower heart chambers (ventricles) periodically have disorganized electrical activity and are unable to effectively pump blood to the body. He received his defibrillator after collapsing with cardiac arrest at Cape Cod the previous Fourth of July.

Thomas' defibrillator gave his heart three other jump-starts that fall and winter—his last one occurring in January 1991. To reduce the frequency of these episodes, his doctor prescribed drug therapy with Tenormin (atenolol), and Thomas has been free of the episodes ever since.

FDA Consumer, April 1994.

The Stats

While most cardiac arrests result from rapid heartbeat (tachycardia), some are due to slowed heartbeat (bradycardia), which is often treated with an implanted pacemaker. The Food and Drug Administration estimates that doctors implant about 15,000 defibrillators and 110,000 pacemakers each year.

Clinical studies submitted to FDA show the newest heart-regulating device—a pacemaker-cardioverter-defibrillator— corrected nearly 98 percent of patients' abnormal heart rhythm or cardiac arrest episodes. Some 400,000 Americans die annually from abnormally fast or irregular heart rhythm, FDA said in announcing approval of the device in February 1993.

The Antiarrhythmics *vs.* Implantable Defibrillators (or AVID) pilot study at the National Heart, Lung, and Blood Institute is examining whether defibrillators or antiarrhythmia drugs are more effective in reducing deaths.

Pacemaking, Naturally

Responsibility for pacing heartbeats, which circulate blood, belongs to the sinus node atop the heart's right atrium (one of two upper chambers). This natural pacemaker's specialized cells fire electrical impulses that cause the atria and their respective ventricles to contract to move the blood in perfect timing.

The impulses travel down the atria, which receive blood through the veins from the body and lungs, and cause their contraction to "top off" the amount of blood in the ventricles. The impulses continue through a conductive pathway into the ventricles and cause their contraction, resulting in the pumping of blood through the arteries to the body and lungs. The right chambers circulate oxygen-depleted blood from the body to the lungs, while the left chambers circulate oxygen-rich blood from the lungs to the body.

Aside from speeding up in situations such as physical activity and slowing during rest or sleep, the normal heart typically completes 72 of these cycles a minute.

Some hearts, however, beat less than 60 times a minute (bradycardia) or race at over 100 a minute (tachycardia). These "arrhythmias" may have any number of causes, such as a birth defect, injury, chemical imbalance, even anti-arrhythmia medication. But the main predisposing factor, according to the American Heart Association, is acquired heart disease. Some arrhythmias aren't serious enough to warrant treatment.

To treat serious arrhythmias, doctors can turn to a permanently implanted artificial pacemaker or defibrillator. (Temporary emergency pacing with an external pacemaker is possible by threading lead wires through a vein to the patient's heart. Emergency defibrillation is possible with external defibrillator paddles.) Alternative treatments are drug therapy and surgical correction.

Artificial Pacemakers

The pulse generator of the artificial pacemaker corrects for a defective sinus node or conduction pathway by emitting rhythmic electrical impulses similar to those of the sinus node. Usually, it's made with a titanium metal case and other materials compatible with the body and powered by a lithium battery system.

The doctor implants the generator under the skin in the upper left part of the chest, attaching it to lead wires threaded to the heart.

Traveling along the wires, the impulses "tickle" the heart, stimulating it to beat at a normal pace, says Donald Dahms, chief of the pacing and electrophysiology devices branch at FDA's Center for Devices and Radiological Health.

The first pacemaker was implanted in 1958. These early devices had only one wire and paced the ventricles at regular intervals. They paced at a single rate prescribed by the doctor—usually 70 beats a minute.

The first advance, around 1976, was a design change that allowed "demand" pacing: A pacemaker would only pace if the patient's heart didn't beat within a given time period.

Then, early in the 1980s, programming capability was introduced. The subsequent development of transmitting by telemetry, a system for sending and receiving electromagnetic signals as radiofrequency, enables the doctor to check and adjust the pacemaker. In addition, simple monitoring can be done over the telephone.

Placing a transmitting wand (called a programming head) on the patient's skin overlying the pacemaker, the doctor can determine voltage, pacing rate, and the status of the wiring and electrodes and can make adjustments to fit the changing needs of the patient. For instance, an increase in voltage output might be needed if the connection to the heart gets bad, Dahms says.

"The problem with the early pacemakers' having only a constant rate," he says, "is when you need a faster rate—if you run, for instance—they can't give it to you. So your heart has to strain to increase its blood output to make up the difference. And if your heart beats on its own, the pacer continues beating, competing with your natural heartbeat." A constant rate also can cause adverse effects, such as dizziness, he says.

By 1983, the first dual-chamber pacemakers entered the market. Using two lead wires, these devices pace the atrium and then the ventricle, when necessary.

"Dual pacing lets you synchronize pacing of both chambers, more like the heart's natural functioning," Dahms says. "If you have a wire pacing away just on the ventricle, your atrium might get out of synch, which reduces your blood output. Without the 'atrial kick' you have less efficient circulation."

Within the next couple of years, firms developed techniques to make single-chamber pacemakers "rate responsive."

These pacemakers contain a sensor to detect the need for increased rate. The simplest ones, Dahms says, gauge response by body movement. Some, however, respond to the person's breathing. Still others base their response on changes in blood temperature. Thus, if a person starts to walk or run, the device senses the activity and increases the heart rate.

Rate-responsive, two-wire, dual-chamber devices became commercially available in 1987.

Many pacemakers automatically provide for a slower heart rate at night or when the person rests. A very few devices are clock-timed to slow at night.

Despite such sophisticated capabilities, miniaturization techniques have allowed pacemakers to become quite tiny in size, some as small as a quarter and less than an ounce in weight. The many companies making pacemakers today offer more than a hundred models.

Pacemakers last four to 12 years. Factors that shorten a pacemaker's life include the requirement to pace every beat, the size of the batteries, dual-chamber pacing, and the tightness of the electrical connection to the heart, which is not completely controllable.

Another use for pacemakers has been to treat heart rates that are too fast, slowing them back to a normal rhythm. But antitachycardia pacing can also pose a problem. If pacing doesn't stop a rapid heartbeat, Dahms says, it may accelerate it, possibly leading to fibrillation.

Defibrillators

Newer than the pacemaker in regulating heartbeats is the implantable defibrillator, made of the same materials but powered by a special higher energy battery.

Implanted under the skin in the upper abdomen, the defibrillator is connected with lead wires to two defibrillation electrodes placed surgically in or around the heart. There must always be two, Dahms says, to provide the electric field needed across the heart.

The defibrillator interrupts the abnormal rhythm, allowing the normal rhythm to resume. The abnormal beating is so rapid and uncoordinated that the heart can only quiver ineffectively.

Sensors inside the generator monitor the heart. If a sensor detects an irregularity, such as fibrillation, the generator is programmed to deliver a strong electric shock directly to the heart. Being kicked in the chest by a horse is how some people describe this jolt.

Others, like Thomas, lose consciousness before they experience the shock.

"I've never felt it," Thomas says. "I'm just a little lightheaded, like when you stand up too quickly. Then I'm unconscious for 5 to 10 seconds. When it's happened at home, my wife has observed my body jerk as though I'm having a seizure."

Although a patient may sometimes be unaware the defibrillator has been activated, this information is stored in the device's memory. During periodic checkups, the doctor can therefore tell how frequently it has gone off and how much shock it has delivered.

FDA approved the first defibrillator in 1985, after clinical trials with the device produced dramatic results. In the trials, the agency announced, the cardiac arrest death rate was under 5 percent a year, down from a 27 to 66 percent annual rate previously reported (before the use of implanted defibrillators) for patients not helped by medication.

These early devices were limited in detection and programming capability and delivered only one level of therapy—a painful, jolting shock. Still, says Dahms, they provided almost certain protection against death from cardiac arrest.

In 1988 and 1989, FDA approved the first cardioverter defibrillators, which offer the programmability of a two-stage shock treatment. The life-saving jolts of these defibrillators continued to be painful, causing significant psychological suffering in some patients with frequent episodes.

337

The newer pacemaker-cardioverter-defibrillator monitors the heart and refrains from delivering a shock if the heart rhythm has returned to normal on its own. Using staged therapy, this first "third-generation" defibrillator measures varying degrees of rapid heartbeat so that it can deliver gentle *pacing* impulses to slow the heart, low-energy *cardioversion* shocks to restore normal rhythm when the pacing is inadequate, or high-energy *defibrillation* shocks to restart the quivering heart.

Some devices also use "biphasic" pulses, which holds promise for extending the life of the device, as well as other possible benefits. (The biphasic wave-form pulse derives its name from the fact it delivers a pulse with a positive and negative polarity.)

Last August, FDA approved a new lead system that can be implanted through a vein, eliminating the need for open-chest surgery when implanting a defibrillator in certain patients. In some of these patients, generators with biphasic pulses are used with the leads.

A defibrillator usually lasts two or three years, depending on how often it has to defibrillate.

Thomas' defibrillator was replaced last September. His concern about being off work for the surgery and uncertainty about whether the replacement, like the first device, would go off several times were soon alleviated. Unlike his first surgery, which required opening the chest to attach the lead system to his heart, this implantation was a minor outpatient procedure under local anesthetic because the leads were already attached to his heart. "It was much easier the second time," he says.

Although today's defibrillators are the size of a deck of cards and weigh about 8 ounces, Dahms says future devices. now in clinical studies, will be small enough for implanting in the upper chest, like pacemakers.

Risks and Precautions

As with anything electronic, glitches can occur in a pacemaker or defibrillator. Among possible causes of malfunction, says Dahms, are circuitry failure, lead breakage, electrode displacement, and scarring around the electrodes. Regular checkups by the doctor every two or three months are crucial so that any problems, including battery depletion, are detected as early as possible.

There's no question that defibrillator failure due to battery depletion could be life-threatening. However, death is extremely rare following pacemaker failure. In almost all pacemaker-battery failures, the underlying natural heartbeat takes over (albeit at a slowed rate) until a new device is implanted or an external pacemaker applied.

Nevertheless, as a precaution for pacemakers as well as defibrillators, FDA requires special labeling specifying a warning period when a battery is about to wear out, to allow for timely replacement. (The warning is detected during medical checkups.)

Extreme electromagnetic interference can cause some devices to malfunction. Someone implanted with a defibrillator, for instance, should avoid airport security scans, because the interference can turn off a device, in which case some devices start beeping. It is inadvisable for patients with pacemakers or defibrillators to undergo magnetic resonance imaging, a diagnostic technique that pictures the body's internal structures.

Some older pacemakers were susceptible to interference from microwave ovens. More recent models are shielded. Patients in doubt about any interference should check with the doctor.

Under FDA regulations required by the tracking provisions of the Safe Medical Devices Act of 1990, manufacturers must track pacemakers and defibrillators from production through distribution to patients. This will speed patient notification if a problem should arise. These regulations went into effect on Aug. 28, 1993.

In addition, a few state laws prohibit driving for a period of time after arrhythmia-induced unconsciousness. While Massachusetts doesn't have such a law, Thomas was under his doctor's orders to not drive for six months following an episode.

Not driving that first year was hard, Thomas says, along with constant anxiety about having an episode. As for today:

"It does tend to give me more perspective, so that little things don't bother me as much. Once in a while it's on my mind. And it impresses upon me how fragile life can be."

Language of the Heart

arrhythmia: abnormal heart rhythm

artificial pacemaker: corrects for a defective sinus node (see "sinus node" entry) or conduction pathway by emitting a series of rhythmic electrical discharges to control the heartbeat

atria: the two upper heart chambers

339

bradycardia: slowed heartbeat, less than 60 beats a minute

cardiac arrest: stopped heart activity

defibrillator: electronic device that helps reestablish normal heartbeat in a malfunctioning heart

fibrillation: rapid, uncoordinated heart muscle contractions; the chamber involved can't pump effectively, so blood flow is compromised

sinus node: the natural pacemaker, whose cells in the top of the right atrium produce electrical impulses that travel to the ventricular muscle, causing the heart to contract

tachycardia: fast heart rate, over 100 beats a minute

ventricles: two lower chambers of the heart

Medic Alert

FDA encourages people implanted with a pacemaker or defibrillator to join the free Medic Alert International Implant Registry by calling (1-800) 344-3226.

Those who enroll will receive a free Medic Alert bracelet or necklace to notify health-care staff of the implant in the event of a medical emergency.

—*by Dixie Farley*

Dixie Farley is a staff writer for FDA Consumer.

Chapter 38

Heart Valve Surgery

Diseases Commonly Affecting Heart Valves

Heart valves may not always work as well as they should. Several things can cause problems with them. A heart valve may not be normal at birth and may need to be repaired right away. A minor defect that exists at birth may not be found but may slightly weaken the heart valve or affect blood flow patterns. As a result, the heart valve will get worse later in life. Diseases such as rheumatic fever or bacterial infections may affect the valve, causing scarring or totally destroying it (as with bacterial endocarditis). The aging process also may weaken or harden heart valves. This happens because of the enormous number of times the delicate valve tissue must flex and move.

The mitral and aortic valves are most commonly affected by diseases that degenerate the valve. The tricuspid valve may be affected if abnormal pressure builds up because other heart valves are diseased. The pulmonary valve also may become abnormal. This is usually related to some deformity present at birth, however.

When disease causes the valve tissues to thicken and harden, the valve fails to open properly and blocks or interferes with blood flow. This blocking process is called *stenosis*. When a heart valve becomes weak or stretched, it may not close properly. If that happens, blood can

---

341

leak back through the opening. This leakage is called *incompetence,* *insufficiency* or *regurgitation.*

Any problem with a heart valve greatly increases your heart's work. That may cause the heart to enlarge to make up for its extra workload. When the heart can no longer do that, heart failure soon follows. Over time the heart muscle is permanently damaged.

Correcting Heart Valve Problems

Some people with diseased heart valves can lead normal lives as long as they get careful medical supervision. Others with more severe heart valve damage, need surgery.

In some cases, operating to repair a person's own valve may relieve the stenosis or leakage. In other cases, the valve is so badly damaged that it must be replaced. The best solution depends on the person's needs. Your doctor will discuss the options and recommend the best way to manage your case.

Heart Valve Repair Operations

Valve stenosis often occurs when the cusps or leaflets are scarred or fused at the edges where they touch each other (*commissures*). A blockage caused when a valve can't open properly may be relieved by cutting with a scalpel. This separates the parts of the valve and helps them move more freely.

Valve incompetence (insufficiency) is often caused by the weakening and lengthening of the valve leaflets. The edges that normally touch (to keep the valve closed) begin to slip past each other (*prolapse*). This lets blood regurgitate through the valve.

As leakage progresses, the whole valve may enlarge or dilate. Restoring the valve to normal functioning then requires remodeling its tissues.

Different approaches can be taken. Removing excess leaflet tissue and sewing the edges may be required. Shortening or connecting suspensory chords is sometimes done. Prosthetic rings are used to narrow a dilated valve and to reinforce valve repairs.

One advantage of valve repair operations is that a person's own valve tissues are used. Thus repair is a more natural way to treat valve failure.

Heart Valve Replacement Operations

Sometimes heart valves are seriously deformed, degenerated or destroyed. When that's the case, repairing them isn't reasonable. Then the old, damaged valve is removed and replaced with a new valve mechanism. The new valve is firmly attached by sewing it to a rim of tissue kept from the person's original valve.

Several types of replacement valve mechanisms are used. They mainly fall into one of two groups: tissue (biologic) valves or mechanical (metal, plastic, etc.) valves.

Biologic tissue valves use animal valves that have been chemically processed for the moving part of the valve. They're mounted in a cloth-covered metal or plastic frame; this makes inserting them into a patient easier.

Another type of tissue valve uses the aortic valve from another person. This valve has been preserved by carefully freezing it using controlled methods (*cryopreservation*). These valves are transplanted directly into a person's aorta.

A tissue valve has the great advantage of being very similar to the natural heart valve it replaces. That's why these valves are well tolerated in the body without special medication. A disadvantage is that they're usually less durable than natural valves. The reason is that even the most scientific methods to preserve them can cause some injury.

Mechanical valves are artificial devices (*prosthetic valves*). They're made of hard and durable metals, carbon ceramics and plastics. A fabric ring made from Dacron or Teflon is used to attach the device to tissues in the patient's heart.

There are different types of mechanical valves. The first ones used a moving part (a ball) held in a cage. This ball-in-cage design has been successful and reliable for many years. Another group of useful prosthetic valves uses a disk that tilts to open and close. The disk is attached to the valve housing by a wire or hook device. Lastly, a third group of mechanical heart valves employ two half disks (bi-leaflet) that tilt to open and close. The leaflets are hinged to the valve housing.

An advantage of mechanical valves is that they're durable, due to the strong materials used in their construction. These materials aren't natural to the body, however, so they may cause blood clots to form. To keep this from happening, medications (*anticoagulants*) are used to slow the rate of blood clotting. Most patients with mechanical valves must take anticoagulant medications every day for the rest of their lives. The effect of the drug on blood clotting also must be checked regularly by a blood test called the *prothrombin time* (pro-time).

Many things must be considered in selecting the best device to use to replace a heart valve. A surgeon will draw upon his or her own experience and knowledge to recommend the valve best suited to each patient's needs. Factors to consider include a patient's age, the valve disease process, the size of the valve to be replaced, and the person's ability and willingness to take anticoagulant medications. The feelings and wishes of the patient are carefully considered in planning the operation.

[The American Heart Association reports that operations to repair or replace heart valves typically last three to five hours. Your operation may take a longer or shorter amount of time depending on the complexity of your individual situation. Your recovery time in the hospital may last one to two weeks.

During your hospital stay, respiratory therapy may be instituted to help keep your lungs clear of fluids. Your doctor may also prescribe elastic stockings to help maintain circulation in your legs.

When you are discharged from the hospital, your doctor will give you instructions about activities such as how much you can exercise or lift and when you can drive your car. You will have to take your temperature on a regular basis and report to your doctor if it becomes elevated.]

Signals and Actions

Repairing heart valves or replacing them with prosthetic valves are very reliable operations. But the truth is, the operations, the remodeled valves, and the artificial valves aren't absolutely perfect. Problems are rare but sometimes do happen. Certain signs and symptoms indicate that a person should call the doctor at once or, if the doctor can't be reached, go to the hospital. It's important to get competent medical advice.

These signs or symptoms call for IMMEDIATE action:

1. Chest pain or tight pressure that doesn't go away after a few minutes.

2. Sudden, severe shortness of breath that isn't related to exercise.

3. Temporary blindness in one eye or noticing a grey curtain coming over an eye.

4. Weakness, clumsiness, or numbness of the face, arm, or leg on one side of your body, even if only temporary.

5. Slurred speech. even if it only lasts a short time.

6. Unusually rapid weight gain, retaining fluid or swelling of the ankles.

7. Fatigue, especially along with a fever that doesn't go away in a few days.

8. Unusual bleeding.

9. Loss of consciousness, even if it's regained shortly after.

10. Sudden change in the normal sound or sensation of your heart valve opening and closing, or an absence of normal sound and sensation of the valve.

11. Sudden disturbing changes in your heartbeat's rate and rhythm.

If any of these warning signs or symptoms occur, **call your doctor right away**. Don't wait until tomorrow! Getting prompt medical attention may save your life if your heart valve fails to perform properly. Your doctor won't mind being bothered even if it turns out there's nothing to worry about.

Have a plan in mind in case of a heart valve emergency:

• Keep your doctor's phone number handy. Carry it with you at all times and keep a copy at home and at work for your family and co-workers to use.

- If your surgery was done at a distant hospital, find out what hospitals close to you can perform open heart surgery in an emergency.

- Make sure members of your family, neighbors and co-workers know *in advance* where to take you if you have a medical emergency related to your heart valve.

- Find out if your area has "911" access to emergency medical services (EMS). If not, it may be a good idea to check with local rescue squads or ambulance services to plan the best course of action in an emergency.

Chapter 39

FDA Cardiovascular Device Actions

Faulty Catheter Prompts New Requirements (3/90)

A "balloon-on-a-wire" device may sound like something frivolous. In fact, it's a new type of life-saving catheter for treating blocked heart arteries. A recent recall of a hazardous model pointed up the unique danger these instruments pose and led FDA to tighten its pre-marketing requirements for all balloon-on-a-wire catheters.

The new balloon-tipped catheter is as thin as paper-clip wire, making it narrow enough to traverse and open clogged coronary arteries, which are very small. FDA learned, however, that in certain models the inflated balloon can wrap around the wire shaft, cutting off the heart's blood supply and preventing removal of the device. In other models, the tip of the catheter can become lodged in the artery, break off, and remain in the heart. In the past, manufacturers could market a balloon-on-a-wire catheter after submitting to FDA a supplement to a previously approved application for a standard balloon catheter. But now, because the agency is aware of the unusual problems associated with these small-diameter catheters, a complete pre-market approval (PMA) application is required.

FDA's more stringent application of PMA rules occurred after C.R. Bard, Inc., of Billerica, Mass., changed its original balloon-on-a-wire catheter, which had been a supplement to the firm's 1980 PMA

FDA Consumer, March 1990, March 1993, May 1993, September 1993, November 1993, November 1994, December 1994.

for its USCI Gruntzig catheter, the first balloon heart catheter ever approved. Bard described some, but not all, of the changes in supplements to the PMA. Apparently minor changes had created a new catheter with new problems, as FDA later discovered.

The Gruntzig and balloon-on-a-wire catheters are variations of a PTCA (percutaneous transluminal coronary angioplasty) catheter—a long, flexible tubular instrument with a balloon at the tip. PTCA catheters are used to treat atherosclerotic disease, in which plaque buildup in the coronary arteries restricts blood flow to the heart. The cardiologist threads the catheter into an artery in the patient's leg, through the blood vessels, to the blocked coronary artery. The balloon is then inflated at the point of blockage to press the obstructing material against the artery wall, opening the artery for resumed blood flow.

On July 15, 1987, Bard submitted a PMA supplement requesting approval to market the USCI Probe I, an ultra-thin PTCA catheter.

"Because of its small size, the Probe I could enter arteries too narrow for a standard PTCA catheter, which is about the size of a cooked spaghetti noodle," says Lynne Reamer, who oversees the review of heart catheters for FDA's Center for Devices and Radiological Health.

Any PTCA catheter can cause complications such as injury to the coronary artery, blood loss, a drop in blood pressure, or heart attack, which may lead to emergency bypass surgery or even death. "Some of these complications were seen in human studies with the Probe I," says Reamer, "but not to a greater degree than with other such catheters."

In clinical trials, Bard found the Probe I could fail if a cardiologist twisted the catheter too far in one direction while trying to navigate the curving heart arteries. The firm therefore relabeled the catheter to limit rotation.

CDRH approved the Probe I in November 1987 and a supplement adding two balloon sizes to the Probe I in March 1988. The following November, Bard submitted a supplement for approval of its USCI Probe II catheter, claiming it was the same as the Probe I except for an added inner tube to allow increased catheter rotation. No mention was made about balloon wrapping with the Probe I.

Meanwhile, Reamer learned that two deaths from the Probe I had been reported to CDRH—one due to balloon rupture, the other to a balloon leak. But these problems were not uncommon with balloon catheters, and the Probe II was approved in January 1989.

CDRH later received documents from other PTCA catheter firms indicating Bard was marketing another catheter, the Probe C. Bard had written its customers March 17, saying it received 33 complaints about Probe II tips breaking and describing in a diagram the differences between the Probe II and a Probe C. Reamer said that, after examining CDRH records and finding nothing about a Probe C, she alerted CDRH's office of compliance and surveillance that Bard might be selling an unapproved catheter.

On April 25, CDRH held the first of many meetings with Bard. CDRH repeatedly stressed that, in issues of patient safety, firms cannot arbitrarily redesign a device and market it without FDA approval. Data gathered at these meetings and at plant visits by investigators from FDA's Boston district office showed that Bard had withheld important facts from FDA, such as that balloon deflation problems with the Probe I were the reason for changing the catheter.

At FDA's recommendation, Bard voluntarily recalled all Probe IIs because the tip failure was excessive for PTCA catheters. Because the Probe C had never been approved by FDA, Bard voluntarily recalled this catheter. The Probe I is the only Bard balloon-on-a-wire catheter still on the market.

Heart Assist Device OK'd (3/93)

The first mechanical circulatory support system was cleared for marketing by FDA on Nov. 20, 1992.

The heart-assist device, manufactured by Abiomed, Inc., of Danvers, Mass., temporarily supports blood circulation in patients with hearts too damaged following heart surgery to pump blood on their own.

The Abiomed BVS 5000 bi-ventricular support system is a computerized console that operates one or two disposable bedside blood pumps, each with two chambers, connected by tubes to the patient's heart. It is intended to reestablish circulation in patients who do not respond to conventional postoperative treatments—drug or intra-aortic balloon pumps. The heart-assist device is disconnected after the heart recovers.

The device is recommended for short-term use in patients whose bodies are large enough to support it. The recommended upper age limit is 75, which was the top age of those participating in clinical studies on the device. The BVS 5000 is not intended for use on patients awaiting heart transplants.

Implantable Defibrillator Combines Three Actions (5/93)

The first implantable device to combine three actions to help the heart beat regularly was approved by FDA last Feb. 11.

The Medtronic PCD (pacer cardioverter defibrillator) Tachyarrhythmia Control System can be electronically programmed to deliver:

- small, swift, "pacing" electrical impulses to restore regular beating to a heart whose rate is too slow (bradycardia) or too rapid (tachycardia)

- stronger "cardioversion" shocks to restore normal rhythm when pacing doesn't stop the irregularity

- a high-energy "defibrillation" shock to restart the heart when the PCD detects heart fibrillation, or quivering.

The PCD has three main parts: the pulse generator, wire leads, and an external programmer.

The pulse generator, about the size of a cassette tape, is implanted under the skin or muscles of the abdomen. It contains a computer and battery that monitor the heart rhythm and deliver electrical stimuli when necessary.

Several wire leads, which carry the electrical impulses, connect the pulse generator to the surface of the heart.

The external programmer allows the doctor to fine-tune the pulse generator to the patient's needs. The programmer's memory bank stores facts, such as the number, types and success of heart-rhythm treatments the patient has received and a record of what the heart was doing during the most recent abnormal episode.

The device is intended for patients with chronic, prolonged abnormal heart rhythm, usually caused by coronary artery or heart muscle disease. Many people who have this kind of heart rhythm will have suffered and survived cardiac arrest or a stopped heart. Nearly 400,000 Americans die annually from abnormally fast or irregular heart rhythm.

In a study of 434 patients implanted with the PCD system, 271 patients together had more than 9,700 episodes of abnormal heart rhythm or cardiac arrest. The device corrected nearly 98 percent of these incidents, thus showing it can prevent sudden death in such patients.

Patients receiving the PCD should be closely followed by their doctors. FDA requires that the manufacturer, Medtronic, Inc., Minneapolis, track the patients and look for unexpected problems. The firm must also study certain aspects of performance, such as the lead system's function and fracture rate and the survival rate of PCD patients compared with that of patients implanted with another approved defibrillator.

New Device for Heart Surgery (9/93)

A new medical device is approved for use during balloon angioplasty to help keep heart arteries from closing again, FDA announced last June 2. This reclosing occurs in 2 to 11 percent of patients.

The Gianturco-Roubin Flex-Stent Coronary Stent is an implantable, tube-shaped stainless steel mesh device about 1 inch long. It remains inside the artery walls as a "scaffold" to improve blood flow.

About 300,000 balloon angioplasties are performed each year in patients with atherosclerosis, a progressive disease in which heart arteries become blocked with fatty plaque, causing chest pain, heart attack, and death.

In balloon angioplasty on the heart, the surgeon threads a balloon-tipped catheter through a leg or arm artery to the heart artery. When the catheter reaches the blockage, the surgeon inflates the balloon to compress the plaque against the artery walls, then deflates it, and withdraws the catheter. If the artery closes or threatens to close, the surgeon withdraws the first balloon catheter and inserts a stented balloon catheter. As this balloon inflates, the stent's mesh scaffold expands, to remain in place and hold the artery open after its balloon catheter is removed.

FDA based its approval on a review of clinical studies of 306 patients at 13 medical centers for two years. The studies showed the stent not only reduced the need for bypass surgery, which is more risky and costly than balloon angioplasty, it also reduced the incidence of heart attack from reclosing arteries during angioplasty.

The Gianturco-Roubin Flex-Stent Coronary Stent is made by Cook Inc. of Bloomington, Ind.

Another stent, the Palmaz Balloon-Expandable Stent, was approved by FDA in 1991 for use on leg arteries and, when other techniques don't work, for blockages of major bile ducts. It's made by Johnson & Johnson Interventional Systems Co. of Warren, N.J.

Defibrillator Device Changes Need for Open-Chest Surgery (11/93)

A medical device approved by FDA Aug. 26 eliminates the need for open-chest surgery when a defibrillator is implanted. The device is called the Endotak Lead System, and is manufactured by Cardiac Pacemakers Inc., of St. Paul, Minn. It is approved for use with the firm's automatic cardioverter defibrillator pulse generator, with which it was tested in clinical trials.

An implanted defibrillator monitors heart rate and, if it detects an extreme irregularity such as heart fibrillation (quivering) or a heart attack in progress, it delivers a strong electrical shock directly to the heart. Until now, defibrillator implantation required open-chest surgery to attach the lead wires that deliver the shock onto the heart muscle. The new device consists of a lead system that can be threaded to the heart through a vein under the collarbone. This technology is already used for pacemakers.

The Endotak system is approved for use in people at high risk of sudden death because they have chronic, recurring or prolonged abnormal heart rhythm, usually as a result of coronary artery or heart muscle disease. Many of these people may already have had a heart attack brought on by an abnormal heartbeat.

FDA based its approval on results of the manufacturer's two-year clinical study of the Endotak Lead System implanted in 400 patients at high risk of heart attack. In the study, 1,815 shocks were delivered in 1,369 instances of rapid heart rhythm or heart attack. In more than 90 percent of the episodes, a single shock corrected the problem.

FDA is requiring the firm to keep track of all patients implanted with the lead system and check for unexpected problems.

Device Approved to Unblock Heart Arteries (11/94)

An implantable medical device that can unblock and keep open previously obstructed heart arteries better in some cases than balloon angioplasty received FDA approval last Aug. 3.

Called the Johnson & Johnson Palmaz-Schatz Balloon-Expandable Stent, the tube-shaped device achieved greater enlargement of arteries in clinical trials than balloon angioplasty and a lower rate of repeat blockage. With the stent, however, patients were more likely to have bleeding and clotting, requiring longer hospital stays.

In balloon angioplasty, a catheter holding a strong balloon is inserted into an arm or leg artery and threaded to the blockage in the coronary artery. The balloon is inflated, compressing plaque against the artery wall to open the artery, and the catheter is removed.

Implanting the stent also requires an angioplasty balloon. Collapsed over the deflated balloon at insertion, the device's stainless-steel mesh "scaffold" expands with inflation of the balloon and then remains permanently in place where the blockage was to hold the artery open after the balloon is removed. The procedure significantly improves blood flow to the heart muscle. The stent is for patients with atherosclerosis who have a short blockage in a large artery. Atherosclerosis is a progressive heart disease in which the heart arteries become blocked with fatty plaque, causing chest pain and heart attacks.

FDA based its approval on safety and effectiveness data from clinical studies of some 2,000 men and women at 48 medical centers in North-America and Europe. An FDA advisory panel recommended approval of the device.

Heart-Assist Device Approved (12/94)

To improve chances of survival for some patients waiting for a heart transplant, FDA last Sept. 30 approved the first implantable heart-assist device.

The Heartmate Implantable Pneumatic Left-Ventricular Assist System helps do the heart's work by pumping blood through the body. It consists of an implanted blood pump connected by a cable to an external computerized console, which powers the pump. The pump remains implanted until the patient receives a donor heart.

The device is approved for use in patients with non-reversible heart failure who are deteriorating so rapidly they are likely to die within 24 to 48 hours. They must also be registered on their hospital's heart transplant list.

An estimated 15,000 to 20,000 people are potential candidates for heart transplants yearly in the United States, but there are only about 2,000 donor hearts. While waiting for a transplant, which can take more than a year, patients currently are treated with drugs or intra-aortic balloon pumps. But these treatments only provide partial help for a short time, and almost half of the waiting patients die.

The pump is implanted in the abdominal cavity and connected to the left ventricle, the main pumping chamber of the heart.

The external console is mounted on a mobile cart and plugged into an electrical outlet. It can also operate on batteries for up to 30 minutes, allowing the patient to move the console during walks or exercise in the hospital.

FDA approved the device on the basis of a review of safety and effectiveness data submitted by the manufacturer, Thermo Cardiosystems Inc. of Woburn, Mass. The data were derived from a long-term clinical study begun in 1985, which included 162 patients at 17 U.S. institutions.

Chapter 40

Questions and Answers about Organ Transplantation

Introduction

Medical advances have made it possible to transplant numerous tissues and organs from one human being into another to improve and save lives. The first corneal transplant was performed in 1905, the first blood transfusion in 1918, the first kidney transplant in 1954, and the first heart transplant in 1967. Now, current medical technology also enables the transplantation of skin, heart-lung combinations, lung, pancreas, liver, bone, and bone marrow.

In 1992, there were 10,210 kidney, 3,059 liver, 2,172 heart, 557 pancreas, 48 heart-lung, and 535 lung transplants performed in the U.S. The number of transplantations has nearly doubled since 1983, due primarily to dramatic increases in the number of heart and liver transplants. However, the number of individuals awaiting transplants also continues to grow.

Did you know that:

- Approximately 24,359 patients were awaiting kidney transplants in September 1993.
- Almost 10 percent of all individuals awaiting liver transplants are age 5 or younger.

U.S. Department of Health & Human Services, Public Health Service, Health Resources and Services Administration, 1993.

- The one-year survival rate for heart transplant recipients is 82 percent.
- One donor, a victim of an automobile accident, recently was responsible for saving the lives of five individuals awaiting transplant surgery.

Please make a decision to become an organ and tissue donor. Discuss your decision with your family and let them know of your desire to become a donor. Then, sign and carry in your wallet a donor card.

You can make a miracle, give the gift of life!

Who Can Donate?

Anyone over the age of 18 can indicate their desire to be an organ donor by signing a donor card or expressing their wishes to family members. Relatives can also donate a deceased family member's organs and tissues, even those family members under the age of 18.

Donation of heart, liver, lung, pancreas, or heart/lung can occur only in the case of brain death. The donation of tissues such as bone, skin, or corneas can occur regardless of age and in almost any cause of death.

Can You Donate an Organ While You Are Still Alive?

Certain kinds of transplants can be done using living donors. For example, almost 25 percent of all kidney transplants are performed with living donors. They are often related to the person needing the transplant, and can live normal lives with just one healthy kidney. Also, there are new methods of transplanting a part of a living adult's liver to a child who needs a liver transplant. Parts of a lung or pancreas from a living donor can also be transplanted.

Can You Still Choose to Donate If You Are Younger Than 18 Years of Age?

Yes, but only with the consent of an adult who is legally responsible for you, such as your parents or legal guardian. The adult or adults should witness your signature on a donor card.

What Can Be Donated?

Organs that can be donated include: KIDNEYS, HEART, LIVER,

LUNGS, and PANCREAS. Some of the tissues that can be donated include: CORNEAS, SKIN, BONE, MIDDLE-EAR, BONE MARROW, and CONNECTIVE TISSUES and BLOOD VESSELS.

Total body donation is also an option. Medical schools, research facilities and other agencies need to study bodies to gain greater understanding of disease mechanisms in humans. This research is vital to saving and improving lives. If you wish to donate your entire body, you should directly contact the facility of your choice to make arrangements.

Why Should You Consider Becoming an Organ/Tissue Donor?

Advances in medical science have made transplant surgery increasingly successful. Transplantation is no longer considered experimental, but rather a desirable treatment option. The major problem is obtaining enough organs for the growing number of Americans needing them. As of September 1993, there were more than 32,000 Americans waiting for organs to become available. And, approximately 1,700 more individuals are added to the waiting list each month. By contrast, in 1992 there were only 4,522 donors in the United States. Even though most donors contribute multiple organs, there still are not enough to meet the need and many people die while waiting for an organ.

Everyone's help is needed to resolve the donor shortage. The best way to assure that more organs and tissues are made available is to sign and carry a donor card and encourage others to do so. It is especially important to let your family know of your wishes to donate if the opportunity arises. It will most likely be a family member who is in a position to see that your wishes are carried out.

How Do You Become a Donor Candidate?

Fill out a donor card and carry it with you in your wallet. Also, most states have some way that you can use your driver's license to indicate your wishes to be a donor. Some states have a donor card on the back of the license; others have a place to check or a colored sticker to put on the license.

It is also extremely important that you let your family know that you want to become an organ and tissue donor at the time of your death. Ask family members to sign your donor card as a witness. When you die, your next-of-kin will be asked to give their consent for you to become a donor. It is very important that they know you want to be a donor because that will make it easier for them to follow through on your wishes.

It would also be useful to tell your family physician and your religious leader that you would like to be a donor. And, it would be a good idea to tell your attorney and indicate in your will that you wish to be a donor.

Below is a little check list for you to use in making it known that you wish to be a donor.

My Donation Check List

- Sign an organ and tissue donor card; ask family members to witness your card.
- Carry the card in your wallet
- Indicate your intent to be donor on your drivers license (If applicable)
- Discuss your wish to donate with: Your family; Your physician; Your religious leader; Your attorney
- Indicate your wish to be a donor in your will
- Encourage others to become donor candidates

What Is Brain Death?

Death occurs in two ways: 1) from cessation of cardio-pulmonary (heart-lung) functioning; and 2) from the cessation of brain functioning.

Brain death occurs when a person has an irreversible, catastrophic brain injury which causes all brain activity to stop permanently. In such cases, the heart and lungs can continue to function if artificial life-support machines are used. However, these functions also will cease when the machines are discontinued. Brain death is an accepted medical, ethical, and legal principle. The standards for determining that someone is brain dead are strict.

Tissue and bone may be useable in either type of death. Organs, however, are useable only in cases where brain death occurs.

What If Members of Your Family Are Opposed to Donation?

You can have an attorney put your request in writing. This document, along with your donor card, may help ensure that your wishes will be honored. In any event, tell your family that you have decided to become a donor in the event of your death.

Are There Religious Objections to Organ/Tissue Donation?

Most major religious groups in the United States approve and support the principles and practices of organ/tissue donation.

Transplantation is consistent with the life preserving traditions of these faiths. However, if you have any doubts, you should discuss them with your spiritual leader.

Is There a Registry of Signed Organ/Tissue Donors? What If You Change Your Mind about Donating?

There is no national registry of those who have indicated their willingness to be organ and tissue donors. If you change your mind, TEAR UP YOUR DONOR CARD. If you have indicated your wishes to be a donor on your driver's license, ask your local office of the Division of Motor Vehicles (DMV) what steps you need to take to revoke your decision.

In all instances, be sure to let your family know whether you wish to donate or not.

Does the Donor's Family Have to Pay for the Cost of Organ Donation?

No. The donor's family neither pays for, nor receives payment for, organ and tissue donation. Hospital expenses incurred before the donation of organs in attempts to save the donor's life and funeral expenses remain the responsibility of the donor's family. All costs related to donation are paid for by the organ procurement program or transplant center.

Will the Quality of Hospital Treatment and Efforts to Save Your Life Be Lessened If Staff Know You Are Willing to Be a Donor?

No. A transplant team does not become involved until other physicians involved in the patient's care have determined that all possible efforts to save the patient's life have failed.

Does Organ Donation Leave the Body Disfigured?

No. The recovery of organs and tissues is conducted in an operating room under the direction of qualified surgeons and neither disfigures the body nor changes the way it looks in a casket.

Is It Permissible to Sell Human Organs?

No. The National Organ Transplant Act (Public Law 98-507) prohibits the sale of human organs. Violators are subject to fines and imprisonment. Among the reasons for this rule is the concern of Congress that buying and selling of organs might lead to inequitable access to donor organs with the wealthy having an unfair advantage.

What Is "Required Request?"

"Required request" is a policy requiring hospitals to systematically and routinely offer the next-of-kin the opportunity to donate their deceased relative's organs and tissues. This policy enables hospitals and health care professionals to play a key role in increasing donation because families might otherwise not be aware of their right to donate. As of 1992, forty-eight states and the District of Columbia had enacted "required request" laws.

The Omnibus Budget Reconciliation Act of 1986 (Public Law 99-509) established additional requirements for hospitals that participate in the Medicare and Medicaid programs. It required each participating hospital to establish written protocols for identification of organ donors and to notify an organ procurement organization designated by the Secretary of Health and Human Services of any potential donors it identifies.

Since January 1988, the Joint Commission for the Accreditation of Healthcare Organizations has required its member hospitals, as a prerequisite for accreditation, to develop policies and procedures on the identification and referral of potential donors.

What Are Organ Procurement Organizations (OPOs)?

OPOs are organizations that coordinate activities relating to organ procurement in a designated service area. Evaluating potential donors, discussing donation with family members, and arranging for the surgical removal of donated organs are some of their primary functions. OPOs also are responsible for preserving the organs and making arrangements for their distribution according to national organ sharing policies established by the Organ Procurement and Transplantation Network and approved by the U.S. Department of Health and Human Services.

In addition, OPOs provide information and education to medical professionals and the general public to encourage organ and tissue donation and increase the availability of organs for transplantation.

How Many Transplant Programs and OPOs Are There in the United States?

As of June 22, 1992 there were 95 liver, 237 kidney, 157 heart, 92 pancreas, 84 heart-lung, and 87 lung transplant programs in the United States. Names and addresses of transplant programs can be obtained from the United Network for Organ Sharing at the following address:

United Network for Organ Sharing
1100 Boulders Parkway, Suite 500
Richmond, Virginia 23225
(804) 330-8500

As of September 1993 there were 67 OPOs certified by the Health Care Financing Administration of the U.S. Department of Health and Human Services. Their names and addresses can be obtained from the Association of Organ Procurement Organizations at the following address:

Association of Organ Procurement Organizations
One Cambridge Court
8110 Gatehouse Road
Suite 101 West
Falls Church, Virginia 22042
(703) 573-2676

What Are the Steps Involved in Organ Donation and Transplantation?

1. A potential donor who has been diagnosed as brain dead must be identified.

361

2. Next-of-kin must be informed of the opportunity to donate their relative's organs and tissues, and must give their permission.

3. An Organ Procurement Organization is contacted to help determine organ acceptability, obtain the family's permission, and match the donor with the most appropriate recipient(s).

4. Organ(s) and tissues are surgically removed from the donor.

5. The donor organs and tissues are taken to the transplant center(s) where the surgery will be performed.

When a potential organ donor is identified by hospital staff and brain death is imminent or present, an organ procurement organization (OPO) is contacted. The OPO is consulted about donor acceptability and often asked to counsel with families to seek consent for donation. If consent is given, a search is made for the most appropriate recipient(s) using a computerized listing of transplant candidates managed by the United Network for Organ Sharing which operates the National Organ Procurement and Transplantation Network.

It is increasingly common for donors and donor families to contribute multiple organs and/or tissues. Therefore, several recipients may be helped by a single donor. When a match is found, the OPO will arrange for the donated organ(s) to be surgically removed, preserved, and transported to the appropriate transplant center(s). A potential recipient(s) is also alerted to the availability of an organ and asked to travel to the transplant center where he or she is prepared for surgery. The recipient's diseased or failing organ is removed and the donated organ is implanted.

How Are Recipients Matched to Donor Organs?

Persons waiting for transplants are listed at the transplant center where they plan to have surgery, and on a national computerized waiting list of potential transplant patients in the United States. Under contract with the Health Resources and Services Administration, the United Network for Organ Sharing (UNOS) located in Richmond, Virginia maintains the national waiting list. UNOS operates the Organ Procurement and Transplantation Network and maintains a 24-

hour telephone service to aid in matching donor organs with patients on the national waiting list and to coordinate efforts with transplant centers.

When donor organs become available, several factors are taken into consideration in identifying the best matched recipient(s). These include medical compatibility of the donor and potential recipient(s) on such characteristics as blood type, weight, and age; urgency of need; and length of time on the waiting list. In general, preference is given to recipients from the same geographic area as the donor because timing is a critical element in the organ procurement process. Hearts can be preserved for up to 6 hours, livers up to 24 hours, and kidneys for 72 hours. Lungs cannot be preserved outside the body for any extended period of time.

Why Should Minorities Be Particularly Concerned about Organ Donation?

Minorities suffer end-stage renal disease (ESRD), a very serious and life-threatening kidney disease, much more frequently than do whites. Asian Americans are three times more likely than whites to develop ESRD; Hispanics are three times as likely; and blacks are twice as likely as whites to develop ESRD.

ESRD is treatable with dialysis, however, dialysis is costly and can result in a poor quality of life for the patient. The preferred treatment of ESRD is kidney transplantation. Transplantation offers the patient "freedom" from dialysis to lead a more normal lifestyle and can successfully cure ESRD for many years.

As with any transplant procedures, it is very important to assure a close match between donor and recipient blood types and genetic make-up. Members of different racial and ethnic groups are usually more genetically similar to members of their own group than they are to others. (For example, blacks are usually more genetically similar to other blacks than they are to whites.) It is important, therefore, to increase the minority donor pool so that good matches can be made as frequently as possible for minority patients.

How Many Organ Transplants Have Been Performed Each Year and What Are the Survival Rates for Each Organ?

[The following table reports on heart, kidney, liver, pancreas, heart/lung, and lung transplants:]

Transplants Performed in the U.S.

	1985	1989	1990	1991	1992	1-Year Graft Surrvival Rate[1]
Heart	719	1,690	2,023	2,125	2,172	81.0%
Kidney	7,695	8,945	9,528	9,949	10,210	90.6%[2]
						78.9%[3]
Liver	602	2,191	2,570	2,954	3,059	66.7%
Pancreas	130	418	530	532	557	72.7%
Heat/Lung	30	67	51	51	48	55.4%
Lung	20	91	190	401	535	65.8%
TOTAL	9,196	13,402	14,892	16,012	16,581	

[1]Survival rates can be measured in two ways:

- the length of time the transplant patient survives after surgery; and
- the length of time the graft (transplanted organ) survives after surgery. In the case of kidney and pancreas transplants, if the graft fails, the patient has a backup form of therapy available (e.g., insulin or dialysis). Failure of other types of transplanted organs, however, results in patient death unless the recipient can receive another transplant. The figures above represent patient survival rates as cited in the Annual Report of the U.S. Scientific Registry of Transplant Recipients and the Organ Procurement and Transplantation Network. These data were gathered from 1988 to 1991.

[2]Donations from live donors
[3]Donations from cadaveric donors

How Many People Are Currently Waiting for Each Organ to Become Available So They Can Have a Transplant?

As of September 1993, the waiting list for donor organs totaled 32,431. The number of people waiting for each organ is listed below.

24,359 kidney
2,765 liver
169 pancreas
877 kidney-pancreas
34 intestine
2,877 heart
199 heart-lung
1,151 lung
32,431 TOTAL

What Is the Average Cost of a Transplant?

Average transplant costs are listed below. Many variables account for the range of costs in transplantation procedures. Such variables may include the type of transplant procedure, post-surgical complications, length of hospital admission, medication requirements, and differences in hospital costs. The range and average for specific procedures are listed below.

Organ	Cost Range	Average Cost
Heart	$50,000 - $287,000	$148,000
Kidney	25,000 - 130,000	51,000
Liver	66,000 - 367,000	235,000
Pancreas	51,000 - 135,000	70,000
Heart/Lung	135,000 - 250,000	210,000

Source: Battelle Institute/Seattle Research Center

Who Pays for Transplant Surgery?

Most transplants are paid for by private health insurance, although the Medicare and Medicaid programs pay for certain transplants for eligible beneficiaries. Coverage for transplants, other than kidneys, by major third party payors is [summarized and] described below.

Percentage of Third Party Payors Providing Some Type of Coverage
for Extra-Renal Transplant Procedures

	Heart	Heart/Lung	Liver[4]	Pancreas
BC/BS[1]	100	72	100	53
HIAA[2]	95	78	95	77
GHAA (HMOs)[3]	73	50	94	38

[1]Blue Cross/Blue Shield Plan; heart and liver data are for 1990; pancreas and heart-lung data are from 1985.

[2]Health Insurance Association of America, 1988 data.

[3]Group Health Association of America, 1989 data.

[4]Data on liver transplant coverage include some members who provide coverage only for children/youth under 18 years of age.

It should be noted that while insurance companies may offer coverage for transplantation, individual employers may or may not elect to include it in their specific packages.

1. Many private insurers, including some health maintenance organizations, now include heart, liver, pancreas, and heart-lung transplantation in their benefit package. Individuals should contact their insurance company to determine if they are covered.

2. Medicare coverage is provided for almost all kidney transplants through the End-State Renal Disease program.

Heart and liver transplant recipients can also be reimbursed by Medicare if the recipient is Medicare eligible and the transplant is performed at a Medicare approved center. Only a small percentage of heart and liver transplant recipients are Medicare eligible.

3. Medicaid coverage for particular organ and tissue transplants is determined by the individual State Medicaid program. For those States providing such coverage, the Federal Government will provide funds on a matching basis. Currently, most States do offer at least partial Medicaid coverage for some transplants.

What Are Immunosuppressive Drugs? Which Are Most Commonly Used to Prevent Rejection of Transplanted Organs?

Immunosuppressive drugs are chemical agents that cause the human organism not to produce antibodies that normally fight off foreign material in the body. The production of these antibodies needs to be thwarted (suppressed) in order to permit the acceptance of a donor organ by the recipient' s body.

The drugs most frequently used for immunosuppressive therapy are cyclosporine, imuran, and prednisone.

Are Immunosuppressive Drugs Covered by Third Party Payors?

In general, Medicare covers drugs administered in an inpatient setting, or as outpatient care incident to physician services. In addition, Medicare provides payment for immunosuppressive drugs for one year from the date of transplant for individuals whose transplant is paid for by Medicare. Forty-seven States offer Medicaid coverage for outpatient immunosuppressive drugs. Between 90-98 percent of independent insurance companies pay for drug therapy.

Can Anything Be Done to Improve Access to a Donor Organ for Those in Critical Need of an Organ Transplant? What about Special Public Appeals?

The primary impediment to transplant surgery for most of the people on the waiting list is a lack of donor organs. Quite simply, the demand far exceeds the supply. Therefore, anything that can be done

367

to increase the level of donation in this country would be helpful to all individuals needing transplants.

Families and attending physicians need to maintain close contact with the transplant team to keep them fully up-to-date on the patient's condition. A family could assist community groups in their ongoing efforts to increase public awareness of the need for organ donation.

While family appeals through the media have had a positive effect on increasing donation overall, efforts do not necessarily result in an organ being made available to the individual for whom the appeal has been made. The decision as to which patient on the waiting list will receive any particular organ is made according to objective criteria which include medical urgency and length on the waiting list, and is not subject to external influences including those that might result in inequitable access to donor organs. Any prejudicial or discriminatory practices in organ allocation are forbidden by the policies governing the operation of the Organ Procurement and Transplantation Network. However, raising the level of organ donation in general will necessarily be of help to all those awaiting transplantation.

Chapter 41

Patient Selection for Heart or Liver Transplantation

In Brief:

- In 1984-85, 86 percent of liver recipients and 80 percent of heart recipients had no contraindications for transplantation, and this rate did not change significantly by 1986-87, despite a rapid growth in the number of transplants and an upward shift in the age distribution of recipients.

- Private insurance covered about 70 percent of heart or liver transplants, public insurance covered 24 percent, and 6 percent of the transplant recipients had no third-party coverage.

- From 1984 to 1987, the mean hospital charges for the stay that included the transplant did not change significantly for either heart or liver transplants, and hospital charges and intensity of inpatient care for nonrecipients did not increase.

Background

One of the most dramatic medical breakthroughs of recent years is the ability to replace diseased organs with healthy ones. Since the early 1980s, heart and liver transplantation has been characterized by

AHCPR Pub. No. 93-0119

improved survival rates, expanded insurance coverage, and lengthening waiting lists, despite the extremely high cost of this treatment. Insurance payers, especially Medicare, have adopted unusually detailed regulations aimed at allocating scarce organs to patients with the best expected health outcomes. (Liver transplantation in adults was not covered by Medicare until 1990.) The actual allocation of organs might differ from outcome-based medical guidelines due to variation in third-party coverage and patient ability to pay, competition among health care organizations, or other influences.

The effect of various factors on patient selection for heart or liver transplants was examined in an analysis of data from a large, nationally representative sample of hospitals, the second Hospital Cost and Utilization Project (HCUP-2). The HCUP-2 data base contains records of all discharges from a national sample of almost 500 hospitals and includes about 10 percent of U.S. transplants that occurred from 1984 to 1987. These data were used to define a class of potential candidates for heart or liver transplants and to analyze how patient characteristics affected the likelihood of receiving a transplant. Indications and contraindications for transplantation were defined by diagnoses associated with survival rates of transplant recipients, and a system of disease staging was used to estimate the effects of illness severity on treatment patterns for transplant recipients and nonrecipients.

Selected Findings

Characteristics of Transplant Recipients

Contraindications. In 1984-85, a high proportion of recipients (86 percent of liver recipients and 80 percent of heart recipients) had no contraindications for transplantation, and changes over time were insignificant, despite rapid growth in the number of procedures. This finding indicates that guidelines for selecting transplant patients without contraindications were followed in most cases.

Age. From 1984 to 1987, there was an upward shift in the age distribution of recipients. For heart transplant recipients, there were more recipients in their 50s and 60s, and a reduced share for persons age 20-40. The proportion of liver transplant recipients who were children declined, while the proportion of older recipients increased.

Insurance Coverage. Private insurance covered about 70 percent of transplants, public insurance covered 24 percent, and 6 percent of the transplant patients had no third-party coverage. The proportion without coverage is somewhat smaller than for all hospital admissions or for a leading diagnosis group with only nonelderly patients.

Hospital Charges for Transplant Recipients

The mean hospital charges for the stay that included the transplant did not change significantly during the 4-year period for either liver or heart transplants (however, a relatively high variance makes such comparisons imprecise). In 1986-87, mean hospital charges were about $138,000 for liver transplants and $59,000 for heart transplants.

Care and Charges for Nonrecipients

Estimates indicate that—for each year and for each organ—there were more than 20 potential candidates who did not receive a heart or liver transplant for every candidate who did receive one.

Hospital charges and intensity of inpatient care for nonrecipients did not increase between 1984 and 1987 (controlling for patient age, sex, insurance class, illness characteristics, and hospital characteristics). This finding would negate the hypothesis that excess demand for transplantation (as seen in lengthening waiting lists) would increase services and charges for evaluating and prolonging the lives of candidates who do not receive transplants. However, charges for nonrecipients were higher at transplant centers than at other hospitals and fell with the size of the program.

Implications

The potential impact of the growing use of organ transplants on health care costs and insurance coverage is an issue of concern to policy planners. One might expect transplantation to have only a modest impact on overall health care expenses because of the limited availability of organs, the current medical practice of reserving transplants for patients without contraindications, and the lack of increased charges to candidates for transplants who do not receive them, despite an imbalance in the demand and supply of transplants.

However, this situation could be altered by further technological advances, such as better retrieval and storage of cadaveric organs, improved mechanical implants, the use of live donor tissues (for example, in bone marrow transplants), or the development of interim techniques that prolong the lives of candidates until organs are available. International comparisons suggest that even in health systems with fixed budgets, life-saving organ transplantation will tend to be a relatively favored form of technological advance.

This issue of *Intramural Research Highlights* is based on the following publication:

> Friedman, B., R.J. Ozminkowski, and Z. Taylor. Excess demand and patient selection for heart or liver transplantation. Chapter 8 in P. Zweifel and H.E. Frech III (eds.), *Health Economics Worldwide* (1991). The Netherlands: Kluwer Academic Publishers.

For further information on the subject of this issue, please call the Division of Provider Studies, (301) 227-8410.

Chapter 42

A Guide to State Organ Transplant Activities in the United States

Introduction

Understanding the Organ Procurement and Transplantation Process

In 1984, Congress passed the National Organ Transplantation Act. Since that time, more than 66,000 organ transplants have been performed in this country. In compliance with the law, a uniform national process for matching organ donors and recipients was created with the establishment of the Organ Procurement and Transplantation Network (OPTN). The United Network for Organ Sharing (UNOS) currently operates the OPTN as well as the Scientific Registry, a research data base designed to follow all transplant recipients, under a contract with the Health Resources and Services Administration of the U.S. Department of Health and Human Services.

A brief summary of the organ procurement and transplantation process follows:

The Pre-Transplant Evaluation

The patient's personal physician makes a referral to the appropriate transplant program where the patient is evaluated and tested.

HRSA Pub. No. 90-747.

Using the specific medical criteria of the transplant center, the patient's suitability as a potential transplant recipient is determined.

Waiting List Placement

The organ transplant center places the potential recipient's name and medical data on the OPTN waiting list which is maintained by UNOS. This computerized waiting list contains the names of all potential organ recipients, as well as the medical data needed to make the best match possible.

Donor Identification

The vast majority of organs for transplantation come from patients who have suffered a sudden traumatic accident resulting in brain death. The names of potential donors are referred to the local organ procurement organization for evaluation. If all legal and medical criteria are met, the family is approached to give consent for donation. If the family consents, the characteristics (i.e. age, blood type and weight) and medical background of the donor are registered with the national waiting list and suitable recipients are identified.

Matching the Donor and Recipient and Allocating the Organ

All patients accepted onto a waiting list for transplantation are registered with UNOS. UNOS maintains a centralized computer network linking all organ procurement organizations and transplant centers. This computer network is accessible 24-hours per day, seven days per week, with organ placement specialists always available to answer calls.

When a donor organ becomes available, the transplant center or organ procurement organization will access the UNOS computer, which generates a list of patients ranked according to UNOS policies. Ranking is based upon medical and scientific criteria. Factors affecting ranking may include tissue match, blood type, length of time on the waiting list and immune status. In the case of heart, heart/lung, liver, lung or pancreas, distance is also considered.

After receiving a printout of the waiting list, the transplant coordinator contacts the transplant team of surgeons and physicians for selection of a patient using the ranking list. Once the patient is contacted, donor and recipient testing can begin and surgery is scheduled.

Recovery, Preservation and Transplantation

Once brain death of the donor has been determined, the organ transplant team is notified and assembled. The donated organs are surgically removed and prepared for transport to the hospital where the transplant will be done. Timing is a critical element in the organ procurement process. Hearts can be preserved for up to six hours, livers up to 24 hours and kidneys up to 72 hours, while lungs can be preserved for only a few hours. Following the transplant, patients are monitored closely by transplant center staff to assure that the best possible outcome for each organ recipient is achieved.

Overview

This section of the report provides an overview of the solid organ transplant and donor services available in the United States today. It describes state government activities, including health insurance programs such as Medicaid, as well as other financial assistance, social service and educational initiatives. It also reviews the role of private organ transplant-related organizations and summarizes the nature and scope of services they offer to the public. Finally, it explains how to use the guidebook to find specific information on programs and resources within each state.

Public Sector Resources

The Medicaid Program

Background. Medicaid is the major state program that assists low income individuals in paying their medical bills. It is a health insurance program jointly financed by the states and the federal government. Each state health department administers its own program and has significant latitude in designing eligibility standards, service coverage and payment rates to health care providers. Medicaid is viewed as the "payor of last resort." That is to say, it will pay for approved medical treatments, such as organ transplants, only if an individual has no other insurance coverage or has exhausted his or her coverage.

Medicaid eligibility is strongly linked to eligibility for the following federal cash assistance programs: Supplemental Security Income (SSI) and Aid to Families with Dependent Children (AFDC). In order to be eligible for SSI, an individual must be either aged, blind or disabled and meet income and resource limits set by the government. For AFDC, an individual must be a member of a family with dependent children and meet income and resource tests.

The Medicaid program provides coverage to numerous groups, but they can all be defined as either categorically needy or medically needy. The "categorically needy" are those persons eligible for the above-mentioned cash assistance programs. At its option, a state can also allow medically needy persons to participate in Medicaid. "Medically needy" individuals have incomes and/or resources that exceed the amounts allowed under a state's categorical program, but have incurred significant medical expenses that would cause them to "spend-down" to meet eligibility levels.

Medicaid provides health insurance protection for numerous medical and health-related services. States are required to cover the following mandatory services for categorically needy recipients: inpatient and outpatient hospital care; physician services; laboratory and X-rays; skilled nursing home care for adults; home health care; care in a rural health clinic; nurse midwife; and family planning services. In addition, states have the discretion to provide over 30 optional services that include such items as: prescription drugs; intermediate nursing home care; health clinic services; and transportation. A state Medicaid program can have a more limited benefits package for its medically needy recipients than for its categorically needy ones, but not vice versa.

MEDICAID and ORGAN TRANSPLANTS. Federal guidelines governing state Medicaid payment of solid organ and tissue transplants have, in the past, been limited. The Consolidated Omnibus Budget Reconciliation Act of 1985 required state Medicaid agencies to develop written policies on the coverage of transplants under their state plans. Traditionally, states have had the option of covering all, some or none of these surgical procedures and their associated costs. At present, states that choose to cover transplants may restrict the facilities or practitioners from whom Medicaid recipients may obtain the services, as long as the restrictions are consistent with accessibility to high quality care and as long as similarly situated individuals are treated alike. In 1987, the Omnibus Budget Reconciliation Act clarified this last point by saying that states may not limit coverage in such a way that the services provided are not reasonable in amount, duration and scope to achieve their purpose. At the same time, Congress made clear that states may require a reasonable expectation of therapeutic benefit from an organ transplant, provided such requirement is applied uniformly.

Under recent federal law, the Omnibus Budget Reconciliation Act of 1989, states will probably have to expand coverage for certain organ transplants for children under 21 years of age. Specifically, Section 6403 of the Act adds a new required service component of the Medicaid program for children. It requires that states pay for treatment to correct or ameliorate defects and physical and mental illnesses and conditions discovered during a Medicaid EPSDT (Early and Periodic Screening, Diagnosis and Treatment) screening examination—whether or not such services are covered under a state's Medicaid plan. While federal regulations to implement this amendment have not yet been issued, it is anticipated that organ transplants will be considered a necessary health care service as long as they: (1) are not considered experimental procedures; (2) are not inconsistent with existing state laws; and (3) are medically necessary.

Medicaid coverage of solid organ transplants varies considerably from state to state. All but one state (Wyoming) pays for at least one type of solid organ transplant. Ten states (Kentucky, Louisiana, Massachusetts, Michigan, Mississippi, North Dakota, Ohio, Pennsylvania, Vermont and Wisconsin) pay for all six solid organ transplant procedures—i.e., heart, heart/lung, kidney, liver, lung and pancreas. Although attention has been given in the popular media to a few instances where states have cut back on their commitments to pay for certain high-cost transplant procedures, the national trend is towards expansion of the transplant benefit.

Medicaid coverage is nearly universal for some transplant surgery, while for other types, coverage is not widespread as yet. Kidney and liver transplants are allowable benefits in virtually every state. Heart transplants are generally available but not as prevalent (covered in 40 states). Coverage for the following procedures is relatively limited: heart/lung (23 states), lung (15 states) and pancreas surgeries (12 states). (Both the Oregon and Washington Medicaid programs provide coverage for pancreas/kidney transplants, but not for a simple pancreas transplant procedure). All but three states (Nevada, New Mexico and Tennessee) also cover organ procurement costs for their Medicaid transplant patients; and every state pays for immunosuppressive drugs.

Most states do not impose significant restrictions on the availability of covered organ transplant services. For example, with the exception of liver transplants, the age of a Medicaid patient is rarely, if ever, a cause for denying coverage for a transplant operation. In the case of liver transplants, 11 states (Alabama, Arizona, Hawaii, Iowa, Minnesota, Montana, New Hampshire, Nevada, Oklahoma, Oregon, and South Dakota) place an absolute age restriction on the benefit, limiting it to children only. States that allow medically needy individuals to participate in their Medicaid programs generally permit them to receive the same organ transplants to which categorically needy individuals are entitled. Finally, several states impose special payment restrictions or caps for organ transplant surgery, as opposed to other types of surgery (Alabama, Arizona, Arkansas, Florida, Kentucky, Missouri, New Hampshire, Pennsylvania, South Carolina and West Virginia).

Most state Medicaid programs follow specific medical criteria to select patients for transplant surgery. The task of determining whether a particular applicant meets these criteria is frequently contracted out to an independent medical advisory committee. States that have not adopted independent medical standards generally accept the decisions of individual physicians and transplant centers on a case-by-case basis.

Typically, the medical selection criteria seek to assure that the transplant procedure under consideration is medically necessary and appropriate and likely to result in prolonged life of improved quality. Well developed criteria require that each applicant's diagnosis, current prognosis and medical history be taken into account. In addition, detailed contraindications of a medical nature are often specified. There are often express prohibitions against approving procedures that are deemed to be experimental. Generally speaking, the patient selection guidelines set by the states confine themselves to medical considerations and do not factor ethical, financial or administrative concerns into the development of policy. Federal regulations prohibit states from making a determination of eligibility for transplants on the basis of race, color, sex, national origin or handicapping condition.

Approximately half of the states have developed their own standards that medical transplant centers must meet in order to qualify as providers under Medicaid. Others have simply adopted the facility standards used in the federal Medicare program for the aged and disabled. Facility guidelines typically set forth the type and extent of institutional support services and resources that are required. The 49 states and the District of Columbia that cover organ transplants under Medicaid all require approved transplant centers to accept the Medicaid rate as payment in full.

State Kidney Programs

In 1972, amendments to the Social Security Act created the federal End-Stage Renal Disease (ESRD) program. This entitlement program covers up to 80% of Medicare allowable costs for those beneficiaries who need kidney dialysis and/or transplants. (In addition to kidney transplants, the Medicare program currently pays for the following transplants for its aged and disabled beneficiaries if warranted by medical necessity: cornea, bone marrow, liver and heart). Prior to this federal initiative, a number of states had already established their own programs to benefit those suffering from end-stage renal disease. Currently, a total of 19 states continue to operate and fund independent kidney programs for their own residents. Each state kidney program requires a participant to be a state resident and have a diagnosis of end-stage renal disease. Most of the programs also require applicants to be: (1) on dialysis; (2) in need of a transplant; or (3) a transplant recipient within the past 12 months. In general, applicants who are eligible for the Medicare or Medicaid programs are not eligible for a state kidney program. However, a few of the programs do provide limited services to applicants eligible for other forms of public assistance. For example, the Texas kidney program pays for those drugs and transportation costs that Medicare does not cover.

One notable difference in eligibility for state kidney programs is the requirement of an income test. Sixteen of the 19 states have such a test and the income ceilings vary greatly. In addition, five states require an assets test.

State expenditures also differ significantly in each program, contingent upon budget priorities, services offered and number of participants. Because all of the existing state kidney programs were established through legislative action, support for them is often sporadic and depends on the annual budget process in which other priorities may override them. All but one of the kidney programs are administered by the department of health or social services.

Services provided by the programs differ greatly. Except for New Jersey, all pay for dialysis and related medical treatment. Sixteen states cover transplant medications, most commonly cyclosporine, while ten cover the cost of kidney transplant surgery (Hawaii, Iowa, Maryland, Missouri, Montana, Nebraska, Pennsylvania, South Dakota, Tennessee and Washington). In addition, some state kidney programs offer financial assistance up to a maximum amount per year per participant. Other states pay for additional items, such as airfare for transplant recipients, organ procurement costs associated with surgery and private health insurance premiums.

State General Assistance-Medical Care Programs

Twenty-two states have medical assistance programs associated with state or county general assistance programs. General assistance programs (also called general relief, home relief and poor relief) serve as the ultimate safety net for people with little or no income who are ineligible for federally supported assistance programs such as AFDC or SSI. In certain instances, they may cover benefits to transplant recipients and, therefore, should be explored as a potential—though limited—resource.

Because these general assistance-medical programs are similar in many ways to the federally assisted Medicaid program, they are often referred to as state-only Medicaid programs. However, they are considerably smaller in size and expenditures than the regular Medicaid programs. Responsibility for the funding and administration of these general assistance-medical programs may be vested entirely with state government or shared with county and city governments.

In most of these 22 states, a recipient of cash assistance from the general assistance program is automatically eligible for services under the medical component. In the remaining states, a general assistance recipient must apply separately for medical assistance. Applicants must meet certain income and assets limits in order to be eligible for general assistance-medical services.

Seventeen of the states with general assistance medical programs cover essentially the same health care services as those provided under Medicaid. Since these states offer inpatient hospital and physician services, the programs should be viewed as potential sources of aid for transplant candidates. However, it should be kept in mind that states sometimes place greater restrictions on the amount and duration of health services under their general assistance-medical programs than they do under Medicaid.

State Health Risk Pools

In 24 states, individuals in poor health or at high-risk of needing medical care have access to state-sponsored health insurance risk pools. Under such programs, health status is in theory eliminated as a barrier to health insurance, since private insurance is available through the pool. The basic design of a risk pool is to guarantee availability of adequate health insurance to all, regardless of physical condition. While the operation of pools varies considerably from state to state, there is a basic pattern. A state generally forms an association of all health insurance companies doing business in the state. One organization is selected to administer the plan under the guidelines for benefits, premiums, deductibles, etc., as set forth in state law.

Individuals applying for pool coverage must be state residents. They must also prove that they have been rejected for similar health insurance coverage by a private insurance company; a few states require proof of rejection by more than one insurer. On the other hand, several states allow automatic acceptance into their risk pools without proof of rejection if the individual is afflicted with certain medical conditions. Many of the state plans do not allow individuals to apply for pool coverage if they are eligible for or receiving Medicare or Medicaid.

Risk pool policies provide a fairly comprehensive package of benefits that include inpatient hospital services, physician services, skilled nursing care, home health care and prescription drugs. Organ transplant surgery of a non-experimental nature is also a covered benefit, except in the Wyoming risk pool.

Before applying for insurance with one of the 16 health risk pools that are fully operational, organ transplant candidates should be aware of the disadvantages. First, private insurance available through the risk pools is expensive. Some form of pre-existing condition restriction is also common, in order to prevent individuals from "gaming" the system by enrolling for insurance only after they need medical care. Most pools have a six-month waiting period for pre-existing conditions, although some states waive this waiting period through payment of a premium surcharge.

State Educational Initiatives

The great majority of state governments do not conduct formal education programs to inform the public about the benefits of organ donation and transplantation. Currently, only seven states have appointed special staff and appropriated funds to maintain an active outreach program on this subject. Most states, however, do engage in passive education efforts through their motor vehicle departments which distribute organ donor cards along with drivers license applications.

Three states (New York, North Carolina and Pennsylvania) have designated staff members within their health departments to coordinate organ donor awareness programs. Staff responsibilities include the development and distribution of pamphlets and public service announcements, maintenance of an information hotline, and, in some cases, coordination with organ transplant related organizations. Tennessee has embarked upon a new program in which it not only engages in public information activities to encourage donation, but is also compiles and maintains an organ and tissue donor registry for state residents.

In three other states (Florida, New Jersey and Virginia), public funds are being used to support private, autonomous statewide councils in public education campaigns. The goal of these councils is to inform the public about the urgent need for an increase in donors. They serve as a coalition of interested member organizations which include providers, public members and organ procurement organizations. In their role as facilitators, the councils assist their members through the development of brochures, video cassettes, public service announcements, speakers bureaus and the like.

Private Sector Resources

Patient Services and Educational Programs

There are a variety of private organizations that provide a range of services to transplant candidates, recipients, organ donors and their families. The goals and activities of these groups are described below. In general, inquiries should be addressed to the national headquarters, which will then make referrals to local chapters as appropriate.

American Association of Kidney Patients, Inc.
1 Davis Boulevard Suite LL-1
Tampa, Florida 33606
(813) 251-0725

The American Association of Kidney Patients, Inc. was formed by people on dialysis or with kidney transplants to help those with kidney failure cope with its physical, mental and emotional impact on their lives. Its direct patient services include mutual support groups and patient advocacy. The 26 local chapters hold regular meetings that offer members a chance to share their experiences and make an impact in their communities. The national office assists with patient complaints and serves as a voice for kidney patients in government and health care circles. It also operates the Dessner Memorial Fund, which makes limited grants to kidney patients. Public education efforts by the chapters and the national office provide information about renal disease and the need for kidney donors through use of AAKP literature, newspaper and magazine articles and public exhibits.

American Association of Tissue Banks
1350 Beverly Road Suite 220-A
McLean, Virginia 22101
(703) 827-9582

The American Association of Tissue Banks is a scientific, non-profit organization founded to facilitate the provision of transplantable tissues of high quality in quantities sufficient to meet national needs. The Association publishes standards to ensure that the conduct of tissue banking meets acceptable norms of technical and ethical performance. Based upon these standards, the AATB inspects and accredits tissue banks nationwide. In addition, the Association established a national Tissue Network composed of accredited facilities designed to help ensure an adequate supply of tissue to requesting hospitals and surgeons. The AATB also supports promotional and educational programs for the purpose of stimulating tissue donation. Membership in AATB is open to individuals who are involved or interested in banking of tissues or organs and who support the objectives and policies of the Association.

American Kidney Fund
6110 Executive Boulevard Suite 1010
Rockville, Maryland 20852
National Toll Free: (800) 638-8299
Maryland Toll Free: (800) 492-8361

The American Kidney Fund is a non-profit, voluntary health organization providing direct financial assistance to kidney disease patients. It provides a limited number of grants and emergency funds to needy dialysis patients, transplant recipients and donors to help cover the cost of such health-related support services as transportation, medications and special dietary needs, as well as insurance premiums and other hidden expenses related to the patient's kidney condition. Since the American Kidney Fund is a"last resort" financial source, applicants should have explored all other possible means of assistance from both private insurers and public sources, including federal, state and county agencies.

The Fund provides information and support for kidney donation and transplantation. It also provides the general public with information on the prevention, symptoms and treatment of kidney disease. Educational materials include brochures, public service announcements, newsletters and audio-visual materials.

American Liver Foundation
1425 Pompton Avenue
Cedar Grove, New Jersey 07009
National Toll Free: (800) 223-0179

The American Liver Foundation is a non-profit, voluntary health agency dedicated to fighting liver disease through research, education and patient self-help groups. Its national office sponsors scientific research, makes referrals to medical professionals, advises families on how to raise funds and serves as a trustee for transplant funds. Its network of 17 chapters nationwide provides support groups for liver patients and their families. The chapters also offer grassroots educational programs to local communities on liver health and disease prevention and carry out organ donor awareness campaigns.

American Organ Transplant Association (AOTA)
2306 Texas Parkway Suite 130
Missouri City, Texas 77489
(713) 261-2682

The Association is a private, non-profit group that provides a number of services to transplant recipients and their families. The Association has a working relationship with 75 transplant centers in 33 states. Individuals should contact hospital staff about the organization and its services. If a particular transplant center is not familiar with AOTA, then the organization should be contacted directly.

384

AOTA provides airfare to and from transplant centers for needy transplant recipients and their families on a limited basis. Bus fare is provided on an unrestricted basis. In many cities nationwide, AOTA also arranges for hotel accommodations for transplant families. In addition, the Association advises on fund-raising in local communities, and can set up and administer transplant trust funds. AOTA publishes a regular newsletter for its members, and also distributes a brochure written by transplant recipients that discusses life after transplantation.

American Red Cross
Services National Offices
4050 Lindell Boulevard
St. Louis, Missouri 63108
National Toll Free: (800) 2-TISSUE

The American Red Cross works directly with health care facilities in collecting, storing and providing donated human tissue such as bone, skin and heart valves. It serves only as a referral agency for solid organ transplant donations. Some 43 Red Cross chapters nationwide are involved in tissue donation services, procurement, distribution and/or public education campaigns. The precise scope of each chapter's activities varies considerably, according to local needs.

Association of Organ Procurement Agencies
1714 Hayes Street
Nashville, Tennessee 37203
(615)327-3756

The Association counts among its members nearly all of the certified organ procurement organizations (OPOs) in the country. The national office refers individuals seeking assistance to the nearest local member.

OPOs are diverse in terms of their functions and capabilities. All are involved in the procurement and distribution of kidneys; most also assist the public with other solid organs and many are involved with tissue and bone donation. All of the OPOs make an effort to inform the public about the benefits and usefulness of organ donation and transplantation. In addition to printed materials and speakers bureaus, most of the larger OPOs employ their own independent education coordinators to develop a host of sophisticated community outreach activities, such as TV spots and minority health education campaigns. A recent trend among the OPO community is the creation of donor family support groups, although relatively few OPOs are active in this area as yet.

Children's Liver Foundation
14245 Ventura Boulevard Suite 201
Sherman Oaks, California 91423
Outside California: (800) 526-1593
California only: (818) 906-3021

The Children's Liver Foundation is a voluntary, nonprofit organization engaged in a variety of activities to assist children suffering from liver disease and their families. Its local chapters serve as a network of referrals to medical and other resources and provide families with emotional support groups. Some of the chapters are also involved in public education campaigns concerning liver disease and transplantation.

Children's Organ Transplant Association
917 South Rogers Street
Bloomington, Indiana 47403
National Toll Free: (800) 366-2682

The Children's Organ Transplant Association is a non-profit charity dedicated to providing assistance to the families of children in need of organ transplants, while also educating the public about the need for organ and tissue donations. COTA's immediate goal is to guarantee that no child is ever excluded from the transplant candidate list because of a lack of funds. To date, the Association has established community volunteer networks in the following states: Florida, Georgia, Indiana, Kansas, Louisiana, Oklahoma, Oregon and Texas. When a need arises in a particular geographic area, COTA staff will go there to establish a network of volunteers, who will be trained to set up various fund-raising events. COTA staff will work with these volunteers to raise money for a specific child. This money is earmarked for that child until his or her needs are met. Any remaining funds will then be placed into a revolving fund to assist other children.

The Association's national office endeavors to increase public awareness in several ways: answering questions through its hotline, writing and distributing printed materials; operating a speakers bureau; and preparing public service announcements.

Children's Transplant Association
P.O. Box 53699
Dallas, Texas 75253
(214) 287-8484

The Association is a private, non-profit organization that assists both children and adults with fund-raising efforts in local communities, and is empowered to set up and administer transplant trust funds. It also provides short-term housing for families of transplant recipients during hospitalization in the cities of Omaha, Nebraska, and Minneapolis, Minnesota. The Association has four local affiliates operating in Louisiana, Minnesota, Nebraska and North Carolina.

The Compassionate Friends, Inc.
P.O. Box 3696
Oak Brook, Illinois 60522-3696
(708) 990-0010

The Compassionate Friends, Inc. is a nationwide self-help organization for families who have experienced the death of a child. All parents are welcome to participate, whatever the age of their child who has died or the cause of death. Participants include families of children who have been organ donors or recipients. Presently, the organization has 628 chapters throughout the United States. Family members contacting the national office will be sent general information on bereavement, a national newsletter and a resource guide. They will also be directed to the closest chapter in their community. Each chapter develops its own local resources, newsletter, library and support groups. Some chapters have established professional advisory committees consisting of physicians, nurses, clergy, social workers, psychologists and others who are available as educational resources.

NAACP Black Donor Education Program
4805 Mt. Hope Drive
Baltimore, Maryland 21215
(301) 358-8900

The NAACP has identified organ donor awareness as a top priority for 1990. It has recently launched a demonstration project in five major cities (Baltimore, Detroit, Memphis, New York and St. Louis). The primary goal is to increase blacks' support of organ donation across the country through educational efforts developed for area schools, churches, community organizations and departments of motor vehicles offices. In addition to counseling on how to implement and sustain an effective donor awareness program, each participating NAACP branch is provided with brochures, videotapes and public service announcements. The grass-roots campaign is being underwritten by the Dow Chemical company.

National Heart Assist and Transplant Fund
P.O. Box 163
519 W. Lancaster Avenue
Haverford, Pennsylvania 19041
(215) 527-5056

The National Heart Assist and Transplant Fund is a private, non-profit organization dedicated to providing financial, social and emotional support to patients needing heart and heart/lung transplants and their families. The Fund offers modest financial support by awarding emergency grants of several hundred dollars to eligible candidates to help offset immediate treatment-related costs such as medications, home care and transportation. It also counsels patients regarding the location and cost of treatment centers, other possible sources of financial assistance and fund-raising opportunities within their communities. It acts as a trustee for locally raised funds to assure professional accountability and appropriate distribution.

The Fund serves as a national clearinghouse to support groups throughout the country that provide social and psychological assistance to patients. It also involves patients and support groups, as well as volunteers, in its public education campaign by providing training, materials, organ donor cards, news releases and public service announcements.

The National Kidney Foundation, Inc.
30 East 33rd Street
New York, New York 10016
National Toll Free: (800) 622-9010

The National Kidney Foundation is a non-profit, voluntary health agency seeking the answer to diseases of the kidney and urinary tract through prevention, treatment and cure. The Foundation is committed to the goal of ensuring that everyone who needs a transplant is able to get one. Its nationwide organ donation program supplies organ donor cards and information about organ and tissue donation to the public. Special public information programs are developed annually to increase public awareness. In addition, its 49 affiliates nationwide provide a variety of services including: support groups for patients and their families; information and referral services; assistance in the purchase of prescription drugs; transportation to and from treatments such as dialysis; and financial aid.

Organ Transplant Fund, Inc.
1420 Union Avenue
P.O. Box 41903
Memphis, Tennessee 38174-1903
(901) 274-6268

The Fund is a private, non-profit group that assists with fundraising efforts in local communities, and maintains emotional support groups for transplant recipients and their families. It also operates a public education program on organ donation and transplantation that includes brochures, videotapes and a speakers bureau. The Fund has three branch offices in Little Rock, Arkansas; Morris, Illinois; and Oklahoma City, Oklahoma.

Transplant Recipients International Organization (TRIO)
244 North Bellefield Avenue
Pittsburgh, Pennsylvania 15213
(412) 687-2210

TRIO is an international, non-profit organization that is structured as an association of member chapters. Within each chapter, individuals who have undergone transplant surgery provide one-on-one counseling for transplant candidates, recipients and their families. In addition to counseling, chapters also coordinate events throughout the year to promote public awareness and to raise funds. The National Office assists the chapters in efforts to promote donor awareness. Educational materials have been developed, including a school-based educational program.

United Network for Organ Sharing, Inc.
1100 Boulders Parkway, Suite 500
P.O. Box 13770
Richmond, Virginia 23225
National Toll Free: (800) 24-DONOR

The National Organ Transplant Act of 1984 mandated the creation of an Organ Procurement and Transplantation Network for the United States. The contract for establishing and administering this system was awarded to the United Network for Organ Sharing, a private, nonprofit organization. UNOS' responsibilities include: (1) maintenance of a national list of patients who need organs and a system to match individuals on the list with available organs; (2) operation of a 24-hour hotline service to assist in matching patients and organs; (3) assisting organ procurement organizations in organ distribution; and (4) developing standards of quality for the acquisition and transportation of donated organs.

In addition to its other responsibilities, UNOS is involved in public education. Its telephone hotline provides general information on transplants, current statistics and referrals to local organ procurement organizations (OPOs). UNOS produces and distributes a series of brochures for patients and their families on such topics as organ donation, transplantation, choosing a transplant center and financing a transplant. It also makes available public service announcements, press releases and video cassettes and operates a national resource library.

UNOS members include transplant centers, OPOs, tissue typing laboratories, voluntary health organizations and members of the public. As of June 1990, the membership included 258 transplant centers throughout the country; 51 independent OPOs and 22 hospital-based OPOs; and 40 independent tissue labs and 101 hospital-based tissue labs.

Will Sampson Transplant Foundation
4710 Greeley Street
Suite 300
Houston, Texas 77006
National Toll Free: (800) 383-LIFE

The Foundation is a non-profit, voluntary organization that functions as a resource center and information clearinghouse. Its staff advise individuals on fund raising in local communities, and make referrals to transplant centers. It also operates a statewide, multi-media public education campaign in support of organ donation.

Organization of Report

This guidebook is divided into two sections. Section A provides a general introduction to the public programs and private organizations that currently assist transplant candidates, recipients and their families. Section B contains state-by-state profiles that describe in more detail the nature of the resources that are available locally in each state to assist residents with organ donation and transplantation. It also explains how to gain access to these programs and who to contact for further information. For example, descriptions of national organizations such as the American Association for Kidney Patients can be found in Section A because they request that the public initially contact their national office and not their local chapters. Organ transplant-related groups that are purely local in scope of operations are listed in Section B. Section B also includes the addresses and phone numbers of the medical transplant centers, tissue typing laboratories and organ procurement organizations that exist in each state.

[To obtain a copy of part B of this report, contact the US Department of Health and Human Services, Public Health Service, Health Resources and Services Administration. Or order #1991-524-456/D06299 from the US Government Printing Office.]

Chapter 43

Advances in Heart-Lung Transplantation at Stanford University

Advances in heart-lung transplantation now make longer and healthier lives possible for patients with end-stage heart and lung disease, say researchers at Stanford University in California.

"In carefully selected patients, heart-lung transplantation holds a high promise of rehabilitation," says Dr. Edward B. Stinson, professor of cardiovascular surgery at Stanford University School of Medicine and director of Stanford's clinical heart-lung and lung transplantation program.

The Stanford transplantation program team performed the first successful combined heart-lung transplantation in the United States in March 1981. Since that time 62 patients have received heart-lung transplants at Stanford, which has become a leader among the 141 centers currently performing heart or heart-lung transplantations in the United States.

According to Dr. Stinson, three types of patients with debilitating heart and lung disease can be considered candidates for heart-lung transplantation. The first category includes patients with severe, untreated congenital heart disease that is complicated by hypertension in the lungs. Patients in the second group have primary pulmonary hypertension complicated by secondary right-sided heart failure caused by the increased blood pressure in the lungs.

NCRR Reporter, October 1989.

A third group, which was recently added to the list of potential heart-lung recipients, includes young adult patients with severe pulmonary disease caused by cystic fibrosis. Several of these patients in the Stanford program were the focus of media attention when they became part of a "domino transplant." Such a transplant involves transplanting a healthy heart and lungs into a cystic fibrosis patient whose original heart is then transplanted into another recipient who needs a heart transplant. Thus the cystic fibrosis patient becomes both a recipient and a living donor during the surgery. The prognosis for the cystic fibrosis patient is improved when the heart and lungs are replaced as a unit, Dr. Stinson explains.

Eight years and 62 transplantations have given the Stanford transplantation research team valuable experience in refining the criteria for the selection of donors and recipients, and in improving the operative techniques and postoperative management of patients with heart-lung transplants. However, the strict selection criteria for heart-lung donors has limited the availability of healthy hearts and lungs that can be transplanted. Donors are generally young, healthy adults who have suffered irreversible brain trauma from car accidents or gunshot wounds. Donors must have blood types that are compatible with those of the recipients and also have compatibility with the recipient's human leukocyte antigens (HLA).

HLA refers to a large group of cell surface proteins, or histocompatibility antigens, that can stimulate an immune response leading to transplant rejection when donor and recipient are mismatched. Donor lungs must also match the shape and size of a recipient's chest cavity and, most important, must be relatively free of bacterial, viral, or fungal infections. Since most potential donors have been maintained on artificial respiration prior to organ transplantation, they often develop severe lung infections that then exclude them as heart-lung donors. In the Stanford program, only one of every ten heart donors is suitable for heart-lung transplantation, according to Dr. Stinson.

The United Network for Organ Sharing (UNOS), a private, nonprofit organization devoted to increasing the number of organs available for transplantation, reports that 221 individuals currently are on the national waiting list for heart-lung transplants. To assist local organ procurement programs, UNOS maintains a 24-hour telephone and computer system that assists in matching donors and recipients and transporting organs. The supply of donors can be expected to increase as more hospitals comply with the 1987 "Required Request" law, which directs hospitals to discuss organ donation with the families of potential organ donors. Dr. Stinson predicts, nevertheless, that the supply of organs for heart-lung transplantation will remain inadequate because of the greater demand created by increasing numbers of transplantation programs and the strict donor criteria that cannot be relaxed without adverse effects on patient survival.

Careful selection of recipients is also a critical factor in the success of heart-lung transplants. Studies conducted during the 8-year course of the Stanford program have shown that recipients with impaired liver function and scarring in the chest area had increased bleeding during surgery, impaired postoperative lung function, increased infection frequency, and a higher rate of postoperative mortality. According to Dr. Stinson, the surgery involved in the transplantation of an entire heart-lung system is more complicated and of greater magnitude than that of a heart transplant. Accordingly, the average 3-week postoperative recovery period for patients also is considerably more complicated than that of patients receiving a heart transplant. In addition, the risk of bacterial, viral, and fungal infections is greater with the transplantation of two organs than it is with one. The Stanford experience has shown that patients who require longer time in surgery, excessive blood transfusions and repeated openings of the chest cavity have the greatest postoperative risk of complications.

Since the risk of organ rejection is higher for lung transplants than for heart transplants, patients undergoing heart-lung transplantation must be given a combination of three antirejection drugs that suppress immune reactions. These drugs, cyclosporine, prednisone, and azathioprine, can cause severe side effects such as depression of the bone marrow's ability to produce red and white blood cells, abnormal kidney function, weight gain, abnormal redistribution of weight, skin fragility, and osteoporosis (bone loss). The patients also may develop accelerated heart disease. Approximately 25 to 30 percent of heart-lung transplant patients have some degree of coronary artery disease in their transplanted heart 5 years after surgery, Dr. Stinson explains. Changes in the immune system of the recipients as well as higher triglyceride levels are thought to play a role in the development of the disease, although the exact mechanism remains unknown, he says.

Despite all of these difficulties, heart-lung transplantation is now "a generally accepted therapeutic option" for patients with extremely severe heart-lung disease that has not improved with conventional medical therapy, Dr. Stinson says. In the 40 years since the first heart-lung transplant was performed on a dog by Russian surgeons, increased sophistication in transplantation techniques has been translated into hope of a longer life for patients who are debilitated by heart and lung disease. Hope has been the motivating force for many of the heart-lung transplant candidates who have relocated their families to the Stanford area as they wait for a suitable donor. During that waiting period, which can last as long as a year, all the Stanford heart-lung transplant candidates participate in a patient support group that includes both patients waiting for and recovering from surgery.

The Stanford experience in refining operative techniques and postoperative care has shown definite results. In 1987, the overall 1-year survival rate of Stanford heart-lung transplant patients was 65 percent, compared to approximately 50 percent for other programs around the world. According to Dr. Stinson, the most recent analysis of survival data from the Stanford group shows that their 1-year survival rate has increased to 71 percent. The 2-, 3-, and 4-year rates are 60, 52, and 48 percent, respectively. For patients who have been crippled by end-stage heart disease such results mean renewed vitality, natural breathing, and the capacity to return to work and become physically active again. After discharge from the hospital, transplant patients return to the regular care of their private physicians who maintain communication with the Stanford research team. All the patients return to Stanford annually for lung function tests, examination of the heart, general physical examination, and blood tests. Heart-lung transplantation will never become as common as heart transplantation, but for a special group of patients it is a real gift of life, Dr. Stinson concludes.

—*by Diane B. Stoy*

Additional reading:

1. Annas, G. J., The paradoxes of organ transplantation. *American Journal of Public Health* 78:621-622, 1988.

2. Gutkind, L., Life after transplantation. *Transplantation Proceedings* 20:1092-1099, 1988.

3. Hardy, J. D., Transplantation of tissues and organs: Review of the first 100 years of the Southern Surgical Association. *Annals of Surgery* 207:776-787, 1988.

4. House, R. M. and Thompson, T. L., Psychiatric aspects of organ transplantation. *Journal of the American Medical Association* 260:535-539, 1988.

5. Taylor, R. M. R. and Salaman, J. R., The obligation to ask for organs. *Lancet* 8592:985-987, 1988.

6. Frist, W. H., Oyer, P. E., Baldwin, J. C., Stinson, E. B., and Shumway, N. E., HLA compatibility and cardiac transplant recipient survival. *Annals of Thoracic Surgery* 44:242-246, 1987.

7. Harjula, A., Baldwin, J. C., Starnes, N. A., Stinson, E. B., Oyer, P. E., Jamieson, S. W., and Shumway, N. E., Proper donor selection for heart-lung transplantation: The Stanford experience. *Journal of Thoracic and Cardiovascular Surgery* 94: 874-880. 1987

The research described in this article was funded in part by the General Clinical Research Centers Program of the NIH Division of Research Resources and by the National Heart, Lung, and Blood Institute.

Part Six

Living With Cardiovascular Disease

Chapter 44

Living with Heart Disease: Is It Heart Failure?

Purpose of This Booklet

If you have heart failure due to reduced pumping power of your heart (left-ventricular systolic dysfunction), this booklet is for you. Understanding your condition and following a few simple guidelines can improve the quality of your life.

This booklet is designed to help you and your family be active partners with your health care team—doctors, nurses, and other professionals. It is your guide to living with heart failure. Share it with your family and other caregivers.

This booklet will tell you how and why heart failure affects your body. It also tells how to respond to symptoms and what to expect from treatment. You need to know as much as you can to improve the quality of your life. Be involved in managing your condition.

What is Heart Failure?

"Heart failure" simply means that your heart's pumping power is weaker than normal. Although it still beats, a weakened heart pumps too little blood rich with oxygen and nutrients to meet the body's needs. Walking, carrying groceries, or climbing stairs can be difficult. You may feel short of breath; the body is not getting all the oxygen it needs.

NIH Pub. No. 94-0614.

For most patients, heart failure is a chronic condition, which means it can be treated and managed, but not cured. If it is a complication of other medical conditions such as blocked coronary arteries or heart valve disease, surgery may help.

Causes of Heart Failure

The most common causes are:

- Coronary artery disease, usually with previous heart attack (myocardial infarction [MI]).
- Heart muscle disorder (cardiomyopathy).
- High blood pressure (hypertension).
- Heart valve disease.

Sometimes the exact cause of heart failure is not found. However, the actual cause is not as important as your heart's reduced pumping power and what can be done about it.

Symptoms

Check your symptoms:

- Difficulty breathing, especially with exertion or when lying flat in bed.
- Waking up breathless at night.
- Frequent dry, hacking cough, especially when lying down.
- Fatigue, weakness.
- Dizziness or fainting.
- Swollen feet, ankles, and legs (edema).
- Nausea, with abdominal swelling, pain, and tenderness.

Other medical problems can cause the same symptoms. A thorough physical exam and a complete health history, plus certain tests, are needed to diagnose heart failure and find its possible causes.

Causes of Symptoms

A healthy heart can increase how much oxygen-rich blood is pumped to vital organs and muscles as it is needed.

When a heart pumps with less power and force than normal, it cannot pump enough blood to organs and muscles. As a result, your body cannot do as much. Blood and fluids may collect or "pool" in the lungs. This can cause breathing problems when you lie down. Fluids can also collect in other parts of the body, swelling the feet, ankles, legs, and abdomen.

Your Health Care Team

Because heart failure is complex, a team of health care professionals is needed for special skills and expertise.

By working with your health care team in learning how to treat your condition, you may live longer and also improve the quality of your life.

Health care providers on the team may include:

- Your **primary care doctor**—the doctor you normally see for health problems. General internists or family physicians normally provide primary care.

- A **cardiologist**, if your primary care doctor believes a heart specialist is needed.

- Other **doctors**, such as surgeons and other specialists, if needed and recommended by your primary care doctor or cardiologist.

- **Clinical nurse specialists and nurse practitioners**, who care for you and are sources of information, education, and counsel.

- **Other health care professionals**, including physician's assistants, nurses, dietitians, physical and occupational therapists, pharmacists, case managers, social workers, and other mental health professionals.

You and your family are important parts of this health care team. Before seeing other members of the health care team, write down your questions. Mark anything in this booklet you don't understand or would like to know more about. Using the list and this booklet, ask your health care provider questions. Tell him or her how you feel about your care. **Be involved in management of your condition.**

Diagnosis and Evaluation

Your health care team will want to know:

- About your symptoms and how long you've had them.

- If you have ever had a heart attack, a heart murmur, or other heart problems. If so, how are these problems being treated?

- About your general health history and status. What other health problems do you have, and how are they being treated? Are your diet, activities, or exercise restricted? Have family members had heart problems?

- About your lifestyle and health habits. What is your daily life like? What do you do to prevent health problems?

- If you use tobacco, alcohol, or illegal drugs.

Be honest and candid. Information you share with health care providers is confidential. Evaluating, treating, and managing heart failure depends on accurate information, including facts that only you and your family can provide.

A health history, physical exam, chest x-ray, and electrocardio-gram (called ECG or EKG) help diagnose heart failure.

Based on your symptoms and first test results, a test is needed to measure the amount of blood pumped from the heart with each beat (the ejection fraction). Patients with suspected heart failure should undergo echocardiography or radionuclide ventriculography to mea-sure the ejection fraction.

Echocardiography uses sound waves to make images of the heart and its chambers. The procedure is safe and does not require en-tering the body with any instruments or devices.

Radionuclide ventriculography is a special test that tracks very low doses of a radioactive substance as it travels through the heart. The radioactive substance is safe and completely leaves the body.

A normal heart pumps one-half (50 percent) or more of the blood in the left ventricle with each heartbeat. With heart failure, the weakened heart may pump two-fifths (40 percent) or less, and less blood is pumped with less force to all parts of your body.

Managing Heart Failure

To manage heart failure, follow the instructions of your health care team. You may reduce symptoms and improve how you feel if you take medicines as prescribed and change how you live.

Work with your health care team to make the best choices and set goals to keep life interesting and enjoyable.

Your management plan consists of:

- Medicines.
- Diet.
- Daily activities.
- Exercise.
- Lifestyle and health habits.
- Family support.

Work with your health care team to learn how to treat your condition. If you do not want to change how you live or take medicines as prescribed, tell your health care provider. Explain your reasons to your health care provider.

Medicines

Importance. Taking medicine every day is vital to treating heart failure. Depending on your symptoms and diagnosis, your doctor may start treatment by prescribing one medicine and then adding others later. Sometimes, treatment will begin with two or more medicines.

It may take several days or weeks to find the right doses of prescribed medicines. Be patient as you and your health care provider work together to find:

- The right medicines for you.
- The right amount of each one.
- The best time of day to take each medicine.

The benefits of these medicines will be lost or reduced if you do not take your medicines as prescribed. Skipping doses or not refilling a medicine's prescription can cause serious problems. Do not take more than the prescribed dose of any medicine.

Be sure to tell your health care provider about other health conditions you have and other medicines you take. These medicines include nonprescription medicines such as aspirin, antacids, and cold remedies.

Side Effects. Any medicine can have unplanned results. If you have any side effects, tell your health care provider right away. He or she can work with you to lessen bothersome effects. If the first medicines prescribed do not work as expected, others are available.

Ask your health care team about side effects caused by taking prescribed medicines with:

- Other prescribed medicines.
- Medicines you can buy without a doctor's prescription (such as aspirin, antacids, and cold remedies).
- Certain foods.

Always report side effects to your health care provider. He or she will know what to do about side effects.

Common Kinds of Medicines. Medicines commonly prescribed for treating heart failure include:

- ACE inhibitors (angiotensin-converting enzyme inhibitors) to make it easier for the heart to pump.
- Diuretics, or "water pills," to help remove excess fluid and salt from the body.
- Digitalis to strengthen each heartbeat, allowing more blood to be pumped.

When other heart or health problems exist with heart failure, your doctor may prescribe additional medicines, such as drugs to lower blood pressure.

ACE inhibitors. ACE inhibitors have been shown to help heart failure patients live longer and feel better. The drugs relax blood vessels and make it easier for the heart to pump. For some people, it may take weeks before they feel better from taking the medicine.

Depending on your initial diagnosis and evaluation, an ACE inhibitor may be the first medicine prescribed. Based on your symptoms, a diuretic and digitalis may be prescribed with the ACE inhibitor or added later.

Captopril, enalapril, lisinopril, and quinapril are generic names for ACE inhibitors now being used for heart failure. Others may be used in the future.

Although most patients take an ACE inhibitor without problems, some patients have side effects. They include:

- Cough.
- Dizziness.
- Skin rash.

Tell your health care provider if any of these symptoms occur.

ACE inhibitors may also produce high potassium levels and affect kidney function. Blood tests are needed to monitor these actions.

If you have any side effects, tell your health care provider right away.

Diuretics. By making you urinate more often, diuretics keep fluid from collecting in your feet, ankles, legs, and abdomen. Skipping doses can cause swelling in these parts of the body and shortness of breath when lying down or during physical activity.

The most commonly used diuretics are hydrochlorothiazide and furosemide (Lasix).

Regular use of some diuretics can lead to the body losing too much potassium and to other imbalances. Blood tests are needed to monitor these levels.

To replace lost potassium, you *may* have to:

- Eat more foods rich in potassium, including bananas and raisins, and drink orange juice and other citrus juices.
- Take a prescribed potassium supplement.

Diuretics may also cause:

- Leg cramps.
- Dizziness or lightheadedness.

407

- Incontinence (accidental urine leakage).
- Gout (a type of arthritis).
- Skin rash.

Tell your health care provider if you have any of these symptoms. (Urinating more often is not a side effect. It is caused by the diuretic.)

Digitalis. Digitalis helps the heart pump more effectively and may improve your ability to exercise. Prescribed as digoxin Lanoxin, digitalis is taken daily by many heart patients.

Digitalis has been proven safe for most patients. If too much digitalis is in your body, you may have:

- Nausea, loss of appetite.
- Mental confusion.
- Blurred or yellow-colored vision.
- Rapid, forceful heartbeat (palpitations).

Tell your health care provider right away if you have these side effects. Do not stop taking digitalis unless told to do so by your health care provider.

Keeping Track of Your Medicines. Having a system can help tell you when to take medicines, especially if you take several each day. Use the form [at the end of this chapter] each day to remind you:

- Which medicines to take each day.
- What each pill looks like.
- When to take them.
- When each medicine was taken.

Make copies of the blank form for future use.

Always carry with you a list giving the doses of each medicine you take. [In an] emergency, this information can help medical workers help you.

Cost of Medicines. The retail cost of medicines varies greatly among different pharmacies. If cost is a problem, ask your health care provider or pharmacist if there is a lower cost and acceptable generic form of your medicine. You can also compare prices of different pharmacies and mail-order prescription services.

If needed, financial assistance may be available through social service agencies where you live. You also may qualify for help through programs established by drug companies.

Let your health care provider know if the cost of medicines is a problem. Your health care team can help you apply for assistance.

Diet

In addition to taking medicines, you must change and then monitor your diet. Because salt (sodium) causes fluid to build up in the body, you must restrict salt intake. If you do not, your feet, ankles, legs, and abdomen may swell, and you may find it hard to breathe. If severe, these symptoms may require hospital treatment.

Your health care provider will tell you how much salt, if any, can be in your diet. You and your family may be asked to see a dietitian, nurse specialist, or other health educator for special diet instructions and counseling. They may also suggest new ways to prepare foods and how to modify family recipes. For example, lemon juice and many spices and herbs can add flavor to unsalted foods.

Be especially aware of foods with "hidden" salt such as frozen or canned foods, cheeses, and processed meats. Foods such as hot dogs, salami, and canned soups often contain a lot of salt. Check the nutrition labels for salt content.

If you drink alcoholic beverages, you may have to stop or have only one drink per day. One drink means a glass of beer or wine, or a mixed drink or cocktail containing no more than 1 ounce of alcohol.

Changing your diet can be complicated and confusing. The goal is to reduce salt, and possibly fat, in your food without sacrificing the pleasure of eating. If you have trouble changing your diet, ask your health care team for help.

Watch your weight. Obtain an accurate scale and weigh yourself each morning after urinating, but before eating breakfast or dressing.

If you gain 3 to 5 pounds since last visiting your health care provider, tell him or her promptly. The weight gain may mean your body is retaining fluid.

Daily Activities

How heart failure affects you depends on how severe it is. Mild heart failure may have little effect on work or recreation. Severe heart

409

failure may restrict what used to be easy. Talk to your health care team about:

- **Work.** Can you still work? Full time or part time?
- **Recreation.** Can you go hiking, play golf, swim, and attend sporting events?
- **Leisure.** Can you travel, work in the garden, and do volunteer work?
- **Sex.** Can you have sexual intercourse?

Involve your family members in discussions about activities. They need to know how to support and help you. This is especially true when what you can do changes over time. Some activities (such as work or recreation) may become more difficult while others do not change.

Do not be afraid of discussing private aspects of your life. Your health care team must rely on what you say to help reduce symptoms and improve the quality of your life.

Heart failure means you may have to change your lifestyle and health habits.

As you learn to live with heart failure, you may discover new satisfactions and pleasures. Changes to daily life can be positive and rewarding. Work restrictions may lead to interesting and enjoyable leisure activities. Recreation may become a valuable part of daily life. Sexual relations can be very enjoyable as you and your partner discover less demanding ways to express and share affection.

Exercise

Exercise regularly within your doctor's guidelines. Many people with heart failure say they feel better when they exercise regularly. Usually you can exercise safely at home or in a supervised rehabilitation setting such as a hospital, health club, recreation center, YMCA, or YWCA.

Exercise includes:

- Walking.
- Cycling.
- Swimming.
- Low-impact aerobic routines.

Your health care provider will advise you about the right kind and amount of exercise. Find out before starting. You may be asked to see a cardiac rehabilitation specialist to help plan and monitor an exercise program. Also, you may need an exercise stress test to see how much you can do safely.

Lifestyle and Health Habits

Your lifestyle reflects attitudes and values. Health habits involve what you do to reduce chances of illness or injury. Heart failure means you may have to change your lifestyle and health habits.

Examine your lifestyle and health habits. The following changes can reduce the symptoms of heart failure and improve the quality of your life:

- Lose weight if you are overweight.
- Do not smoke or chew tobacco.
- Eliminate or reduce alcohol.
- Do not use illegal drugs.

You should also:

- Avoid exercise that exceeds your exercise guidelines.
- Avoid coming in contact with people who have colds.
- Get a flu and pneumonia shot.

You may want to make other changes too, such as learning how to reduce stress. Work with your health care team to decide which choices are best.

Family Support

Your family can be a great source of support and encouragement. As much as possible, include family members in all decisions that affect you. These decisions involve your lifestyle and your ability to work and earn a living. Support by family members can be especially important as you adjust to lifestyle changes and if you face emotional difficulties. Let family members know how they can help.

Family members can help you:

- Keep track of medicines.

- Prepare special meals.
- Exercise.
- Find more information on treating heart failure.
- Join a support group.

The diagnosis of heart failure may affect your family as much as you. Family support can help you change your lifestyle and health habits.

Chest Pain (Angina)

Some people have chest pain (angina) in addition to heart failure symptoms. Angina is caused by blockage in the coronary arteries. When angina is a symptom, a test called **cardiac angiography** (heart catheterization with angiography) may be needed.

In this diagnostic procedure, fluid is injected into the coronary arteries through a long, thin tube called a catheter. Special x-rays show where and how much arteries are blocked. Ask your health care provider about expected benefits and risks of the procedure before agreeing to it.

The results of cardiac angiography are usually used to help health care providers plan your care. Treatment may include surgery. Cardiac angiography may not be needed if you do not want heart surgery. Ask your health care provider how information from the procedure will affect your care.

Heart Surgery

If a heart valve problem or coronary artery disease is suspected as the cause of your heart failure, you may be asked to consider heart surgery. Detailed information should be provided. You should know what may result from heart surgery. You should know its:

- Benefits.
- Risks, including the risks of doing nothing.
- Alternatives, including their benefits and risks.
- Total cost and how much is paid by insurance.

Before deciding to have surgery, ask for a second opinion from another health care provider. Health insurance often requires a second opinion before surgery.

If heart surgery is a realistic choice for you, seek an experienced surgeon and hospital for the surgery. Ask for information about their success rates and costs before selecting a surgeon and hospital.

Heart Valve Surgery

Repairing or replacing one or more heart valves may be needed if heart failure is caused by heart valve problems. This surgery is common and has proven to be successful in many cases.

Coronary Artery Bypass Graft Surgery and Angioplasty

Coronary artery bypass graft (CABG) surgery is major surgery. In it, veins or arteries from other parts of the body are used to bypass blocked coronary arteries on the heart to restore more normal blood flow to the heart. As a muscle, the heart needs its own blood supply for nourishment so it can pump blood throughout the body.

An alternative to CABG surgery is angioplasty (or PTCA, percutaneous transluminal coronary angioplasty). In this major procedure, a catheter (long, thin tube) is inserted into the arteries on the heart. Inflating the small balloon on the catheter's tip expands the coronary artery and crushes the blockage, restoring blood flow.

Current research indicates that CABG surgery may benefit many people with angina (chest pain) and worsening heart failure resulting from coronary artery disease. The long-term benefits of angioplasty for such patients have not been established by research.

After heart surgery, you must follow a plan for managing and monitoring your heart health.

Heart Transplant Surgery

Heart transplantation is considered only in cases of very severe heart failure. Heart transplants are only performed in specialized centers.

Monitoring Your Progress

Managing heart failure requires keeping track of symptoms and monitoring how well you follow instructions of your health care team. Report changes in your health to your health care provider.

Your Responsibilities

As part of your health care team, you should:

- Monitor your general health and report any changes in how you feel.
- Report changes in your symptoms.
- Take medicines as prescribed and report any side effects.
- Follow your guidelines for activities and exercise, and report when you are not able to do an activity or exercise easily.
- Follow a prescribed diet.
- Report any sudden weight changes.

Family Responsibilities

Your family is part of your health care team. Ask family members for help in monitoring your condition. They should know when to report new symptoms, or a change in symptoms, to your health care provider if you do not.

When calling the health care provider's office, your family should:

- Say you are being treated for heart failure.
- Describe your symptoms.
- Describe what has already been done to bring relief or comfort.
- Give the names and amounts of medicines you take.

The Future

Ask your primary care doctor to explain how heart failure is likely to affect your life. Many people adjust to limits imposed by heart failure and still lead active lives.

Although a sudden change in symptoms is not expected, certain activities may become harder because you are tired and short of breath. If your symptoms do change suddenly, call your health care provider right away.

Emergencies

In an emergency, such as if your heart or breathing stops, acceptance of medical care and treatment is assumed. However, you have a right to accept or refuse any medical care and treatment in advance. You can direct that you do not want emergency medical workers to restore the heartbeat or use special equipment to breathe for you.

Specific instructions for family members and others may be needed so they will know how to react in a medical emergency. A legal document called an advance directive lets others know what to do in a medical emergency. This document states what lifesaving measures you want taken if you cannot think clearly or speak for yourself.

Advance directives include these legal documents:

- Living wills.
- Medical durable power of attorney.
- "No cardiopulmonary resuscitation" (CPR) instructions.
- Substitute decisionmakers (medical proxies).

If you do not have an advance directive, discuss your medical care and treatment wishes with your family and health care team before preparing one. Ask your health care team or attorney for more information about advance directives. These decisions may be difficult. Your health care team will help you understand how these decisions may affect you. Individual State laws govern the content and use of advance directives.

Support Groups and Counseling

Diagnosis of heart failure can generate a wide range of feelings. You and your family should express these feelings to your health care team. Seek help in dealing with feelings that cause problems.

In addition to professional counseling, local support groups can be a source of help. These groups offer the chance for you to talk about your feelings with other heart patients and families during regular meetings. Support groups may also offer educational programs about heart problems.

415

Ask your health care team about support groups where you live. If no support group exists, your health care team may help you start one.

Many people adjust to limits imposed by heart failure and still lead active lives.

For more information about support groups for heart patients and their families, contact:

The Mended Hearts, Inc.
7272 Greenville Avenue
Dallas, TX 75231
(214) 706-1442

The Coronary Club, Inc.
9500 Euclid Avenue, E-37
Cleveland, OH 44195
(216) 444-3690

How to Use Your Weekly Medicine Record

Use a weekly medicine record [like the one shown in Figure 44.1] to keep track of what medicines to take every day, when to take them, and when you took them.

Write your name and the date, starting on Sunday, at the top of the record.

Each numbered row is for one medicine. Write the name and dose (amount) of each medicine under the first column. For example: **Lanoxin .25 mg.** The medicine's name and dose appear on the label of the medicine container.

In the second column, write the size, shape, and color of the pill. For example: **Small, round, white pill.**

In the third column, write when to take the medicine. For example: **Before breakfast.**

When you take a medicine, place an **x** in the column for the day of the week. If you take a medicine more than once a day, mark it each time.

Make copies of the form. Use it every day.

416

Weekly Medicine Record

Your Name _____

Week of _____

Name of Medicine and Dose	Size, Shape, and Color of Pill	When to Take	Place an X after each medicine when taken						
			Sun	Mon	Tues	Wed	Thur	Fri	Sat
1									
2									
3									
4									

Figure 44.1.

Additional Resources

If you want more information about heart failure and its treatment, bookstores and your local public library have helpful books and articles about the subject. Hospitals and health care providers may also have booklets, brochures, videotapes, and audiotapes about heart failure for patients. You may also contact:

The American Heart Association
7272 Greenville Avenue
Dallas, TX 75231-4596
(800) AHA-USA1 (242-8721)

National Heart, Lung, and Blood Institute Information Center
Public Health Service
P.O. Box 30105
Bethesda, MD 20824
(301) 251-1222

For More Information

Information in this booklet was taken from *Heart Failure: Evaluation and Care of Patients With Left-Ventricular Systolic Dysfunction. Clinical Practice Guideline*. The guideline was developed by a private, non-Federal expert panel of physicians, nurses, pharmacists, and consumers. Development of the guideline was sponsored by the Agency for Health Care Policy and Research (AHCPR), an agency of the U.S. Public Health Service. Other guidelines on common health problems have been issued and are under development for release in the future.

For more information on guidelines and to receive more copies of this booklet, call toll free (800) 358-9295 or write to:

AHCPR Publications Clearinghouse
P.O. Box 8547
Silver Spring, MD 20907

Chapter 45

Managing Unstable Angina

What Is Unstable Angina?

Unstable angina is a type of coronary artery disease. The coronary arteries bring oxygen-rich blood to your heart. Because your heart is a muscle it needs oxygen to work well. In coronary artery disease one or more of these arteries may be partially or even completely blocked.

The type of coronary artery disease you have usually depends on the amount of blockage in your arteries. A heart attack, called a myocardial infarction, means the heart muscle has been damaged by not getting enough blood. Stable angina usually does not damage the heart. Unstable angina is worse than stable angina and may progress to a heart attack if not treated.

Angina is caused by a lack of oxygen in the heart muscle. The symptoms of angina include pain or discomfort in the chest, arms, back, neck, or jaw. Sometimes, anginal pain may feel like a tightness or crushing sensation, or it may be a stabbing pain or seem like numbness. Some people mistake anginal pain as indigestion or gas pain.

Having either stable or unstable angina does not always mean you will have a heart attack. But, unstable angina can be serious and should be treated by a doctor.

NIH Pub. No. 94-0604

Purpose of This Booklet

The purpose of this booklet is to describe unstable angina and how it relates to other heart conditions, answer some common questions about this condition, and describe the main types of treatments available.

This booklet is written for people who have been told they have unstable angina, have been treated before for coronary artery disease, or think they might have coronary artery disease. It is also for people with a family member or friend who has unstable angina or stable angina.

This booklet also suggests some questions to ask your doctor, as well as the best time to ask them.

How Are Stable and Unstable Angina Different?

Anginal discomfort may be different for different people. Some people have anginal discomfort when they over-exert themselves (for example, when they shovel snow). Other people feel anginal pain when they get very upset or excited. Over time, they can usually tell which activities will give them discomfort. Usually, the discomfort will go away in a few minutes. This type of chest discomfort is called stable angina.

Stable angina attacks usually have a regular pattern. But in some people the pattern of angina is different—it becomes unstable.

People with unstable angina include those who:

- Have anginal discomfort when they are resting or that awakens them from sleep.
- Suddenly develop moderate or severe discomfort on exertion when they have never had angina before.
- Have a marked increase in the frequency or severity of their discomfort.

Unstable angina is more serious than stable angina because the risk of having a heart attack is greater.

What Causes Unstable Angina?

In coronary artery disease, blockages—made up of fats, such as cholesterol, and other debris—form on the inside walls of the coronary arteries. In patients who have stable angina, the blockages may not seriously block the flow of blood.

In unstable angina, the blockages may be large. Sometimes, the blockage cracks open. When this happens, your body tries to heal the crack in the blockage by making a blood clot around the damage. If the clot is big enough to block the artery, the clot will keep blood flow from getting through. This can cause a heart attack.

Do I Need to See a Doctor?

This may depend on whether or not your doctor has ever told you that you have coronary artery disease.

If you have chest pain like that described in the section "Chest Pain Can Be An Emergency, " you should call an ambulance and then your doctor.

People Without Known Coronary Artery Disease

Many people do not know if they have heart disease. Any new or severe chest discomfort that is not related to an injury, such as a pulled muscle, could be unstable angina or a heart attack.

Unstable angina is not dangerous to most people who get medical care right away, but it can be very serious if it is not treated. Even anginal pain that goes away with rest can be serious. Only your doctor will be able to tell how serious it is and what should be done.

People with Known Coronary Artery Disease

If you have coronary artery disease, your past symptoms are the best guide to whether you should call your doctor about new symptoms. Call your doctor if the discomfort you are having is more severe or lasts longer than the discomfort you have had before, has begun to happen more frequently or with less effort, or happens when you are resting or asleep.

Chest Pain Can Be an Emergency

Here are some signs that your angina is very serious and you should go to the hospital right away:

421

- Pain or discomfort that is very bad, gets worse, and lasts longer than 20 minutes.
- Pain or discomfort along with weakness, feeling sick to your stomach, or fainting.
- Pain or discomfort that does not go away when you take three nitroglycerin tablets.
- Pain or discomfort that is worse than you have ever had before.

If you live in an area where ambulance service is not quickly available, have someone drive you to the nearest hospital. You should not drive yourself to the hospital.

It is a good idea to talk with your family, friends, or neighbors about your heart condition and have them read this booklet. They should be familiar with warning signs that signal when you should go to the hospital. You also may want to tell them which medicines you are taking and where you keep them.

What Will Happen in the Emergency Room?

At your hospital emergency room, the doctors and nurses will decide if you have unstable angina. If you do have unstable angina, they will give you medicines through a vein in your arm to stop your pain and prevent injury to your heart. These medicines will help prevent blood clots and help your heart work more easily. You probably will be given oxygen to help you breathe and get more oxygen in your blood.

The doctors and nurses will ask how you are feeling and if the medicines have stopped your discomfort. It is important to tell them how you really feel. If the medicines do not stop your discomfort, there are other things they can do to help you.

These things need to be done quickly. The doctors and nurses may not be able to explain everything as it is happening. There will be time for you to ask questions after your doctor finds out how serious your condition is.

What Is an Electrocardiogram?

When you are in the emergency room you may have an electrocardiogram, called an ECG or EKG. An ECG records on paper the electrical activity of your heart beat. The ECG may show your doctor if your heart muscle is getting enough oxygen-rich blood.

Will I Have to Stay in the Hospital?

Your ECG, past medical history, and the nature of your pain tell your doctor how serious your problem is.

If your doctor does not consider your condition to be serious enough to admit you to the hospital, he or she may make an appointment to see you in a day or two for more tests. If your chest discomfort comes back before this appointment and is like that described in "Chest Pain Can Be an Emergency" you should return immediately to the hospital.

It is not easy to accurately diagnose unstable angina, and your doctor may need to see you more than once to be sure.

If your doctor suggests admission to a hospital, you may be put in a regular bed or in an intensive care unit. In either case, treatment will continue while your doctor does more tests.

The tests you have will depend on how serious your condition is and how well the medicines control your discomfort.

What Tests Will I Have?

There is more than one kind of test your doctor can do to decide how badly your coronary arteries are blocked. Some of these tests are usually done while you are in the hospital. Other tests can be done in the hospital, but you do not have to stay overnight. Some tests can be done in your doctor's office.

Stress Tests

You may have an exercise tolerance test. In this test you will be asked to ride a stationary bicycle or walk on a treadmill while a doctor takes an ECG. Your doctor may give you an injection of a radioactive drug that shows up on special cameras. This allows your doctor to make pictures of how your heart moves and the way your blood flows.

This test will let the doctor see the changes that take place in your heart when you exercise. Trained personnel or the doctor will watch your condition by asking how you are feeling during the test. Be sure to follow their instructions carefully and tell them exactly how you feel.

If you have other health problems, you may be given another kind of stress test that does not use exercise. If you have this test, you will be given a special type of drug that makes your heart beat faster and opens your coronary arteries. An ECG will be taken at the same time. This test gives the doctor the same type of information as the exercise tolerance test.

The exercise tolerance test or other stress test will help your doctor tell how well your heart is functioning. Although stress tests are useful, they cannot tell your doctor exactly where your arteries are blocked or how bad the blockages may be. Also, these tests are accurate no more than 90 percent of the time. In some cases, doctors will want to do a cardiac catheterization.

Cardiac Catheterization

An angiogram or cardiac catheterization (sometimes called a cath) lets the doctor see the coronary arteries. A thin tube, called a catheter, is placed in an artery in either your arm or leg. The catheter is threaded up to your heart while your doctor watches on a screen.

The catheter will measure the blood pressure in your heart to see how well it is pumping blood. Then, a liquid is injected through the catheter into the artery, and x-rays are taken. The x-rays allow the doctor to see how much blockage there is and where it is located.

Cardiac catheterization is a test and not a treatment for unstable angina. A treatment called angioplasty looks and feels a lot like cardiac catheterization. Angioplasty is described [in a separate section below].

What Can These Tests Show?

Stress testing may help your doctor decide how much of the heart could be in danger from blockages in your arteries. An angiogram shows how severe the blockages are and where they are. If you are told that you have single, two, or three-vessel disease, it means that one, two, or three of the major coronary arteries have a blockage. Your doctor may also talk about the percentage of blockage in the vessel.

The number of blocked arteries and the percentage of blockage are used to measure the severity of your coronary artery disease. Generally, the greater the number of vessels that are blocked, the higher the percentage of blockage, and the more poorly your heart pumps blood, the more severe the disease.

These tests will give your doctor a lot of information about your condition. At this point, he or she can start to give you more information about how serious your condition is and the types of treatment available.

Treatment of Unstable Angina

After your tests, you and your doctor can decide on which treatment you should have. The treatment that is best for you will depend on the results of your tests, whether or not you are still having discomfort, and your own preferences. In general you will have three choices: medical therapy, angioplasty, or bypass surgery.

Medical Therapy

You may have been given medicine in the hospital or emergency room. Some of these medicines, such as heparin which is used to decrease blood clotting, are given to you only in the hospital.

Many other medicines used to treat unstable angina can be taken at home. They come in the form of pills or creams that you can use by yourself.

Many people do very well on medicine alone. If you decide to use medicine to treat your unstable angina, and it does not control all your discomfort, you can still have bypass surgery or angioplasty later.

Almost everyone who has unstable angina will be given some type of medicine. The nurses or doctors caring for you will explain how and when to take all your medicines.

Several types of medicine can help to relieve the discomfort of unstable angina. Many of these drugs also make it easier for the heart to work. Medical therapy may be used alone or in combination with the other treatments described later in this booklet.

Medical therapy alone also may be the right treatment for people with other illnesses and people who do not want to have surgery or other procedures.

Medical therapy alone may benefit patients who:

- Have a blockage or blockages in only one vessel
- Have a less severe blockage
- Do not have severe anginal discomfort
- Have stabilized in the hospital

Here are some questions to ask your doctor about medical treatment.

- What side effects will I have from the medicine?
- Will I have to take medicine for the rest of my life?

Some people have uncomfortable side effects from the medicine, but most people feel better because they have less anginal discomfort. If you do have a reaction to a medicine, be sure to tell your doctor about it. Often the reaction goes away or becomes less severe with time. If not, your doctor may be able to change your medicine to make you more comfortable.

Remember, none of these drugs removes any of the blockages from your arteries. They do relieve anginal discomfort by bringing more blood to your heart or by making it easier for your heart to work.

Some of the most common medicines given to patients with unstable angina include aspirin, nitrates, and beta blockers.

Aspirin

How it works: Most people think of aspirin as something to relieve a headache or a fever. But aspirin also can prevent blood clots from forming. These are the same kind of blood clots that can block the coronary arteries and cause a heart attack.

Research in patients with unstable angina has proven that taking an aspirin every day reduces the risk of heart attack or death. Acetaminophen (for example, Tylenol®) and ibuprofen (for example, Advil®) are not the same as aspirin and should not be used in place of aspirin.

Side effects: Most patients with unstable angina will be told to take aspirin every day. Your doctor will tell you how much to take. When coated or buffered aspirin is used there are few major side effects. Aspirin should not be used if you are allergic to it or if you have had an ulcer or any other bleeding problem.

Nitrates

How they work: Nitrates (usually nitroglycerin and isosorbide) are used to open blood vessels. Nitrates increase blood flow to the heart muscle and the blood vessels and make it easier for the heart to work. Nitrates can relieve most anginal discomfort very quickly.

Nitrates come in tablets that you put under your tongue or a different type of tablet that you swallow, as a patch that you wear on your skin, or as a cream that you apply on your skin.

Nitrate tablets, cream, and patches all have a limited shelf life after which they will no longer work. Ask your pharmacist how long they will last and when you should replace them.

Nitrate cream and patches are for maintenance therapy only. If you are using a nitrate patch or cream, you should still use nitrate tablets if you have anginal discomfort.

Take one nitroglycerin tablet as soon as you feel discomfort. If the discomfort does not go away in 5 minutes, take a second tablet. If the discomfort does not go away after 5 more minutes, take a third tablet.

If the discomfort has not gone away after taking three tablets in 15 minutes, go to the hospital immediately. Do not wait!

Persistent discomfort that does not go away could be a sign that you are having a heart attack. You should see a doctor immediately.

Side effects: You may feel dizzy or lightheaded right after taking nitrates. Patients are usually told to take nitrate tablets while sitting down. Some people may also get a headache when they take nitrates.

Beta Blockers

How they work: This drug decreases the amount of work your heart has to do and the amount of oxygen your heart needs.

Side effects: Beta blockers are very powerful drugs that can have many side effects. About 10 percent of patients taking beta blockers will feel tired or dizzy. Depression, diarrhea, or skin rash may also happen in about 5 percent of patients. Mental confusion, headaches, heartburn, and shortness of breath are much less common.

Angioplasty

This procedure is done like an angiogram. A thin tube called a catheter is inserted into an artery in the groin and threaded up to the blocked artery. This catheter has a very small balloon attached on the end. When the catheter gets to the blockage, the doctor inflates the balloon. When the balloon is deflated, the blockage should be open enough for the blood to get through, stopping the anginal discomfort.

Benefits and Risks of Angioplasty

Possible benefits

- Relieve anginal pain
- Increase activity/exercise
- Allow return to former activities
- Reduce amount of medicine
- Decrease anxiety/fear

Possible risks

- Worsened angina
- Emergency bypass surgery
- Heart attack
- Damage to the artery
- Re-blockage of the artery
- Death

Questions to ask your doctor about angioplasty include:

- Will I need additional angioplasty or bypass surgery in the future?
- What will it feel like to have angioplasty?
- What is the chance that I might die during the angioplasty procedure or have other problems?

Bypass Surgery

Surgery is usually recommended for patients who have severe blockages in the left main coronary artery or disease in several vessels. Surgery is also an option when medicines do not control anginal symptoms.

Coronary artery bypass surgery can be a very effective way to increase the amount of blood getting to your heart and stop your discomfort.

In this operation, a piece of a vein, usually from your leg or an artery from your chest, is removed and used to "bypass" the section of your artery that has the most blockage. One end of the blood vessel is placed into your aorta. The aorta is the artery that supplies all the blood going out of your heart into your body. The other end is sewn into the artery below the blocked section to bypass the blockage.

Here are some questions to ask your doctor about bypass surgery:

- What will it feel like to have bypass surgery?
- Is it normal to be afraid of having surgery?
- What is the chance that I might die during surgery or have other problems?
- Will I need more surgery in the future?

Benefits and Risks of Coronary Artery Bypass Surgery

Possible benefits

- Prolong life
- Relieve anginal pain
- Increase activity/exercise
- Allow return to former activities
- Reduce need for medicine
- Decrease anxiety/fear

Possible risks

- Bleeding, requiring more surgery
- Wound infection
- Stroke
- Blood clots
- Organ failure (liver, kidney, lung)
- Heart attack
- Death

Angioplasty or Bypass Surgery?

Both angioplasty and bypass surgery are designed to do the same thing. They both can increase the supply of blood to your heart muscle. Depending on the severity of your disease, you may have a choice between the two.

How will you know which one is right for you? Your doctor will help you make this decision. But in general, angioplasty:

- Is not as major a procedure as bypass surgery.
- Results in a shorter hospital stay.
- Will allow you to return to normal activities sooner.

You should also know that:

- In about 2 to 5 percent of cases, angioplasty does not work, and emergency bypass surgery will be necessary.
- About 40 percent of the time, the arteries become blocked again within 6 months of the angioplasty. If this happens, you may have to have angioplasty again or have bypass surgery.

Talking with Your Health Care Team

Some people think that their doctors are too busy to answer questions. Other people do not know how to ask their questions. But talking with the doctors, nurses, and other health care providers is an important part of your care.

Your questions are important, and the people taking care of you should make the time to answer your questions and listen to what you have to say. Your preferences for the type of treatment you receive are very important.

You may feel more comfortable if a family member or friend is there when you talk to your doctors, nurses, and other health care providers. This person can help to make sure that you understand what is happening, ask questions, and tell the doctor your concerns and preferences for care.

Here are some questions to ask your doctor before you decide what the best treatment might be for you.

- Am I a candidate for medical treatment, angioplasty, or bypass surgery?
- What are the chances that my arteries will become blocked again if I have angioplasty or bypass surgery? How soon might this happen?
- Will I have to change my job or retire?
- How soon can I resume my normal activities? What about resuming sexual activity?
- How much will my treatment cost?
- Do I have to go on a low-sodium or low-fat diet? If so, for how long?

• Will I have a heart attack? Will I always have chest pain?

Can Blockages Come Back?

Neither angioplasty nor bypass surgery is a cure for coronary artery disease. Blockages continue to build up on artery walls even after angioplasty or bypass surgery.

Both angioplasty and bypass surgery can be repeated if the arteries become blocked again. The only way to stop coronary artery disease is to prevent the blockages from building up.

Although doctors do not know for sure why blockages form, they do know, from studies of large numbers of patients, that some people are more likely to have blocked arteries than others.

Your doctor may recommend that you attend a cardiac rehabilitation program. These programs usually are offered by local hospitals and very often they are covered by insurance. In a rehabilitation program, nurses, exercise specialists, and doctors will help you to change behaviors that put you at higher risk. They will also teach you how to exercise safely and help you gain confidence in your ability to live with heart disease.

Preventing Blockages

The best way to prevent blockages from forming is to:

• Take aspirin every day
• Stop smoking
• Eat foods that are lower in fat
• Keep weight down
• Increase physical activity
• Control blood pressure if it is high
• Lower stress

Living with Coronary Artery Disease

It is normal for you to worry about your health and your future. But, you should know that most people with unstable angina do not have heart attacks. Usually, angina becomes more stable within 8 weeks. In fact, people who are treated for their unstable angina can live productive lives for many years.

431

Coronary artery disease does not go away. Your behavior and lifestyle will affect your condition. This is why it is so important to follow the advice of your doctor and the other health care professionals who treat you.

Every year, thousands of people are told they have coronary artery disease. This may come as a shock, especially if they have never felt ill before. Often, they become anxious about their future and wonder if they will still be able to take care of their families or other responsibilities. It is normal to feel a loss of control, as if something has taken over your life.

Doctors, nurses, members of the clergy, and counselors all have experience in helping people with coronary artery disease. They can help you and your family. It is important to talk about how you feel, not just physically, but emotionally.

The best way to feel like you are in control is to learn more about coronary artery disease—what it is and the choices you have. When you see your doctor or other health care provider, be prepared to ask questions.

How Can I Learn More about Unstable Angina?

Organizations that can provide additional information include:

American Heart Association
7272 Greenville Avenue
Dallas, TX 75231-4596
Phone: (800) AHA-USA1

National Heart, Lung, and Blood Institute Information Center
P.O. Box 30105
Bethesda, MD 20824
Phone: (301) 251-1222

The Mended Hearts, Inc.
7272 Greenville Avenue
Dallas, TX 75231-4596
Phone: (214) 373-6300

For Further Information

The information in this booklet was based on the *Clinical Practice Guideline on Unstable Angina*. The guideline was developed by a private-sector panel of experts, including physicians, surgeons, nurses, and people with unstable angina.

Support for this guideline was provided by the Agency for Health Care Policy and Research and the National Heart, Lung, and Blood Institute. Other guidelines on common health problems are available, and more are being developed.

For more information on guidelines or to receive another copy of this booklet, call toll free (800) 358-9295 or write to:

Agency for Health Care Policy and Research
Publications Clearinghouse
P.O. Box 8547
Silver Spring, MD 20907

Chapter 46

Living with Your Pacemaker

An artificial pacemaker works in about the same way as your heart's natural pacemaker. It's a small unit that uses batteries to produce the electrical impulses that make your heart pump. The impulses flow through tiny wires to your heart, and are timed to flow at regular intervals just as impulses from your heart's natural pacemaker would normally do. With the help of an artificial pacemaker your heart should pump almost as well as it did before problems developed.

Significant technological advances have taken place in recent years in pacemakers. Modern pacemakers last much longer than earlier models; some, in fact, are nuclear-powered. As with any electronic device, your artificial pacemaker will require some care. The batteries, for example, will wear down over time and will need to be replaced. As the batteries wear down, your pacemaker will slow down, but it won't stop. The first warning that the batteries are wearing out will be a change in your pulse rate. If your pulse suddenly drops to 40 or 50 beats per minute, tell your doctor.

Here are some guidelines for pacemakers and pulse counts:

- If your pacemaker is beating regularly and at its proper rate, you can be assured it's okay.

Excerpts from American Heart Association Pub. No. 50-1003 (CP). Used by Permission. Editor's comments are bracketed.

- If your pacemaker is beating within the accepted rate but it has an occasional irregularity, don't worry. Occasionally your own heart's natural pacemaker competes with the manmade pacemaker.
- If your pulse rate suddenly drops to the 40s or 50s (usually within the first few months after it was installed), **call your doctor immediately**. A wire may be broken or there may be some other problem.
- If your pacemaker is installed for a fast-slow type of heartbeat and your pulse is rapid and irregular (above 100 beats per minute), **call your doctor for further instructions**.
- If your pacemaker is beating faster than it should be, but below 100, don't be alarmed. Before you leave the hospital, discuss the specific maximum heart rate above your pacemaker rate that's acceptable. Discussing this with your doctor early in your treatment will keep you from worrying unnecessarily.

[Other things that you will have to do if you have an artificial pacemaker include:]

- Take prescribed medications.
- Follow all instructions regarding diet and physical activity.
- Avoid causing pressure over the area of your chest where your pacemaker was inserted.
- Tell doctors and others that you have a pacemaker.
- Always carry your identification card. [You can obtain an pacemaker identification card by contacting your local American Heart Association or by calling 1-800-AHA-USA1.]
- Keep all appointments with your doctor.

[The American Heart Association also directs you to] report to your doctor if: a) You have difficulty breathing; b) You begin to gain weight and your legs and ankles swell; c) You faint, blackout or have dizzy spells.

[For more information about the heart's normal function see Chapter 1; for information about arrhythmias in adults see Chapter 6; for information about heart rhythm abnormalities in children refer to Chapter 22.]

Chapter 47

How to Take Your Medicine

Beta Blocker Drugs

Conditions These Drugs Treat

All beta blockers are used to treat high blood pressure. Many are also used to prevent the heart-related chest pain or pressure associated with angina pectoris (a condition often occurring during exertion where too little blood reaches the heart). Atenolol, metoprolol, timolol, and propranolol are used to improve survival after a heart attack. Propranolol is used to treat heart rhythm problems, other specific heart conditions, migraine headaches, and tremors. Beta blockers can be used for other conditions as determined by your doctor.

Beta blockers cannot cure these conditions. However, by blocking certain receptors in the body, beta blockers lower and regulate the heartbeat and lessen the heart's workload.

While taking beta blockers, it is important that you continue any diet and exercise program prescribed by your doctor, as these are often important parts of the therapy for the conditions being treated.

How to Take

Beta blockers can be taken either with food or on an empty stomach.

FDA Consumer, December 1990 and May 1991.

If you are taking an extended-release product such as Inderal LAR (propranolol), swallow it whole. Don't chew it or crush it in any way.

If you are taking the concentrated solution of propranolol, always use the dropper provided. You can mix the solution with water or any other beverage (or, if you prefer, pudding or applesauce). After taking a dose, rinse the glass with some liquid and drink that liquid as well to be sure that the entire dose is taken.

Be sure to take the right number of tablets or capsules for each dose. Taking your medicine at the same time each day will help you remember to take it regularly.

Missed Doses

Do not suddenly stop taking a beta blocker without first talking to your doctor. Your condition could worsen if you stop taking this medicine or miss many doses.

If you miss a dose, take it as soon as you remember. If you take the beta blocker once a day, you can take it up to eight hours before the next scheduled dose. If you take the medication more often than once a day, you can take it up to four hours before the next scheduled dose. Ask your doctor or pharmacist if you have questions.

Never take two doses at the same time.

Always have enough of your beta blocker medicine to last over weekends, holiday periods, and when you travel.

Relief of Symptoms

For conditions such as high blood pressure, angina, heart rhythm disturbances, or tremors, some effects can be seen immediately and usually peak within a week. If treating migraine headaches, it may take up to six weeks before the full effects occur. For any of these conditions, the dosage of the beta blocker may need to be adjusted by your doctor when you first begin taking it. Also, the appropriate dosage can vary greatly among people, depending on individual response.

Since many of the conditions that beta blockers treat are chronic, you may have to take this medicine for the rest of your life.

Side Effects and Risks

Common side effects include slowed heartbeat, tiredness, nausea, diarrhea, constipation, and decreased sexual ability. Other mild side effects can include difficulty sleeping or nightmares, headache, drowsiness, and numbness or tingling of the fingers, toes or scalp. Also, if you have diabetes, beta blockers can obscure some of the signs of low blood sugar, such as tremors or rapid heartbeat. Check with your doctor if any of these side effects seems troublesome or if you have any questions.

More serious reactions can sometimes occur with beta blockers. These include the following:

- the beginning or worsening of heart failure. Symptoms of this include shortness of breath (especially on exertion), coughing, weakness, weight gain, and swelling of feet, ankles, or lower legs.

- severe wheezing or difficulty breathing, especially in people who have or have had asthma, chronic bronchitis, emphysema, or other breathing conditions. Because beta blockers can trigger or worsen these conditions, make sure your doctor knows about them.

- an extremely slow heartbeat (less than 50 beats per minute)

- cold hands and feet or blue fingernails, which could mean reduced circulation to these areas

- confusion, hallucinations or depression. If any of these or other serious reactions occur, call your doctor immediately.

Precautions and Warnings

If you suddenly stop taking a beta blocker, you could worsen your condition and experience potentially dangerous side effects, such as chest pain, fast or irregular heartbeat, high blood pressure, and headaches. Always check with your doctor before discontinuing a beta blocker.

Consult with your doctor if you think you could become pregnant or plan to breast-feed while on a beta blocker.

Learn how the medicine affects you. Don't drive or operate machines if this medicine makes you drowsy, dizzy or lightheaded. If you are taking labetalol, dizziness or lightheadedness can occur when getting up from sitting or lying down. If this happens, sit up slowly, placing your legs over the side of the bed or couch, and stay there for a few minutes before trying to stand.

Before any surgery or dental work, tell the physician or dentist that you are taking beta blockers. Tell your physician if you are taking or considering taking any other prescription or nonprescription medication.

Drinking alcohol while on beta blockers can sometimes increase the chance of side effects such as dizziness or tiredness.

Generic Names

- acebutolol
- atenolol
- betaxolol
- carteolol
- labetalol
- metoprolol
- nadolol
- penbutolol
- pindolol
- propranolol
- timolol

Drug Tips

Don't store drugs in the bathroom medicine cabinet. Heat and humidity may cause the medicine to lose its effectiveness. Keep all medicines, even those with child-resistant caps, out of the reach of children. Remember, the caps are child-resistant, not child-proof. Discard medicines that have reached the expiration date.

—by Igor Cerney

Igor Cerney is on the staff of FDA's Drug Labeling, Education and Research Branch.

Angiotensin-Converting Enzyme Inhibitors

Conditions These Drugs Treat

All angiotensin-converting enzyme (ACE) inhibitors are used to treat high blood pressure. In addition, captopril and enalapril are used to treat heart failure, usually only after other medications, such as digitalis, have been tried. ACE inhibitors can be used for other conditions as determined by your doctor.

How to Take

Captopril should be taken on an empty stomach one hour before meals. All other ACE inhibitors can be taken without regard to meals.

ACE inhibitors are potent medicines that treat but do not cure chronic conditions such as high blood pressure. That is why it is important to take the ACE inhibitor regularly and make sure you're taking the right amount. Taking doses at the same time each day will help you remember to take the drug regularly. Continue any diet and exercise program prescribed by your doctor.

Missed Doses

If you miss a dose, take it as soon as you remember. As a rough guideline, estimate the number of hours between when you should have taken your missed dose and when your next dose is scheduled (if you take it twice a day, for instance, the time between doses is 12 hours). If you have passed the halfway point (which is six hours in this example), do not take the missed dose. Instead, continue with your next regularly scheduled dose. Do not take two doses at the same time.

Relief of Symptoms

ACE inhibitors begin to work immediately after the first dose. However, a few weeks may be needed before the full effects occur. The dosage of the ACE inhibitor may need to be adjusted by your doctor when you first begin taking it.

Side Effects and Risks

Fatigue, dizziness, headache, insomnia, nausea, vomiting, and diarrhea are all common side effects. These are all usually mild.

Loss of the taste sense can occur, especially with captopril. Taste usually returns within two to three months, even if you are still on the medication. Sometimes slight weight loss can accompany the loss of taste.

Some people develop a persistent dry cough while taking ACE inhibitors. The cough usually does not go away unless the medication is stopped. If this side effect occurs and is bothersome, you should discuss it with your doctor.

ACE inhibitors can cause dizziness, lightheadedness, or even fainting, usually during the first few days. These effects are due to lowered blood pressure and occur mostly when getting up from sitting or prone position. Consult your doctor if these symptoms persist, especially if fainting occurs. Sometimes changes in the dosage of the ACE inhibitor or other medications can ease these symptoms.

A mild, sometimes itchy, skin rash can occur and may be accompanied by fever or joint pains. This usually happens within the first four weeks of beginning an ACE inhibitor, especially captopril. Consult your doctor if this occurs since dosage changes or other medications can help clear the rash.

More serious but infrequent reactions that sometimes occur with ACE inhibitors are:

- *Fever and chills.* Although rare, ACE inhibitors (mostly captopril) can cause a decrease in certain white blood cells, increasing susceptibility to infections. Common symptoms include fever, chills, sore throat, and mouth sores. If these symptoms occur, contact your doctor immediately. The lowered cell count is usually reversible.

- *Allergic reaction.* This is evidenced by sudden difficulty in swallowing or breathing; hoarseness; flushed or pale complexion; and swelling of the face, mouth, hands, or feet. Stop taking the medication immediately, and call your doctor or seek emergency help if the symptoms are severe.

- *Chest (heart-related) pain, rapid or pounding heartbeat.* These symptoms tend to occur most often when you first start taking an ACE inhibitor.

If these serious reactions or other new symptoms occur, contact your doctor immediately.

Precautions and Warnings

Do not stop taking an ACE inhibitor on your own.

ACE inhibitors can sometimes cause a reversible decrease in kidney function. Your doctor may periodically check your kidney function by either blood or urine tests while you are on the medication. If you notice your feet or ankles swelling or weight gain, notify your doctor.

Exercising in hot weather, excessive perspiration, vomiting, or diarrhea can lead to loss of fluid (dehydration) and intensify the ability of ACE inhibitors to lower blood pressure. Low blood pressure could lead to severe dizziness or even fainting. Consult your physician if any of these conditions occurs.

ACE inhibitors can occasionally cause the body to retain too much potassium. Rarely, potassium excess in the body can cause confusion, irregular heartbeat, weakness in the legs, nervousness, or tingling in the hands, feet or lips. If any of these occurs, contact your doctor immediately. Also, consult your doctor before using any salt substitutes, since many of these contain potassium.

Diabetic patients who test their urine for acetone should be aware that captopril can cause a false-positive reading.

Animal studies show ACE inhibitors may cause problems during pregnancy. In a few human reports, some babies of mothers taking ACE inhibitors have been born with very low blood pressure. Let your doctor know if you are or intend to become pregnant while on an ACE inhibitor.

Captopril is secreted into breast milk. It is not known if either enalapril or lisinopril gets into breast milk. In general, breast-feeding is not recommended while taking these drugs unless directed by a doctor.

Common Names

- captopril (Capoten)
- enalapril (Vasotec)
- lisinopril (Prinivil, Zestril)

443

- ramipril (Altace)

—by Igor Cerney

Chapter 48

Dental Care for
Adults with Heart Disease

If you have heart disease, you need special consideration when you get dental treatment.

Several heart problems require you and your dentist to take special precautions. These include:

Heart Attack

Until a person has completely recovered from a heart attack, only emergency dental care should be performed.

Irregular Heartbeat

Minor irregularities of the heartbeat ordinarily aren't affected by dental treatment. Certain serious heartbeat irregularities treated by drugs or a pacemaker may be affected by dental procedures or by drugs used in dental treatment, however. Check with your physician about the specifics of your condition.

Heart Failure

If you're taking medication for heart failure, it's especially important to maintain good dental health. Dental infection associated with

Excerpts from American Heart Association Pub. No. 50-1002 (SA). Used by Permission. Editor's comments are bracketed.

445

severe pain or high fever can seriously increase your heart's workload and interfere with the beneficial effects of these medications.

Angina Pectoris

If you're subject to angina, tell your dentist what's likely to trigger an attack. And carry a fresh supply of nitroglycerine or other comparable medicine to your dental appointment. If the stress of a dental procedure causes an attack of angina, postpone the procedure until a later date if possible.

Heart Murmur [and Other Problems that May Require the Use of Antibiotics]

Structural abnormalities in the heart make the valves or lining of the heart more susceptible to serious infection (infective or bacterial endocarditis) when bacteria enter the bloodstream. And bacteria can enter the bloodstream from any dental procedure that causes bleeding. Consequently, if you have a significant murmur, special precautions during your dental treatment will be required. Antibiotics may be used to prevent infection.

[Other conditions that may require antibiotic treatment to prevent infection include:

- Artificial Heart Valves
- Heart Pacemaker, and
- Vascular Surgery]

Chapter 49

Sex and Heart Disease

Sex After a Heart Attack or Heart Surgery

If you're like most people, there's no reason why you can't resume sexual activity as soon as you feel ready. Still, just to be sure, check with your doctor or rehabilitation nurse first.

A heart patient's interest in sex can be affected by such factors as age and how long a relationship has lasted. Previous sex drive and sexual satisfaction also can play a significant role. Usually both men and women resume sexual activities within a few weeks after a heart attack or heart surgery.

Intercourse takes slightly more energy than other sexual activities. Consequently, most doctors suggest that you wait until you feel stronger before you resume sexual relations. People who've had a heart attack are usually able to resume sex about four weeks after the attack. People who've had heart surgery may reach this point two to three weeks after they leave the hospital.

If you're not sure whether you're ready for sex, a doctor may give you an exercise test to check your physical capacity.

Excerpts from American Heart Association Pub. No. 50-1020 (CP). Used by Permission. Editor's comments are bracketed.

Will Medicines Affect Sex?

Many medicines prescribed for heart problems can affect sexual desire and performance. These include blood pressure medicines, fluid pills, tranquilizers, antidepressants and some medications used for chest pain or irregular heartbeat.

Such medications may affect sex drive and normal sexual function. Possible male sexual problems include the inability to achieve or maintain an erection (impotence). Some men also may have premature ejaculations or none at all. Possible sexual problems of women include decreased vaginal fluid for lubrication, which can make intercourse more painful. Some women may become unable to be sexually aroused (frigidity) or unable to have orgasm (orgasmic dysfunction). Also, medicines may cause the desire for sex to wane.

However, such changes may not be due to the medicine. Other possible causes should be investigated and treated.

If a sexual problem occurs, don't stop taking your medication. Instead, consult your doctor. Try not to feel shy or inhibited when you discuss the problem. Often a change in drug type or dosage can remedy it.

Preparing for Sex

Couples can prepare for sex in several ways. First, you can improve and maintain your physical condition. [Diet, exercise, and smoking cessation are important aspects to consider. **Part Seven—Lifestyle Choices for a Healthier Cardiovascular System** offers suggestions to help you, but you will also want to consult with your doctor before embarking on a new diet or exercise program.]

Another way to prepare for sex is to become tolerant of your emotions. Sometimes after the stress of a heart attack or surgery and hospitalization, you or your partner may feel vulnerable. Expect that you may each have good and bad days and positive and negative feelings about yourselves. That's normal.

Try to keep things in perspective. You and your partner should strive to be flexible and patient with one another. A good sense of humor can help a lot.

The third thing couples can do is to adjust their sexual expectations. Even though you may have had a good sexual relationship before your heart problem, you may be afraid to resume sexual relations because of your emotional and physical responses or potential problems. These are normal concerns, but don't let them stop you from enjoying each other again.

Finally, avoid the temptation to rush your sexual recovery to prove that things are "back to normal." If you and your partner have sex before you're ready for it, any fears you have won't go away. In fact, they may cause even more problems.

Couples shouldn't expect too much at first. Almost everyone has some trouble adjusting to sex after a heart attack or heart surgery. There's no risk if you, as a couple, approach sex slowly and patiently and allow it to happen.

Resuming sex often leads to a closer relationship, because it lets you rekindle tenderness and romance.

Guidelines for Resuming Sex

- Choose a time when you're both rested, relaxed and free from stress.

- It's best to wait one to three hours after eating a full meal before having sex.

- Try to select a familiar, peaceful setting where you'll be free from interruptions.

- Take medications before having sexual relations if they're prescribed by your doctor.

Changing sexual positions to put less strain on the heart is rarely necessary. However, people who've had heart surgery and still feel some discomfort from the incision may want to lie on their side facing their partner or with their partner in front or behind. These positions put less pressure on the chest wall and make breathing easier.

If you have a hard time breathing, you and your partner may prefer to sit in a chair facing each other.

The rehabilitation nurse or doctor should help you discuss your sexual preferences and explore alternatives.

Some couples, because of fear, cardiac symptoms or sexual dysfunction, may not be interested in intercourse or other sexual activities. They can still build a satisfying relationship with expressions of affection, cuddling and caressing.

What If You Experience Symptoms During Sex?

Everyone's heart beats faster and harder during sex than at rest. Breathing is faster and more labored, and the skin becomes flushed and moist. These reactions are normal.

Angina symptoms that show the heart can't handle the workload include:

- a feeling of pressure, pain or discomfort in the jaw, neck, arm, chest or stomach;
- marked shortness of breath; and
- excessively rapid or irregular heartbeats.

If you have any of these symptoms during sex, tell your partner, reduce your activity, rest and take medicine if your doctor has prescribed it. Nitroglycerine tablets, repeated three times over 12-15 minutes, may bring relief. When the symptoms go away, you and your partner may resume sexual activity. If the symptoms aren't relieved by medicine, or if they recur after resuming sex, seek medical help. If you have difficulty sleeping or resting after intercourse; notice a change in the location, frequency, or severity of angina; or are overly tired, discuss these symptoms with your doctor. You may need to make a small change in your daily routine or medication.

Chapter 50

Improving Your Blood Cholesterol Levels: What You Need To Do

Take Action: Here's How

Now that you understand why you should lower your high blood cholesterol, this [chapter] details how to do it. It covers:

- Action steps to take and the benefits to expect
- Specific guidelines for diets to lower high blood cholesterol
- Practical ways to change eating habits
- Tips to increase your physical activity

[It] also describes medicines for lowering high blood cholesterol. Medicines may become necessary for those who cannot lower their blood cholesterol through diet and exercise.

Three Steps to Reducing High Blood Cholesterol Levels

Three steps can help you reduce your high blood cholesterol:

1. Follow the Step I or Step II diet. These diets are described [below]. Your doctor will first recommend one or the other. The diets contain all the daily nutrients you need and em-

Taken from NIH Pub. No. 93-2922.

phasize eating foods that are low in saturated fat, total fat, and cholesterol, and high in starch and fiber. You will probably be asked to follow the Step I diet first to see if it brings your blood cholesterol levels down sufficiently. If not, you may have to move to the Step II diet. If you already have coronary heart disease or a very high LDL level, your doctor may recommend starting with the Step II diet.

2. Be more physically active.

3. Lose weight if you are overweight.

Fortunately, these three steps work together. For example:

• Eating less fat, especially saturated fat, also may help you decrease the amount of cholesterol and calories you eat. Why? Foods high in fat and saturated fat are high in calories and often high in cholesterol. In fact, all fats both saturated and unsaturated fat have more than twice as many calories as either carbohydrate or protein. They provide 9 calories per gram and the other two provide 4 calories per gram.

• Being more physically active helps burn more calories, which helps in weight loss. It may also help you lower your LDL-cholesterol and raise your HDL-cholesterol, as well as improve the health of your heart and lungs.

• Losing excess weight if you are overweight can help lower your LDL-cholesterol and increase your HDL-cholesterol.

How Low Will You Go?

By closely following your diet, being more physically active, and watching your progress with regular checkups, you can lower your blood cholesterol level. How much your cholesterol levels change depends on:

• How much fat, especially saturated fat, and how much cholesterol you ate before you changed your diet;
• How closely you follow the changes; and

452

- How your body responds to these changes. Usually the higher your blood cholesterol is to begin with, the more the levels go down. However, sometimes due to heredity, levels will not change enough no matter how well you change your habits.

For example: Your total blood cholesterol level is 240 mg/dL, and you are eating a diet high in saturated fat and cholesterol. By going on the Step I diet, you could reduce your cholesterol level by 5-35 mg/dL; and 5-15 mg/dL more, if you then go on Step II. Over time, you may reduce your cholesterol level by 10-50 mg/dL or even more. This drop will slow the fatty buildup in your arteries and reduce your risk of illness and death from heart attack. In fact, studies have shown that, in adults with high blood cholesterol levels, for each 1 percent reduction in total cholesterol levels, there is a 2 percent reduction in the risk of heart attack. So if you reduce your cholesterol level by 10 percent (for example, from 240 mg/dL to 216 mg/dL), your risk of heart disease could drop by 20 percent. And many people will get even more of a drop in their cholesterol level.

Learn About the Step I and Step II Diets

Step I Diet

On the Step I diet, you should eat:

- 8-10 percent of the day's total calories from saturated fat.
- 30 percent or less of the day's total calories from fat.
- Less than 300 milligrams of dietary cholesterol a day.
- Just enough calories to achieve and maintain a healthy weight. (You may want to ask your doctor or registered dietitian what is a reasonable calorie level for you.)

Step II Diet

On the Step II diet, you should eat:

- Less than 7 percent of the day's total calories from saturated fat.
- 30 percent or less of the day's total calories from fat.
- Less than 200 milligrams of dietary cholesterol a day.

• Just enough calories to achieve and maintain a healthy weight. (You may want to ask your doctor or registered dietitian what is a reasonable calorie level for you.)

Practical Ways to Change Your Diet.

Here are some tips on how to choose foods for the Step I and Step II diets. For more help, write for *Step by Step: Eating To Lower Your High Blood Cholesterol* (see [section titled "Get More Information]).
To cut back on saturated fats, choose:

• Poultry, fish, and lean cuts of meat more often. Remove the skin from chicken and trim the fat from meat.

• Skim or 1 percent milk, instead of 2 percent or whole milk.

• Cheeses with no more than 3 grams of fat per ounce (these include low-fat cottage cheese or other low-fat cheeses). Cut down on full-fat processed, natural, and hard cheeses (like American, brie, and cheddar).

• Liquid vegetable oils that are high in unsaturated fat (these include canola, corn, olive, and safflower oil). Use tub or liquid margarines that list liquid vegetable oil as the first ingredient (instead of lard and hydrogenated vegetable shortening, which are high in saturated fat). Choose products that are lowest in saturated fat on the label.

• Fewer commercially prepared and processed foods made with saturated or hydrogenated fats or oils (like cakes, cookies, and crackers). Read food labels to choose products low in saturated fats.

• Foods high in starch and fiber, instead of foods high in saturated fats.

Cutting back on saturated fat helps you to control dietary cholesterol as well. Two additional points to remember when cutting back on dietary cholesterol are:

• Eat less organ meat (such as liver, brain, and kidney).

- Eat fewer egg yolks as whole eggs or in prepared foods (try substituting two egg whites for each whole egg in recipes, or using an egg substitute).

To include more foods high in starch and fiber, choose:

- More whole grain breads and cereals, pasta, rice, and dry peas and beans.

- More vegetables and fruits.

Make Physical Activity Work for You

Regular physical activity by itself may help reduce deaths from heart disease by:

- lowering LDL levels
- raising HDL levels
- lowering high blood pressure
- lowering triglyceride levels
- reducing excess weight
- improving the fitness of your heart and lungs

If you have been inactive for a long time, start with low-to-moderate level activities such as walking, taking the stairs instead of the elevator, gardening, housework, dancing, or exercising at home. Begin by doing the activity for a few minutes most days, then work up to a longer program—at least 30 minutes per day, 3 or 4 days a week. This can include regular aerobic activities such as brisk walking, jogging, swimming, bicycling, or playing tennis.

If you have heart disease or have had a heart attack, talk with your doctor before starting an activity to be sure you are following a safe program that works for you. Otherwise you may experience chest pain or further heart damage. If you have chest pain, feel faint or light-headed, or become extremely out of breath while exercising, stop the activity at once and tell your doctor as soon as possible.

Lose Weight If You Are Overweight

Two action steps are key.

- Eat fewer calories (cutting back on the fat you eat will really help)
- Burn more calories by becoming more physically active

You May Need To Take Medicine

If you have successfully changed your eating habits for at least 6-12 months, and your LDL-cholesterol level is still too high, you may need to take medicine. Some people will need to take medicine from the start of their treatment because of a very high LDL level or the presence of heart disease.

If your doctor prescribes medicine, you also will need to:

- Follow your cholesterol-lowering diet
- Lose weight if overweight
- Be more physically active
- Stop smoking

Taking all these steps together may lessen the amount of medicine you need, or make the medicine work better. And that reduces your risk of heart disease.

Medicines Your Doctor May Prescribe

Several types of medicine can help lower blood cholesterol levels. These include:

- Major Drugs: Bile acid sequestrants (cholestyramine and colestipol); Nicotinic acid; HMG CoA reductase inhibitors or "statins" (e.g., lovastatin, pravastatin, and simvastatin)

- Other Drugs: Fibric acid derivatives (gemfibrozil); Probucol

In addition, if you are a woman going through or past menopause, your doctor may talk with you about estrogens. Sometimes called Estrogen Replacement Therapy, this can lower blood cholesterol levels, and may make it unnecessary to take a cholesterol-lowering drug.

Drugs that lower blood cholesterol work in different ways. Some may work for you while others may not. Before the doctor prescribes any medicine, be sure to state what other medicines you are taking. And once a medicine is prescribed, take it exactly the way your doctor tells you to. If you have any side effects from a medicine, tell your doctor right away. The amount or type of drug can be changed to reduce or stop unwanted side effects. *Whatever medicine you take, continue to follow the Step I or Step II diet and to be more physically active. This will help keep the dose of medicine as low as possible.*

Ask Your Health Professionals

In addition to your doctor, other health professionals can help you control your blood cholesterol levels. These persons include:

- Registered dietitians (R.D.) or qualified nutritionists, who can explain food plans and show you how to make changes in what you eat. They can give you advice on shopping for and preparing foods, and eating out. They also can help you set goals for changing the way you eat, so you can successfully lower your high blood cholesterol without making big changes all at once in your eating habits or in your lifestyle. To find a Registered Dietitian contact: The National Center for Nutrition and Dietetics' Consumer Nutrition Hotline 1-800-366-1655; Your local hospital or health department; or your doctor.

- The nurse in your doctors office, who also may be able to answer questions about your high blood cholesterol or your diet.

- Lipid specialists, who are doctors with an expertise in treating high blood cholesterol and similar conditions. In special cases, you may be referred to a lipid specialist if the treatment your doctor is prescribing does not successfully lower your blood cholesterol levels.

- Your doctor, who can answer your questions about the medicines you are taking. Be sure to tell your doctor about everything you are taking and if you feel different after you take any of them.

- Pharmacists, who are aware of the best ways to take medicines to lessen side effects and of the latest research on drugs.

Get More Information

The National Cholesterol Education Program (NCEP), coordinated by the National Heart, Lung, and Blood Institute has a pamphlet called *Step by Step: Eating to Lower Your High Blood Cholesterol.* This pamphlet gives details on how to change your eating habits in order to lower your blood cholesterol levels. The NCEP also has booklets for children with high blood cholesterol levels and their parents. In addition, the NHLBI has a booklet, *Exercise and Your Heart*, and a resource list of agencies and organizations able to answer questions on cholesterol and the other risk factors for heart disease. For these and other materials, write:

National Cholesterol Education Program
NHLBI Information Center
PO Box 30105
Bethesda, Maryland 20824-0105

The American Heart Association can also provide you with additional information. Contact your local American Heart Association or call 1-800-AHA-USA1 (1-800-242-8721).

Glossary

Atherosclerosis: A type of "hardening of the arteries" in which cholesterol, fat, and other substances in the blood build up in the walls of arteries. As the process continues, the arteries to the heart may narrow, cutting down the flow of oxygen-rich blood and nutrients to the heart.

Bile Acid Sequestrants: One type of cholesterol-lowering medication, including cholestyramine and colestipol. The sequestrants bind with cholesterol-containing bile acids in the intestines and remove them in bowel movements.

Calories: Units of measurement that represent the amount of energy the body is able to get from foods. Different nutrients in foods provide different amounts of calories. Carbohydrates and protein provide about 4 calories per gram, while fat (both saturated and unsaturated) yields about 9 calories per gram.

Carbohydrate: One of the nutrients that supply calories to the body. Carbohydrates may be simple or complex. Complex carbohydrates are also called starch and fiber, which come from plants and can be found in whole-grain breads, cereals, pasta, rice, dried peas and beans, corn, lima beans, fruits, and vegetables.

Cholesterol: A soft, waxy substance. The body makes enough cholesterol to meet its needs. Cholesterol is used in the manufacture of hormones, bile acid, and vitamin D. It is present in all parts of the body, including the nervous system, muscle, skin, liver, intestines, and heart.

- *Blood cholesterol*: Cholesterol circulating in the bloodstream. It is made in the liver and absorbed from the food you eat. The blood carries it for use by all parts of the body. A high level of blood cholesterol leads to atherosclerosis and an increased risk of heart disease.

- *Dietary cholesterol*: Cholesterol in the food you eat. It is present only in foods of animal origin, not those of plant origin. Dietary cholesterol, like dietary saturated fat, raises blood cholesterol, which increases the risk for heart disease.

Estrogen Replacement Therapy (ERT): Treatment with the hormone estrogen, which has many effects, one of which is cholesterol lowering. It includes different amounts of estrogen and progestin, two hormones produced normally by women who have menstrual periods. ERT is given only to women who have gone through menopause. ERT may help prevent heart disease by lowering blood cholesterol levels, especially LDL.

Fat: One of the nutrients that supply calories to the body. The body needs only small amounts of fat. Foods contain different types of fat, which have different effects on blood cholesterol levels. These include:

- *Total fat*: The sum of the saturated, monounsaturated, and polyunsaturated fats present in food. All foods have a varying mix of these three types.

- *Saturated fat*: A type of fat found in greatest amounts in foods from animals, such as fatty cuts of meat, poultry with the skin, whole-milk dairy products, lard, and in some vegetable oils, including coconut, palm kernel, and palm oils. Saturated fat raises blood cholesterol more than anything else eaten.

- *Unsaturated fat*: A type of fat that is usually liquid at refrigerator temperature. Monounsaturated fat and polyunsaturated fat are two kinds of unsaturated fat. When used in place of saturated fat, monounsaturated and polyunsaturated fats help to lower blood cholesterol levels.

- *Monounsaturated fat:* An unsaturated fat that is found in greatest amounts in foods from plants, including olive and canola oil.

- *Polyunsaturated fat*: An unsaturated fat found in greatest amounts in foods from plants, including safflower, sunflower, corn, and soybean oils.

Fibric Acid Derivatives: One type of cholesterol-lowering drug. It includes gemfibrozil. The fibric acids lower triglycerides and raise HDLs.

HMG CoA Reductase Inhibitors: See "Statins."

Lipids: Fatty substances, including cholesterol and triglycerides, that are present in blood and body tissues.

Lipoproteins: Protein-coated packages that carry fat and cholesterol through the bloodstream. Lipoproteins are classified according to their density.

- *High-density lipoprotein (HDL)*: Lipoproteins that contain a small amount of cholesterol and carry cholesterol away from body cells and tissues to the liver for excretion from the body. A low level of HDL increases the risk of heart disease, so the higher the HDL level, the better. HDL is sometimes called the "good" cholesterol.

- *Low-density lipoprotein (LDL)*: Lipoproteins that contain most of the cholesterol in the blood. LDL, the "bad" cholesterol, carries cholesterol to the tissues of the body including the arteries. For this reason, a high level of LDL increases the risk of heart disease.

Lipoprotein Profile: A test that uses blood from the arm to measure your total, HDL-, and LDL-cholesterol, and triglyceride levels. The test requires a fast for 9-12 hours beforehand. Nothing can be consumed but water, or coffee or tea with no cream or sugar.

Milligram (mg): A unit of weight equal to one-thousandth of a gram. There are about 28,350 mg in 1 ounce. Dietary cholesterol is measured in milligrams.

Milligrams/Deciliter (mg/dL): The measure used to express cholesterol and triglyceride levels in the blood. It stands for the weight of cholesterol in milligrams in a deciliter of blood. A deciliter is one-tenth of a liter or about one-tenth of a quart.

Nicotinic Acid: A cholesterol-lowering medicine that reduces total and LDL-cholesterol and triglyceride levels and also raises HDL-cholesterol levels. This is the same substance as Niacin or vitamin B1, but in doses that lower cholesterol, it should only be used with your doctor's supervision.

Risk Factor: A habit, trait, or condition in a person that is associated with an increased chance (or risk) for a disease.

Statins: One type of cholesterol-lowering drug that includes lovastatin, pravastatin, and simvastatin. These drugs lower LDL levels by limiting the amount of cholesterol the body can make.

Triglycerides: Lipids carried through the bloodstream to tissues. Most of the body's fat tissue is in the form of triglycerides, stored for use as energy. Triglycerides are obtained primarily from fat in foods.

Chapter 51

Facts about Potassium

Potassium is a mineral your body must have to grow and maintain itself. It is necessary to keep a normal water balance between the cells and body fluids; it also plays an essential role in allowing nerves to respond to stimulation and muscles to contract. Potassium is also necessary for enzymes in cells to function properly.

[The abbreviation for potassium, K, is derived from the word] kalium, the Latin name for potassium.

Potassium is measured in milligrams (mg). One thousand milligrams make one gram; five grams of some food items make one teaspoon. Sometimes the term milliequivalents (abbreviated mEq) is used. One mEq equals about 40 milligrams.

Different foods contain different amounts of potassium. Meats, legumes, vegetables and fruit are usually good sources. Some foods that do not contain a lot of potassium *can* be good sources, if they are eaten often and in large amounts.

Why Do Some People Need More Potassium?

Certain heart diseases cause people to retain sodium and water. When medication is given to correct this, urination increases and sometimes a potassium deficiency results. Physicians often recom-

Excerpts from American Heart Association Pub. No. 50-1006 (CP). Used by Permission. Editor's comments are bracketed.

mend eating more high-potassium foods to overcome this. Additional potassium also may be prescribed as a medicine.

The recommended amount of potassium varies. Your physician or dietitian is the best person to decide how much supplemental potassium you need. Often 2,000 milligrams (51 mEq) of additional potassium is advised, however. Some foods high in potassium are also high in calories. If you are overweight, it may not be healthy for you to simply increase the amount of food you eat.

[Sometimes people are concerned that food costs will increase if they eat more foods that are high in potassium.] Often you can eat better foods without increasing the amount you spend for food. For example, depending on the season and your location, you might find that obtaining 400 milligrams (10 mEqs) of potassium from a cup of orange or grapefruit juice or a medium banana costs a lot less than getting the same amount of potassium from certain other foods.

[If you are striving to increase your potassium intake, pay attention to how foods are processed.] Some kinds of processing remove large amounts of potassium. For example, since this mineral dissolves in water, food loses potassium when it's exposed to water during blanching or cooking. It follows that raw food or food cooked in its skin (such as potatoes) contains more potassium than foods prepared differently. Mashed potatoes made from "instant" potatoes have about the same amount of potassium as fresh potatoes.

[Examples of foods that are low in calories and that are classified as "Very Good Sources" of potassium by the American Heart Association include:

- Bananas
- Cantaloupes
- Grapefruit juice
- Honeydew melons
- Molasses
- Nectarines
- Orange juice
- Potatoes]

Chapter 52

Treatment of
High Blood Pressure

Goal

The goal of treating patients with hypertension is to prevent morbidity and mortality associated with high blood pressure and to control blood pressure by the least intrusive means possible. This should be accomplished by achieving and maintaining arterial pressure below 140 mm Hg SBP [systolic blood pressure] and 90 mm Hg DBP [diastolic blood pressure], while concurrently controlling other modifiable cardiovascular risk factors. Further reduction to levels of 130/85 mm Hg may be pursued, with due regard for cardiovascular function, especially in older persons. How far the DBP should be reduced below 85 mm Hg is unclear.

Lifestyle Modifications

Lifestyle modifications (previously termed nonpharmacologic therapy)—which include weight reduction, increased physical activity, and moderation of dietary sodium and alcohol intake—are used as definitive or adjunctive therapy for hypertension. They offer some hope for prevention of the disease. They are effective in lowering the blood pressure of many people who follow them, and they can also reduce other risk factors for premature CVD. Their capacity to reduce morbidity or mortality in those with elevated blood pressure has not been

Taken from NIH Pub. No. 93-1088.

465

conclusively documented. However, because of their ability to improve the cardiovascular risk profile, lifestyle modification interventions, properly used, offer multiple benefits at little cost and with minimal risk. Even when not adequate in themselves to control hypertension, they may reduce the number and doses of antihypertensive medications needed to manage the condition. Lifestyle modifications are particularly helpful in the large proportion of hypertensive patients who have additional risk factors for premature CVD, especially dyslipidemia or diabetes. Therefore, clinicians should vigorously encourage their patients to adopt these lifestyle modifications.

Tobacco Avoidance

Although unrelated to hypertension, cigarette smoking is a major risk factor for CVD, and avoidance of tobacco is essential. Everyone, especially hypertensive patients, should be strongly advised not to smoke. Repetitive counseling, including referral to effective smoking cessation programs, should be provided. Those who continue to smoke may not receive the full degree of protection against CVD from antihypertensive therapy. The nicotine patch or nicotine chewing gum in conjunction with patient counseling may assist the clinician in promoting smoking cessation. Smoking cessation information is available from voluntary health associations and the NHLBI Information Center (P.O. Box 30105, Bethesda, Maryland 20824-0105).

Weight Reduction

Excess body weight is correlated closely with increased blood pressure. The deposition of excess fat in the upper body (truncal or abdominal), as evidenced by an increased waist-to-hip ratio above 0.85 in women and 0.95 in men, has also been correlated with hypertension, dyslipidemia, diabetes, and increased coronary heart disease mortality.

Weight reduction reduces blood pressure in a large proportion of hypertensive individuals who are more than 10 percent above ideal weight. A reduction in blood pressure usually occurs early during a weight loss program, often with as small a weight loss as 10 pounds. Weight reduction of overweight hypertensive patients enhances the blood pressure lowering effect of concurrent antihypertensive agents and can significantly reduce concomitant cardiovascular risk factors.

Therefore, all hypertensive patients who are above their ideal weight should initially be placed on an individualized, monitored weight reduction program involving caloric restriction and increased caloric expenditure by regular physical activity. In overweight patients with stage 1 hypertension, an attempt to control blood pressure with weight loss and other lifestyle modifications should be tried for at least 3 to 6 months prior to initiating pharmacologic therapy. If pharmacologic therapy is needed, the weight loss program should continue to be pursued vigorously. While recidivism is common and can be discouraging, the long-term goal of attenuating age-related weight gain should be kept in mind.

Moderation of Alcohol Intake

Excessive alcohol intake can raise blood pressure and cause resistance to antihypertensive therapy. A detailed history of current alcohol consumption should be elicited. Hypertensive patients who drink alcohol-containing beverages should be counseled to limit their daily intake to 1 ounce of ethanol (2 ounces of 100 proof whiskey, 8 ounces of wine, or 24 ounces of beer). Significant hypertension may develop during withdrawal from heavy alcohol consumption, but the pressor effect of alcohol withdrawal reverses a few days after alcohol consumption is reduced.

Physical Activity

Regular aerobic physical activity, adequate to achieve at least a moderate level of physical fitness, may be beneficial both for prevention and treatment of hypertension. It can also enhance weight loss and functional health status and reduce the risk for CVD and all-cause mortality. Sedentary and unfit normotensive individuals have a 20 to 50 percent increased risk of developing hypertension during followup when compared with their more active and fit peers.

Regular aerobic physical activity can reduce SBP in hypertensive patients by approximately 10 mm Hg. Effective lowering of blood pressure can be achieved with only moderately intense physical activity (40 to 60 percent of VO_{2max}). Therefore, physical activity need not be complicated or expensive; and, for most sedentary patients, moderate activity such as 30 to 45 minutes of brisk walking three to five times per week will be beneficial. The majority of patients with uncomplicated hypertension can safely increase their level of physical activity without an extensive medical or physical fitness evaluation. Patients with known cardiac disease or other serious health problems need a more thorough examination, often including an electrocardiogram-monitored exercise test, and may need to be referred to medically supervised rehabilitative exercise programs.

Moderation of Dietary Sodium

Epidemiologic observations and clinical trials support an association between dietary sodium intake and blood pressure. Based on linear regression analysis, within populations, a 100 mmol per day lower average sodium intake was associated with a 2.2 mm Hg lower SBP in 10,000 people, and a 5 to 10 mm Hg lower SBP in multiple other studies involving 47,000 participants. Furthermore, a 100 mmol per day lower sodium intake was associated with a 9 mm Hg attenuation of the rise of SBP between the ages of 25 and 55 years.

Multiple therapeutic trials document a reduction of blood pressure in response to reduced sodium intake. In short-term trials, moderate sodium restriction in hypertensive individuals on average has been shown to reduce SBP by 4.9 mm Hg and DBP by 2.6 mm Hg. In trials involving people aged 50 to 59 and lasting 5 weeks or longer, a 50 mmol per day reduction of sodium intake was associated with an average of a 7 mm Hg reduction in SBP in hypertensive persons and a 5 mm Hg reduction in normotensive people.

The impact of dietary sodium on blood pressure depends on the provision of sodium as the chloride salt. Individuals vary in their blood pressure response to changes in dietary sodium chloride. Blacks, older people, and patients with hypertension are more sensitive to changes in dietary sodium chloride.

Because the average American consumption of sodium is in excess of 150 mmol per day, moderate dietary sodium chloride reduction to a level of less than 100 mmol per day (less than 6 grams sodium chloride or less than 2.3 grams sodium per day) is recommended. With appropriate counseling, this is an achievable diet. Blood pressure may be controlled by this degree of sodium chloride restriction in some patients with stage 1 hypertension; in those patients who still need drug therapy, the medication requirements may be decreased.

Potassium

A high dietary potassium intake may protect against developing hypertension, and potassium deficiency may increase blood pressure and induce ventricular ectopy. Therefore, normal plasma concentrations of potassium should be maintained, preferably from food sources. If hypokalemia occurs during diuretic therapy, additional potassium may be needed either from potassium-containing salt substitutes, potassium supplements, or use of a potassium-sparing diuretic. Potassium chloride supplements and potassium-sparing diuretics must be used with caution in patients susceptible to hyperkalemia.

Calcium

In many but not all epidemiologic studies, there is an inverse association between dietary calcium and blood pressure. Calcium deficiency is associated with an increased prevalence of hypertension, and a low calcium intake may amplify the effects of a high sodium intake on blood pressure. An increased calcium intake may lower blood pressure in some patients with hypertension; but the overall effect is minimal, and there is no way to predict which patients will benefit. Therefore, there is currently no rationale for recommending calcium intakes in excess of the recommended daily allowance of 20 to 30 mmol (800 to 1,200 mg) in an attempt to lower blood pressure.

Magnesium

There is suggestive evidence of an association between lower dietary magnesium intake and higher blood pressures. However, there are currently no convincing data to justify recommending an increased magnesium intake in an effort to lower blood pressure.

Other Dietary Factors

Dietary fats. In randomized controlled studies, diets varying in total fat and proportions of saturated to unsaturated fats have had little, if any, effect on blood pressure. Although large amounts of omega-3 fatty acids may lower blood pressure, they may be associated with multiple adverse effects and are not recommended for treatment or prevention of high blood pressure. Nevertheless, dyslipidemia is a major independent risk factor for coronary artery disease; therefore, dietary and, if necessary, drug therapy for dyslipidemia is an important adjunct to the antihypertensive regimen.

Caffeine. Caffeine may acutely raise the blood pressure, but tolerance to this pressor effect rapidly develops. Therefore, unless cardiac or other forms of excessive sensitivity to caffeine are present, no limitation of consumption of caffeine-containing beverages is needed.

Dietary carbohydrates and protein. No consistent effects on blood pressure have been demonstrated in controlled trials of varying proportions of carbohydrate or protein in the diet.

Garlic or onion. No effects on blood pressure of increased amounts of garlic or onion have been found in controlled trials.

Relaxation and Biofeedback

Stress can raise blood pressure acutely and may contribute to the cause of hypertension, but the role of stress management techniques in treating patients with elevated blood pressure is uncertain. Relaxation therapies and biofeedback have been studied in short-term and long-term controlled trials with little effect beyond that seen in the control groups. Therefore, although stress management is an appealing concept, the available literature does not support the use of relaxation therapies for definitive therapy or prevention of hypertension.

Summary

Lifestyle modifications useful in managing hypertensive patients [are summarized below:]

- Lose weight if overweight.
- Limit alcohol intake to no more than 1 ounce of ethanol per day (24 ounces of beer, 8 ounces of wine, or 2 ounces of 100 proof whiskey).
- Exercise (aerobic) regularly.
- Reduce sodium intake to less than 100 mmol per day (<2.3 grams of sodium or <6 grams of sodium chloride).
- Maintain adequate dietary potassium, calcium, and magnesium intake.
- Stop smoking and reduce dietary saturated fat and cholesterol intake for overall cardiovascular health. Reducing fat intake also helps reduce caloric intake—important for control of weight and Type II diabetes.

The modifications also may be useful in preventing blood pressures from rising and protecting cardiovascular health in those with high normal blood pressures.

Pharmacologic Treatment

The decision to initiate pharmacologic treatment in individual patients requires consideration of several factors: severity of blood pressure elevation, TOD [target-organ disease], and presence of other conditions and risk factors.

Efficacy

Reducing blood pressure with drugs clearly decreases the incidence of cardiovascular mortality and morbidity. Protection has been demonstrated for stroke, coronary events, congestive heart failure, progression to more severe hypertension, and all-cause mortality. Meta-analysis of 14 randomized trials has indicated a 42 percent reduction in stroke from a 5 to 6 mm Hg lowering of DBP. This reduction in stroke rate was highly consistent with long-term observational studies that predicted 35 to 40 percent reductions with this blood pressure difference. The same long-term analyses predicted a 20 to 25 percent reduction in the rate of CHD; however, the observed reduction from the 14 pooled trial results was 14 percent during periods of 4 to 6 years. Several explanations but little conclusive evidence have been presented to account for the less than expected reduction in CHD events in these trials. This meta-analysis did not include new data from three recent clinical trials on hypertension control in older persons. The Systolic Hypertension in the Elderly Program (SHEP), the Swedish Trial in Old Patients with Hypertension (STOP-Hypertension), and the Medical Research Council (MRC) Trial, demonstrated a 27 percent, 13 percent, and 19 percent reduction of CHD events, respectively.

Stage 1 and Stage 2 Hypertension

If blood pressure remains at or above 140/90 mm Hg during a 3- to 6-month period despite vigorous encouragement of lifestyle modifications, antihypertensive medications should be started, especially in individuals with TOD [target-organ disease] and/or other known risk

471

factors for CVD. In the absence of TOD and other major risk factors, some physicians may elect to withhold antihypertensive drug therapy from patients with DBP in the 90 to 94 mm Hg range and SBP in the 140 to 149 mm Hg range. In these patients, careful followup is indicated at 3- to 6-month intervals because blood pressure may rise to higher levels, and cardiac and vascular changes may occur. Clinical trial data strongly suggest that antihypertensive drug therapy should be initiated before the development of TOD.

Initial drug therapy is monotherapy for stage 1 and stage 2 hypertension; that is, start with a single drug. Because diuretics and beta-blockers have been shown to reduce cardiovascular morbidity and mortality in controlled clinical trials, these two classes of drugs are preferred for initial drug therapy. The alternative drugs—calcium antagonists, angiotensin converting enzyme (ACE) inhibitors, alpha$_1$-receptor blockers, and the alpha-beta blocker—are equally effective in reducing blood pressure. Although these alternative drugs have potentially important benefits, they have not been used in long-term controlled trials to demonstrate their efficacy in reducing morbidity and mortality and therefore should be reserved for special indications or when diuretics and beta-blockers have proved unacceptable or ineffective. There is an urgent need to evaluate the effectiveness of ACE inhibitors, calcium antagonists, and alpha$_1$-receptor blockers in reducing long-term cardiovascular morbidity and mortality.

Other factors that should be considered in the selection of drugs are the cost of medication, metabolic and subjective side effects, and drug-drug interactions.

Supplemental antihypertensive agents such as the direct-acting smooth muscle vasodilators, the alpha$_2$-agonists, and the peripherally acting adrenergic neuron antagonists are not well suited for initial monotherapy. The direct-acting smooth muscle vasodilators (e.g., hydralazine, minoxidil) often induce reflex sympathetic stimulation of the cardiovascular system and fluid retention. Alpha$_2$-agonists and peripheral acting adrenergic antagonists produce annoying side effects in a large number of patients.

Special Considerations

Also to be considered in the selection of initial therapy are demographic characteristics, concomitant diseases that may be beneficially or adversely affected by the antihypertensive agent chosen, and the use of other drugs that may lead to drug interactions.

Demographics. In general, blacks are more responsive to diuretics and calcium antagonists than to beta-blockers or ACE inhibitors. Older persons with hypertension are generally responsive to all classes of drugs. Gender has not been found to determine drug responsiveness. In any event, gender, age, or race does not provide sufficient reason to avoid any drug class, particularly if it is needed for other therapeutic benefits because efficacy differences can usually be overcome with the addition of a diuretic or another agent.

Concomitant diseases and therapies. Antihypertensive drugs may worsen some diseases while improving others. For example, beta-blockers may worsen asthma, diabetes, and peripheral ischemia, but they may improve angina pectoris, certain cardiac dysrhythmias, and migraine headaches, and they have proven to prolong life after myocardial infarction. Selection of an antihypertensive agent that also treats a coexisting disease may simplify therapeutic regimens and reduce costs.

Quality of life. Antihypertensive drugs may cause undesirable symptoms. For example, many of these agents may impair sexual function, centrally acting drugs may impair mental acuity, and beta-blockers may reduce exercise tolerance.

Physiologic and biochemical measurements. Some clinicians have found certain physiologic and biochemical measurements (e.g., body weight, heart rate, plasma renin activity, resting electrocardiographic tracing, and hemodynamic parameters) to be helpful in choosing specific therapy.

Economic considerations. The cost of therapy may be a barrier to controlling hypertension. Treatment costs include not only the price of drugs but also the expense of routine or special laboratory tests, supplemental therapies, office visits, and time lost from work for visits to physicians' offices.

Dosage and Followup

The lowest dosage... should be selected to protect the patient from adverse effects, although it may not immediately control the blood pressure. If blood pressure remains uncontrolled, the lowest dose should be given for several weeks before it is increased to the next dosage level. It must be recognized that it may take months to control hypertension adequately while avoiding adverse effects of therapy. Most antihypertensive medications can be given once or twice daily, and this should be the goal in order to improve patient adherence. Adherence improves substantially as prescribed dose frequency decreases.

If, after 1 to 3 months, the response to initial therapy is inadequate, the patient is not experiencing significant side effects, and adherence to therapy is adequate, three options for subsequent therapy should be considered:

- Increase the dose of the first drug to or toward maximal levels;
- Substitute an agent from another class;
- Add a second drug from another class.

Combining antihypertensive drugs with different modes of action will often allow smaller doses of drugs to be used to achieve control, thereby minimizing the potential for dose-dependent side effects. If a diuretic is not chosen as the first drug, it will be useful as a second step agent because its addition usually enhances the effects of other agents. If addition of a second agent produces satisfactory blood pressure control, an attempt to withdraw the first agent may be considered because monotherapy with virtually all agents provides blood pressure control for at least half of all patients.

Before proceeding to each successive treatment step, clinicians should address possible reasons for lack of responsiveness to therapy, including those listed [below].

Nonadherence to therapy

- Cost of medication
- Instructions not clear and/or not given to the patient in writing
- Inadequate or no patient education
- Lack of involvement of the patient in the treatment plan
- Side effects of medication
- Organic brain syndrome (e.g., memory deficit)
- Inconvenient dosing

Drug-related causes

- Doses too low

474

- Inappropriate combinations (e.g., two centrally acting adrenergic inhibitors)
- Rapid inactivation (e.g., hydralazine)
- Drug interactions: Nonsteroidal anti-inflammatory drugs; Oral contraceptives; Sympathomimetics; Antidepressants; Adrenal steroids; Nasal decongestants; Licorice-containing substances (e.g., chewing tobacco); Cocaine; Cyclosporine; Erythropoietin

Associated conditions

- Increasing obesity
- Alcohol intake more than 1 ounce of ethanol a day

Secondary hypertension

- Renal insufficiency
- Renovascular hypertension
- Pheochromocytoma
- Primary aldosteronism

Volume overload

- Inadequate diuretic therapy
- Excess sodium intake
- Fluid retention from reduction of blood pressure
- Progressive renal damage

Pseudohypertension

After blood pressure is reduced to goal level and maintenance doses of antihypertensive drugs are stabilized, substituting comparable combination tablets may simplify patients' regimens and promote adherence to a comprehensive antihypertensive treatment program.

Stage 3 and Stage 4 Hypertension

Although similar general approaches are advocated for all patients with hypertension, modification may be appropriate for those with DBP of 110 mm Hg or higher and/or SBP 180 mm Hg or higher.

475

Although some patients may respond adequately to only one drug, it is often necessary to add a second or third agent after a short interval if control is not achieved. The intervals between changes in the regimen should be decreased, and the maximum dose of some drugs may be increased. In some patients it may be necessary to start treatment with more than one agent. Patients with average DBP of 120 mm Hg or greater require more immediate therapy and, if significant TOD is present, may require hospitalization and consultation.

Isolated Systolic Hypertension

Isolated systolic hypertension frequently occurs in older persons and is discussed in more detail in the Hypertension in the Older Patients section. When isolated systolic hypertension occurs in adolescents and young adults, it often indicates a hyperdynamic circulation and may predict future diastolic elevation. Lifestyle modifications should be used in an attempt to lower isolated systolic hypertension. However, when the SBP is consistently 160 mm Hg or greater and the DBP is less than 90 mm Hg despite lifestyle modification, antihypertensive drug treatment is indicated for older patients and should be considered for younger patients.

Step Down Therapy

Sound patient management should include attempts to decrease the dosage or number of antihypertensive drugs while maintaining lifestyle modifications. In general, complete cessation of an antihypertensive treatment program is not indicated. However, after blood pressure has been effectively controlled for 1 year and at least four visits, it may be possible to reduce antihypertensive drug therapy in a deliberate, slow, and progressive manner. Step-down therapy is especially successful in patients who are also following lifestyle treatment recommendations: a higher percentage maintain normal blood pressure levels with less or no medication. Patients whose drugs have been discontinued should have regular followup because blood pressure usually rises again to hypertensive levels, sometimes months or years after discontinuance, especially in the absence of sustained improvements in lifestyle.

J-Curve Hypothesis

Concerns have been raised that lowering DBP too much may increase risk for coronary disease possibly by lowering diastolic perfusion pressure in the coronary circulation—the so-called "J-curve" hypothesis. This concern may be more relevant to hypertensive patients with preexisting coronary disease. No data support a similar relationship of blood pressure reduction to adverse effects on cerebral or renal function. Regardless of the presence or absence of a J-curve, available evidence supports the reduction of diastolic and systolic blood pressure at all ages to the levels achieved in clinical trials—usually less than 90 mm Hg DBP, and 140-160 mm Hg in isolated systolic hypertension.

Resistant Hypertension

Hypertension should be considered resistant if the blood pressure in an adherent patient cannot be reduced to less than 160/100 mm Hg by an adequate and appropriate triple-drug regimen prescribed in nearly maximal doses when the pretreatment blood pressure was greater than 180/115 mm Hg. If the pretreatment blood pressure was less than 180/115 mm Hg, resistance should be defined as failure to achieve normotension (less than 140/90 mm Hg) on a similar regimen. An adequate and appropriate regimen should include at least three different pharmacologic agents, including a diuretic plus two of the following classes of drugs: beta-adrenergic blocker or another anti-adrenergic agent, direct vasodilator, calcium antagonist, or ACE inhibitor.

For older patients with isolated systolic hypertension, resistance in an adherent patient is defined as failure of an adequate triple-drug regimen to reduce systolic blood pressure to less than 170 mm Hg if pretreatment systolic pressure was greater than 200 mm Hg or to less than 160 mm Hg and by at least 10 mm Hg if pretreatment systolic blood pressure was 160 to 200 mm Hg.

If goal blood pressure cannot be achieved without intolerable side effects, even suboptimal reduction of blood pressure will contribute to decreased morbidity and mortality.

Hypertensive Crises: Emergencies and Urgencies

Hypertensive emergencies are those situations that require immediate blood pressure reduction (not necessarily to normal ranges) to prevent or limit target-organ disease. Examples include hypertensive encephalopathy, intracranial hemorrhage, acute left ventricular failure with pulmonary edema, dissecting aortic aneurysm, eclampsia or severe hypertension associated with pregnancy, unstable angina pectoris, and acute myocardial infarction. Hypertensive urgencies are those situations in which it is desirable to reduce blood pressure within 24 hours. Hypertensive urgencies include accelerated or malignant hypertension without severe symptoms or progressive target-organ complications and severe perioperative hypertension.

Although most hypertensive emergencies are treated initially with parenteral administration of an appropriate agent, oral administration of selected agents may also be associated with rapid reduction in blood pressure. There is no clearly defined clinical advantage for sublingual over oral administration of nifedipine or captopril.

When treating the hypertensive urgency or emergency, it is desirable to choose agents that enable a controlled reduction in blood pressure over 30 minutes to several hours. Elevated blood pressure alone, in the absence of symptoms or evident target-organ disease, rarely requires emergency therapy. The risks of overly aggressive intervention in any hypertensive crisis must always be considered. Even the administration of oral agents for hypertensive urgencies has resulted in myocardial ischemia and cerebral hypoperfusion.

Long Term Adherence to Therapy

Followup Visits

Achieving and maintaining target blood pressure with the lowest possible dosage of medication requires ongoing patient followup and may involve dosage adjustments. Patients with stage 1 hypertension without TOD [target-organ disease] should generally be seen within 1 to 2 months following the initiation of therapy to determine the adequacy of blood pressure control, the degree of patient adherence, and the presence of adverse effects. Associated medical problems, including TOD, other major risk factors, and laboratory test abnormalities will also play a part in determining the frequency of patient followup. Once stabilized, followup at 3- to 6-month intervals (depending on the patient's status) is generally appropriate. Monitoring should include blood pressure measurements in the supine or sitting positions and after standing quietly for 2 minutes. Patient education should be an important feature of followup visits.

Planned Patient Education Programs

Poor adherence to long-term treatment, both lifestyle modifications and pharmacologic therapy, has been identified as the major reason for inadequate control of high blood pressure. Planned patient education programs may significantly improve adherence to treatment schedules, improve blood pressure control, and decrease hypertension-related morbidity and mortality. Combinations of patient education intervention strategies are likely to achieve the greatest improvement in long-term adherence and are usually aimed at improving patient understanding of specific therapies and treatment goals, correcting misconceptions, adjusting the therapeutic interventions to patients' lifestyles, and enhancing family or other social support.

Strategies to Improve Adherence to Therapy and Control of High Blood Pressure

The choice and application of specific strategies will depend on individual patient characteristics, severity of specific diseases, and co-morbidities. It is not expected that all strategies would be applied any one time, nor to all patients, as prioritization should occur on an individual basis. It is recommended to review patient progress and effectiveness of the approaches at followup visits. Over time, the patient's needs may change and behavioral and pharmacological approaches may need to be altered. [The list below] outlines a series of strategies to enhance adherence to treatment. They are designed to provide guidance at the initial, as well as followup visits.

Educate about conditions and treatment:

- Assess patient's understanding and acceptance of the diagnosis and expectations of being in care.
- Discuss patient's concerns and clarify misunderstandings.
- Inform patient of blood pressure level.
- Agree with patient on a goal blood pressure.
- Inform patient about recommended treatment and provide specific written information.
- Elicit concerns and questions and provide opportunities for patient to state specific behaviors to carry out treatment recommendations.

- Emphasize need to continue treatment, that patient cannot tell if blood pressure is elevated, and that control does not mean cure.

Individualize the regimen:

- Include patient in decision making.
- Simplify the regimen.
- Incorporate treatment into patient's daily lifestyle.
- Set, with the patient, realistic short-term objectives for specific components of the treatment plan.
- Encourage discussion of side effects and concerns.
- Encourage self-monitoring.
- Minimize cost of therapy.
- Indicate you will ask about adherence at next visit.
- When weight loss is established as a treatment goal, discourage quick weight loss regimens, fasting or unscientific methods, since these are associated with weight cycling which may increase cardiovascular morbidity and mortality.

Provide reinforcement:

- Provide feedback regarding blood pressure level.
- Ask about behaviors to achieve blood pressure control.
- Give positive feedback for behavioral and blood pressure improvement.
- Hold exit interviews to clarify regimen.
- Make appointment for next visit before patient leaves the office.
- Use appointment reminders and contact patients to confirm appointments.
- Schedule more frequent visits to counsel nonadherent patients.
- Contact and follow up patients who missed appointments.
- Consider clinician-patient contracts.

Promote social support:

- Educate family members to be part of the blood pressure control process and provide daily reinforcement.

- Suggest small group activities to enhance mutual support and motivation.

Collaborate with other professionals:

- Draw upon complementary skills and knowledge of nurses, pharmacists, dietitians, optometrists, dentists, and physician assistants.
- Refer patients for more intensive counseling.

Special Populations and Situations

Hypertension in African Americans and Other Racial and Ethnic Minorities

The frequency of hypertension in African Americans is among the highest in the world, and hypertension is the major health problem of adult African Americans. Blacks develop hypertension at an earlier age; and, at any decade of life, hypertension is more severe in blacks than in whites. As much as 30 percent of all deaths in hypertensive black men and 20 percent of all deaths in hypertensive black women may be attributable to high blood pressure. This earlier onset, higher prevalence, and greater severity of hypertension in blacks than in whites is accompanied by a 1.3-fold greater rate of nonfatal stroke, a 1.8-fold greater rate of fatal stroke, a 1.5-fold greater rate of heart disease deaths, and a 5-fold greater rate of end-stage renal disease.

Available evidence indicates that at similar starting blood pressure levels, blacks, when provided equal access to adequate therapy, will achieve similar overall blood pressure declines and may experience a lower incidence of CVD than whites.

Because of the high prevalence of salt sensitivity, obesity, and cigarette smoking in blacks, lifestyle modifications are particularly important. The control of obesity is of particular importance because blacks have twice the prevalence of non-insulin-dependent diabetes mellitus.

In blacks, diuretics have been proven in controlled trials to reduce hypertensive morbidity and mortality; thus, diuretics should be the agent of first choice in the absence of other conditions that prohibit their use. Monotherapy with beta-blockers or ACE inhibitors is less effective in blacks; but calcium antagonists, alpha$_1$-receptor blockers, and the alpha-beta blocker are as effective in blacks as in whites. Because of the greater rate of severe hypertension in blacks, more black patients will require multidrug therapy, and clinicians should not hesitate to use the most powerful agents, including minoxidil, especially in those with impaired renal function.

Little information is available on whether other racial and ethnic groups—including Native Americans, Asians and Pacific Islanders, and Hispanics—respond differently from whites to antihypertensive medications or lifestyle modifications. Further studies are needed to better understand the factors influencing the control of hypertension in these groups.

Hypertension in Children

According to the "Report of the Second Task Force on Blood Pressure Control in Children," hypertension in children is defined as average systolic and/or diastolic blood pressure equal to or greater than the 95th percentile for age on at least three occasions [see Figure 52.1]. In many of the childhood cases, significant and severe hypertension may have an identifiable underlying cause. Children who have slight or periodic blood pressure elevation frequently exhibit other risk factors for future CVD that usually persist into adult life and often cluster within families. All clinicians who care for children age 3 through adolescence should be encouraged to measure blood pressure once a year, when the child is well. This is especially true in children who have a hypertensive parent. Likewise, the parents of children who exhibit elevated pressures should also be screened.

The "Report of the Second Task Force on Blood Pressure Control in Children" offers a comprehensive approach to the detection, evaluation, and treatment of high blood pressure in children. This report provides normative data on blood pressure from more than 70,000 white, black, and Mexican-American children. [Figure 52.1] depicts the levels of blood pressure in childhood that have been used to diagnose hypertension. These levels are different from those levels found in adults because percentile levels are used in classification of blood pressure levels in children and adolescents.

Children, like adults, require repeated measurements with proper equipment to determine the level of blood pressure accurately. The widest cuff that will comfortably encircle the arm without covering the antecubital fossa should be used. For infants in whom the ac-

	High Normal 90-94th Percentile (mm Hg)	Significant Hypertension 95-99th Percentile (mm Hg)	Severe Hypertension > 99th Percentile (mm Hg)
Newborns			
7 days		SBP 96-105	SBP ≥ 106
8-30 days		SBP 104-109	SBP ≥ 110
Infants	SBP 104-111	SBP 112-117	SBP ≥ 118
(≤2 years)	DBP 70-73	DBP 74-81	DBP ≥ 82
Children	SBP 108-115	SBP 116-123	SBP ≥ 124
(3-5 years)	DBP 70-75	DBP 76-83	DBP ≥ 84
Children	SBP 114-121	SBP 122-129	SBP ≥ 130
(6-9 years)	DBP 74-77	DBP 78-85	DBP ≥ 86
Children	SBP 122-125	SBP 126-133	SBP ≥ 134
(10-12 years)	DBP 78-81	DBP 82-89	DBP ≥ 90
Children	SBP 130-135	SBP 136-143	SBP ≥ 144
(13-15 years)	DBP 80-85	DBP 86-91	DBP ≥ 92
Adolescents	SBP 136-141	SBP 142-149	SBP ≥ 150
(16-18 years)	DBP 84-91	DBP 92-97	DBP ≥ 98

* *This classification table is adapted from the "Report of the Second Task Force on Blood Pressure Control in Children—1987."[73] Note that adult classifications differ.*

Figure 52.1. Classification of Hypertension in the Young by Age Group

curacy of measurements by auscultation is uncertain, an electronic device using a Doppler technique can be used.

The higher the blood pressure and the younger the child, the greater the possibility of secondary hypertension. Attention should also be given to risk factor assessment including family history, obesity, diet, and physical activity. In adolescents, use of alcohol, cocaine, or other addictive substances should be considered as a possible cause of the elevated blood pressure. Laboratory tests for young patients are generally similar to those recommended for adults. However, efforts to arrive at a diagnosis of secondary hypertension should be more thorough in a child.

The underlying cause, severity, or complications of hypertension in children will determine the degree and types of intervention required. Therapy should reduce blood pressure without causing adverse effects that limit adherence or impair normal growth and development. Lifestyle modifications can be introduced as initial treatments, but may be insufficient therapy when there is severe hypertension or when there is a demonstrated cause. Weight reduction in obese children often lowers blood pressure. Antihypertensive drug therapy should usually be reserved for patients with levels of blood pressure above the 99th percentile or with significantly elevated blood pressure that responds inadequately to lifestyle modifications or is associated with TOD. As with adults, children with insulin-dependent diabetes mellitus and with primary renal disease may benefit from pharmacologic antihypertensive therapy at any level of hypertension in order to prevent or delay progression of renal insufficiency. Pharmacologic agents generally used for adults are also effective in young persons.

Uncomplicated elevated blood pressure, by itself, should not be a reason to restrict asymptomatic children from participating in physical activities, particularly because exercise may both prevent and relieve hypertension. Use of steroid hormones for the purpose of body building should be strongly discouraged.

Hypertension in Women

The long-term and large clinical trials of antihypertensive treatment have included both men and women but have not clearly demonstrated gender differences in blood pressure response and outcomes. Because the rate of cardiovascular events in middle-aged women is much lower than in men, these trials had limited ability to distinguish the degree of benefit from treatments between men and women. Recent trials in older persons reinforce the conclusion to support a similar approach to the management of hypertension in men and women. Therefore, at this time there are insufficient data to support a different approach to the management of hypertension in women, but further study is warranted.

Hypertension Associated with Oral Contraceptives

Most women taking oral contraceptives experience a small but detectable increase in both SBP and DBP, usually within the normal range. Hypertension has been reported to be two to three times more common in women taking oral contraceptive pills for 5 years or longer than in those not taking oral contraceptives. The risk appears to increase with age, with duration of use, and perhaps with increased body mass. Women age 35 and older who smoke cigarettes should be strongly counseled to stop smoking. If they continue to smoke, they should be discouraged from using oral contraceptives because most of the cardiovascular deaths attributable to oral contraceptive use have been in such women. Since many of the studies of blood pressure and oral contraceptives involved higher doses of both estrogen and progesterone than are presently in use, the current incidence of oral-contraceptive-induced hypertension is probably less than reported earlier. Nonetheless, in a small number of patients, oral contraceptives may cause accelerated or malignant hypertension.

The mechanism of the increase in blood pressure remains unclear. If hypertension develops in a woman taking oral contraceptives, it is advisable to stop the pill. The blood pressure will normalize in most cases within a few months. If it persists and the risks of pregnancy are considered to be greater than the risks of stage 1 hypertension, and other contraceptive methods are not suitable, it may be necessary to continue the pill in spite of the elevation in blood pressure. Lifestyle modifications and antihypertensive medication should be used to normalize blood pressure, and patients should be carefully monitored.

Hypertension in Pregnancy

Hypertension during pregnancy may result in life-threatening consequences for both mother and fetus. The "NHBPEP Working Group Report on High Blood Pressure in Pregnancy" recommends a simple classification of four diagnostic categories: (1) chronic hypertension, (2) preeclampsia-eclampsia, (3) chronic hypertension with superimposed preeclampsia, or (4) transient hypertension. The report emphasizes the importance of differentiating hypertension that antedates pregnancy from a pregnancy-specific condition that is characterized by poor perfusion of many organs and usually has increased blood pressure as one of its features. In the former condition, elevated blood pressure is the cardinal pathophysiologic feature, whereas in the latter, increased blood pressure is important primarily as a sign of the underlying disorder.

Criteria. The criteria for diagnosing hypertension in pregnancy are SBP increases of 30 mm Hg or greater and DBP increases (Korotkoff phase V) of 15 mm Hg or greater compared with the average of values prior to 20 weeks gestation. When prior blood pressures are not known, a reading of 140/90 mm Hg or above is considered abnormal.

Chronic Hypertension. Chronic hypertension is hypertension that is present and observable before pregnancy or that is diagnosed before the 20th week of gestation. The goal of treatment of chronic hypertension in pregnancy is to minimize the short-term risks to the mother of elevated blood pressure while avoiding therapy that compromises fetal well-being. Diuretics or any other antihypertensive drugs except ACE inhibitors may be continued if taken prior to pregnancy. ACE inhibitors should be avoided because serious neonatal problems, including renal failure and death, have been reported when mothers have taken these agents during the last two trimesters. For women who were not on antihypertensive therapy when they became pregnant or those whose antihypertensive therapy was stopped in early stages of pregnancy, increased rest or stopping work may be helpful when DBP is between 90 and 100 mm Hg. Moderate sodium restriction should only be considered if it was useful prior to pregnancy. Antihypertensive drug therapy is reserved for patients with DBP greater than or equal to 100 mm Hg. Aggressive antihypertensive therapy is discouraged because of the concern for maintaining adequate uteroplacental blood flow.

Methyldopa has been most extensively evaluated in pregnancy and is therefore recommended. Beta-blockers compare favorably with methyldopa with respect to efficacy and are considered safe in the latter part of pregnancy, but their use early in pregnancy may be associated with growth retardation of the fetus.

Preeclampsia. The pregnancy-specific condition, preeclampsia, is increased blood pressure accompanied by proteinuria, edema or both, and at times, abnormalities of coagulation and liver function. Preeclampsia may progress rapidly to a convulsive phase, eclampsia. Preeclampsia occurs primarily in primigravidas and after the 20th week of gestation.

Therapy for preeclampsia consists of hospitalization with bed rest, control of blood pressure, seizure prophylaxis when signs of impending eclampsia are present, and timely delivery. If preeclampsia develops before the fetus is mature, then the physician must carefully consider both the maternal and fetal health, and decide whether postponement of delivery is safe. Delivery is indicated, regardless of gestational age, when there are signs of fetal distress, uncontrollable hypertension in the mother, evidence of deteriorating renal or hepaticfunction, epigastric pain, or signs of impending eclampsia (e.g., headache, visual disturbance, and hyperreflexia).

The decision to use antihypertensive drugs should be based on maternal safety because there is no clear-cut fetal benefit of lowering blood pressure, and such treatment does not cure or reverse preeclampsia. Although there is disagreement regarding what level of blood pressure should be treated, most authorities would begin therapy when DBP is greater than or equal to 100 mm Hg. If delivery is not anticipated in 24 hours, an oral agent is preferable, and methyldopa is the drug of choice. Hydralazine, calcium antagonists, alpha-beta blockers, or beta-blockers are reasonable additions or alternatives.

When delivery is imminent, a parenteral antihypertensive agent is preferable. Intravenous hydralazine is effective and has been used safely in pregnancy. Limited data are available on the use of diazoxide, labetalol, and clonidine. Potent diuretics such as furosemide are generally not advisable.

Encouraging preliminary data involving 13 small trials suggest that low-dose aspirin may prevent preeclampsia by reversing the imbalance between prostacyclin and thromboxane that may be responsible for some of the manifestations of this disease. While recommendations for the general pregnant population are not warranted, low-dose aspirin (approximately 60 mg) may be useful in high risk patients, e.g., patients whose previous pregnancies were complicated by preeclampsia of early onset, those who may be at risk for recurrent fetal death or severe fetal growth retardation due to placental insufficiency, or those with poor obstetrical histories.

Estrogen Replacement Therapy and Blood Pressure

The presence of hypertension is not a contraindication to postmenopausal estrogen replacement therapy; and, in fact, such treatment may have a beneficial effect on blood pressure as well as on overall cardiovascular risk. However, because a few women may experience a rise in blood pressure attributable to estrogen therapy, it is recommended that all women treated with hormonal replacement have their blood pressures monitored more frequently after such therapy is instituted. The effects of transdermal estrogen and of progestogen in addition to estrogen replacement on blood pressure in postmenopausal women have not been documented.

Hypertension in Older Patients

Hypertension is present in approximately 60 percent of non-Hispanic whites, 71 percent of non-Hispanic blacks, and 61 percent of Mexican Americans 60 years or older (NHANES III). Systolic hypertension is a well-established independent risk factor for CHD, stroke, and CVD. The prevalence of isolated systolic hypertension (ISH) (defined as SBP of 140 mm Hg or greater with a DBP less than 90 mm Hg) increases after age 60.

In older patients, the sudden onset of hypertension suggests the presence of secondary hypertension, particularly occlusive atherosclerotic renovascular disease. Pseudohypertension is sometimes encountered in elderly patients who have such rigid brachial arteries that they cannot be compressed by the sphygmomanometer cuff, giving falsely high readings. This should be suspected when TOD is absent in spite of high blood pressures and can be confirmed when the pulseless radial artery is palpable even though the sphygmomanometer cuff is inflated to pressures high enough to occlude the brachial artery (Osler's sign).

The value of treating hypertension in older patients has now been established. SHEP compared treatment with a low-dose diuretic, chlorthalidone, and, if needed, atenolol or reserpine to treatment with placebo in patients with baseline average SBP 160 mm Hg or greater and DBP less than 90 mm Hg. The results after an average of 4.5 years clearly favored active treatment, with 36 percent fewer fatal and nonfatal strokes and 27 percent fewer fatal and nonfatal myocardial infarctions in actively treated patients compared with placebo treated. Benefit was evident across all age, race, sex, and blood pressure subgroups, and active treatment was well tolerated. Data from other clinical trials indicate that older patients who have DBP of 90 mm Hg or greater will also benefit from antihypertensive therapy.

Therefore, the initial goal of therapy is to reduce the SBP to less than 160 mm Hg for those with a SBP greater than 180 mm Hg and to lower blood pressure by 20 mm Hg for those with SBP between 160 and 179 mm Hg. If this is well tolerated, it may be appropriate to reduce the blood pressure even further. At ISH levels of 140 to 160 mm

Hg, lifestyle modifications may be adjunctive or definitive therapy. In general, goals of therapy for DBP in older persons are similar to those for the general population.

Antihypertensive drug therapy should be carried out more cautiously in older patients. Older patients may be more sensitive to volume depletion and sympathetic inhibition than are younger individuals because older individuals may have impaired cardiovascular reflexes that make them more susceptible to hypotension. For this reason, blood pressure should always be measured in the standing as well as seated (or supine) positions, and antihypertensive treatment should be initiated with smaller doses than usual. Increases in dosage also should be smaller and spaced at longer intervals than might be appropriate for younger patients. Drugs that have a propensity to cause orthostatic hypotension (e.g., guanethidine monosulfate, guanadrel sulfate, alpha$_1$-receptor blockers, and labetalol) should be used with caution. All classes of antihypertensive drugs have been shown to be effective in lowering blood pressure in older patients. However, only diuretics and beta-blockers have been used in controlled trials that have shown a reduction in cardiovascular morbidity and mortality.

Patients with Hypertension and Coexisting Cardiovascular Diseases

Patients with Cerebrovascular Disease

The presence of clinically evident cerebrovascular disease is an indication for antihypertensive treatment. Immediately after the occurrence of an ischemic cerebral infarction, it may be appropriate to withhold treatment (unless the blood pressure is very high) until the situation has been stabilized. Even when treatment has been temporarily withheld, the eventual goal is to reduce blood pressure gradually with avoidance of orthostatic hypotension.

Severe hypertension that appears in the course of an acute stroke poses a difficult therapeutic problem. Some data suggest that DBP in excess of 120 mm Hg warrants cautious treatment, particularly when the hypertension is accompanied by a complication such as congestive heart failure.

Patients With Coronary Artery Disease

Hypertension in patients with coronary artery disease should be treated. The incidence of angina pectoris or myocardial infarction does not increase when elevated blood pressures are carefully reduced, and many patients experience a decrease in symptoms with pressure reduction. In the Multiple Risk Factor Intervention Trial (MRFIT), men with abnormal stress tests benefited substantially from risk factor reductions. Among MRFIT men with abnormal stress tests who were hypertensives at baseline, risk of CHD was significantly higher for usual care than for special intervention participants. As with patients having cerebrovascular disease, blood pressure should be reduced gradually to avoid hypotensive episodes. Beta-blockers or calcium antagonists (especially those that reduce heart rate) may be specifically useful in patients with angina pectoris. For those who have had a myocardial infarction, non-ISA (non-intrinsic sympathomimetic activity) beta-blockers are the drugs of choice because they have been shown to reduce the risk of a subsequent event and sudden death.

Patients with Cardiac Failure

Control of elevated arterial pressure can improve myocardial function, prevent cardiac failure, and reduce mortality. ACE inhibitors, when used alone or in combination with digitalis or diuretics in patients with congestive failure, are effective in reducing mortality due to progressive congestive heart failure. The use of ACE inhibitors may decrease mortality even more than other vasodilator therapy.

Patients With Left Ventricular Hypertrophy

Left ventricular hypertrophy (LVH) permits cardiac adaptation to the increased afterload imposed by elevated blood pressure. However, LVH represents a major independent risk factor for cardiac death, myocardial infarction, and other morbid events, and control of elevated blood pressure should prevent LVH.

Echocardiography is the most sensitive and specific way to diagnose LVH, but its use is limited by cost. The electrocardiogram remains of value not only for detecting LVH but also for identifying evidence of myocardial ischemia or cardiac dysrhythmias.

All major drug classes, with the exception of direct-acting vasodilators, may reduce left ventricular mass and wall thickness, as may weight loss, and decrease of dietary salt intake. It is not known whether reversal of hypertension-induced cardiac hypertrophy improves the independent risk of cardiovascular morbidity and mortality associated with LVH. However, the presence of LVH is an indication for effective blood pressure control.

Patients with Peripheral Vascular Diseases

Hypertension is a major risk factor for the development of carotid atherosclerosis, arteriosclerosis obliterans, intermittent claudication, and aneurysms, including dissecting aneurysms; however, it is not known whether antihypertensive therapy will alter the course of the diseases. Arterial hypertrophy and atherosclerosis may further increase SBP and the pulse pressure. Effective control of pressure and other atherogenic factors may help retard or even reverse the stiffening of arteries.

Patients with Hypertension and Other Coexisting Diseases

Patients with Renal Disease

The hypertension of chronic renal failure is largely volume dependent due to retention of sodium and water. Thus, relatively large doses of diuretics are often needed as part of the treatment regimen. A loop diuretic (furosemide, bumetanide, ethacrynic acid) or metolazone or indapamide is usually necessary to accomplish a significant diuresis when the serum creatinine level has reached 221 μmol/ L (2.5 mg/dL) or more. Potassium supplements and potassium-sparing diuretics are relatively contraindicated in the presence of even mild renal insufficiency.

All of the commonly used classes of antihypertensive drugs are usually effective in lowering blood pressure in patients with renal disease. In those whose hypertension has become resistant to multiple drug therapy that includes large doses of loop diuretics, minoxidil may be needed. In animal experiments as well as short-term clinical trials of small subsets of selected patients with diabetic nephropathy, ACE inhibitors have been shown to reduce proteinuria and slow progression of renal disease. However, acute renal failure can be precipitated by ACE inhibitors in hypertensive patients with bilateral renal artery stenosis, renal artery stenosis to a solitary kidney, and preexisting re-

491

nal disease. Hyperkalemia is a definite risk in azotemic patients receiving ACE inhibitors, especially those who have diabetic renal disease or those using nonsteroidal anti-inflammatory drugs. Therefore, serum creatinine and potassium levels should be monitored carefully before and after initiation of ACE inhibitors in patients who have renal insufficiency.

Controlling high blood pressure clearly preserves renal function. Aggressive control of hypertension also prevents or slows the progression of renal failure. It is unclear whether any antihypertensive agent is preferred in this regard. It has been suggested that blood pressure should be reduced to 130/85 mm Hg or less to provide adequate protection of renal function in hypertensive patients.

Dietary protein and phosphate restriction are appropriate nondrug therapies that may preserve renal function and should be implemented early in the course of renal insufficiency. In the advanced stages of renal insufficiency, hypertension often becomes relatively resistant to multiple drug therapy, and adequate control requires either chronic dialysis or renal transplantation.

Patients with Diabetes Mellitus

Patients with hypertension and diabetes mellitus are especially vulnerable to cardiovascular complications; therefore, the control of hypertension and dyslipidemia as well as cessation of cigarette smoking are particularly important. For these patients the blood pressure goal should be 130/85 mm Hg or less. Lifestyle modifications are beneficial for control of hyperglycemia, dyslipidemia, and hypertension, which often coexist in obese patients with insulin resistance.

No antihypertensive agent is specifically contraindicated for use in the diabetic population, but caution is needed with most drugs. Diuretic-induced hypokalemia may worsen glucose tolerance; beta-blockers may worsen glucose tolerance, mask the symptoms of and prolong recovery from hypoglycemia; alpha$_1$-receptor blockers may aggravate postural hypotension; ACE inhibitors may induce hyperkalemia.

The potentially beneficial effect of ACE inhibitors on proteinuria and renal function in patients with diabetic renal disease is discussed in the previous section.

The syndrome of insulin resistance very closely parallels Type II diabetes mellitus. Hypertension, dyslipidemia, hyperinsulinemia, glucose intolerance, and, frequently, upper body obesity compose this syndrome. Insulin resistance can be improved by weight loss and exercise. Short-term studies in small numbers of patients have shown that alpha$_1$-receptor blockers and ACE inhibitors decrease insulin resistance.

Patients With Dyslipidemia

The common coexistence of hypercholesterolemia and hypertension mandates effective management of both conditions. Since lifestyle modifications are the first approach to treatment of both conditions, great emphasis must be placed on control of overweight, reduction of cholesterol and saturated fat intake, and increased physical activity in patients with elevated lipids and hypertension.

If lifestyle modifications are not successful in controlling blood pressure, drug therapy must be added. Thiazide and loop diuretics can induce at least short-term small increases in levels of total plasma cholesterol, triglycerides, and low-density lipoprotein cholesterol. Several studies have suggested that this dyslipidemic effect may decrease or disappear with long-term therapy. Dietary modifications may reduce or eliminate these effects.

Beta-blockers may increase levels of plasma triglycerides and reduce those of high-density lipoprotein cholesterol. Despite this effect, non-ISA beta-blockers are the only agents that have been shown to decrease, in those with previous myocardial infarction, the rate of sudden death, overall mortality, and recurrent myocardial infarction. Beta-blockers with intrinsic sympathomimetic activity or labetalol have little or no adverse effect on lipids, but these agents have not been demonstrated to have a cardioprotective effect after a myocardial infarction.

The alpha$_1$-receptor blockers and the central adrenergic agonists may decrease serum cholesterol concentration to a slight degree, especially in the low-density lipoprotein subfraction. Therefore, these agents may offer an advantage in managing hypertensive patients with dyslipidemia. ACE inhibitors and calcium antagonists have no adverse effects on levels of serum lipids and lipoprotein.

Patients With Chronic Airways Disease or Bronchial Asthma

In hypertensive patients with chronic obstructive pulmonary disease (COPD)—including chronic bronchitis, emphysema, and/or asthma—beta-adrenergic blocking drugs can worsen bronchoconstriction and are therefore relatively contraindicated. Calcium antagonists do not cause bronchial constriction but in rare cases can cause or aggravate hypoxemia by dilating the pulmonary arterial circulation, thereby worsening the mismatch between regional ventilation and regional perfusion. ACE inhibitors can cause cough, which may be more significant when it complicates COPD. Recognizing these limitations, all antihypertensive agents, except beta-blockers and the alpha-beta blocker, can be used in hypertensive patients who have COPD.

Methylxanthines (theophylline) and corticosteroids often used in managing COPD can worsen hypertension; in addition, methylxanthines cause tachycardia and are arrhythmogenic. Beta-adrenergic agonists used to treat COPD are not as likely as methylxanthines to worsen hypertension, but they do cause tachycardia and can be arrhythmogenic.

Over-the-counter asthma preparations may contain ephedrine as a bronchodilator, and over-the-counter common cold preparations frequently contain phenylpropanolamine or pseudoephedrine as a vaso-constrictor, all of which can increase blood pressure and heart rate.

Patients With Gout

Hyperuricemia is a frequent finding, even in untreated patients with hypertension, and may reflect a decrease in renal blood flow. In addition, all of the commonly used diuretics, including the potassium-sparing class, can increase serum uric acid and induce acute gout. Body mass and serum uric acid are closely correlated; weight loss can produce a fall in serum uric acid in overweight hypertensive patients even with diuretic treatment. For patients with poorly controlled gout, diuretics should be avoided (or used intermittently). Diuretic-induced hyperuricemia does not require treatment in the absence of gout or urate stones.

Patients Undergoing Surgery

Surgical candidates who are adequately controlling their blood pressure with medication should be maintained on their regimen until the time of surgery, and therapy should be reinstated as soon as possible after surgery. If oral intake must be interrupted, parenteral therapy with diuretics, adrenergic inhibitors, vasodilators, ACE inhibitors, calcium antagonists, or transdermal clonidine may be used to

494

prevent the rebound hypertension that may follow sudden discontinuation of some of the adrenergic-inhibiting agents.

Adequate potassium supplementation should be provided to correct hypokalemia well in advance of surgery. A brief course of intravenous potassium just prior to surgery may not be sufficient to correct longstanding hypokalemia. In all cases, anesthesiologists must be aware of the patient's medication status. Patients with hypertension whose blood pressure has been controlled on medication usually tolerate anesthesia better than do those whose pressures are poorly controlled.

Miscellaneous Causes for Increased Blood Pressure

Cocaine

Cocaine, like the amphetamines, increases release of norepinephrine and prevents neuronal re-uptake of norepinephrine. As a result, it induces acute hypertension, tachycardia, tremor, and seizures and produces coronary artery vasoconstriction. Cocaine is also associated with ischemic and hemorrhagic cerebrovascular strokes in young adults. The onset of symptoms, especially severe headache, often occurs within 1 hour of using the drug. The treatment of choice is alpha-adrenergic inhibition (e.g., phentolamine). A beta-blocker should be used for complicating cardiac dysrhythmias induced by the catecholamine excess.

Lithotripsy

Extracorporeal shock wave lithotripsy (ESWL) can cause localized vascular injury that may be associated with transient decreases in renal blood flow and glomerular filtration rate in the treated kidney, transient proteinuria, and slight elevation of diastolic blood pressure. Acute hypertension following ESWL has been reported but is exceedingly uncommon. The procedure can also cause subcapsular and perirenal hematomas and fluid collection, with the incidence of bleeding higher in patients with hypertension. There is little or no evidence, however, that these complications of ESWL lead to permanent renal damage or hypertension, but there is some concern that they may lead to capsular and perirenal scarring. There are no data to suggest specifically that patients with existing hypertension are made worse by the procedure.

Cyclosporine

Cyclosporine causes vasoconstriction mediated in part by stimulation of the sympathetic nervous system and imbalance in the production of eicosanoids such as prostacyclin and thromboxane. Vasoconstriction of the afferent arteriole leads to reduction in renal blood flow and glomerular filtration rate, resulting in increased reabsorption of sodium, water, and urea. Cyclosporine also has direct nephrotoxicity manifested histologically by nephrosclerosis and interstitial fibrosis. Acute nephrotoxicity usually reverses promptly with intravenous fluids and temporary discontinuation or reduction in the dose of cyclosporine.

The vasoconstrictive and salt-retaining properties of cyclosporine lead to hypertension in 50 to 70 percent of transplant recipients receiving the drug and in 20 percent of patients receiving the drug for other reasons. Diuretics are an effective therapy, but they exaggerate prerenal azotemia and may precipitate gout. Calcium antagonists and labetalol are effective, as are central alpha-agonists such as clonidine. Diltiazem, nicardipine, and verapamil should be used with caution as they increase cyclosporine blood levels, but they may be given if the interaction is appreciated.

Erythropoietin

Recombinant human erythropoietin (rHuEPO) increases blood pressure in one-third of patients with end-stage renal disease. In most cases this necessitates initiation or increase of antihypertensive therapy. The mechanism of hypertension related to rHuEPO remains uncertain. It is not related to the dose of rHuEPO or to the final hematocrit level achieved or to the rate of increase of hematocrit. It is associated with an increase in systemic vascular resistance due largely to an increase in blood viscosity and reversal of hypoxic vasodilatation. Acute elevation in blood pressure during therapy with rHuEPO occasionally results in hypertensive encephalopathy and seizures. Frequent blood pressure monitoring during the first 4 months of treatment is mandatory. If conventional antihypertensive therapy does not control hypertension, the dose of rHuEPO should be reduced or therapy temporarily discontinued.

Chapter 53

High Blood Pressure in Pregnancy

Introduction

The hypertensive disorders during pregnancy are important causes of maternal death throughout the world, and most of these deaths are attributed to eclampsia. The hypertensive disorders also extensively contribute to stillbirths and neonatal morbidity and mortality. Hypertensive expectant mothers (or gravidas) are predisposed to the development of potentially lethal complications, notably abruptio placentae, disseminated intravascular coagulation (DIC), cerebral hemorrhage, hepatic failure, and acute renal failure.

The prevalence of chronic hypertension in pregnancy (that is, in those hypertensive women who become pregnant) is not known. It differs widely in different geographic areas but is probably present in 1 to 5 percent of all pregnancies. The number of women who become hypertensive during pregnancy (preeclamptic) is also unclear, but one estimate from an indigent population is calculated to be about 13 percent, and incidences ranging from 10 to 20 percent have been noted in nulliparous women.

The purpose of this report is to provide guidance to the practicing physician in 1) managing hypertensive patients who become pregnant (hypertension that is present and observable prior to pregnancy or diagnosed before the 20th week of gestation) and 2) managing preg-

NIH Publication No. 91-3029 and *FDA Consumer*, June 1992..

nant patients who become hypertensive (the pregnancy-specific condition termed preeclampsia). This report expands on the recommendations of *The 1988 Report of the Joint National Committee on Detection, Evaluation, and Treatment of High Blood Pressure* (JNC IV).

Executive Summary

High blood pressure complicates almost 10 percent of all pregnancies, and the incidence is higher if the women are nulliparous or carrying multiple fetuses. Causes of hypertension in pregnancy are multiple, and many current and previously used classification systems are elaborate and confusing, due in part to difficulty in making an etiological diagnosis by clinical criteria alone. The consensus group recommends the schema proposed by the American College of Obstetrics and Gynecologists in 1972, which has been in wide use for some time, is practical and concise, and considers hypertension associated with gestation in only four categories: I. chronic hypertension (of whatever cause, but mainly essential in nature); II. preeclampsia; III. preeclampsia superimposed upon chronic hypertension; and IV. transient hypertension.

Preeclampsia (pure or superimposed) represents the greatest danger for the fetus and is associated with life-threatening maternal syndromes, while transient hypertension is a fairly benign disorder characterized by mild to moderate elevations of blood pressure late in pregnancy which return to normal postpartum. Essential hypertension, too, is usually well tolerated if elevations remain (with or without therapy) below diastolic levels of 100 mm Hg (phase V), but complications such as midtrimester loss, growth retardation, and abruption may occur more frequently. (Diastolic blood pressure, in this document, is defined as the onset of Korotkoff phase V—disappearance of sound.) Because the preeclamptic syndromes and essential hypertension comprise over three-quarters of the hypertensive disorders in pregnancy, this document focuses on the presentation, pathophysiology, and management of these diseases.

Preeclampsia, a disease peculiar to pregnancy, mainly in nulliparas, presents primarily after gestational week 20, most frequently near term. Signs helpful in its diagnosis are presence of proteinuria, edema (especially if of recent and rapid onset), and any of the following: hemoconcentration, hypoalbuminemia, hepatic function and/or coagulation abnormalities, and increased urate levels. The predictive value of raised serum iron, low antithrombin III, and hypocalciuria are under investigation.

A major pathophysiological feature of this disease is a marked increase in peripheral resistance. This vasospasm is due, in part, to exaggerated vascular responsiveness to circulating angiotensin II and catecholamines (and possibly an imbalance between thromboxane and prostacyclin production). Prior to intervention, cardiac output is often decreased, pulmonary capillary wedge pressure is normal or low, and intravascular volume is below that of normal pregnant women. Renal hemodynamics also decrease due, in part, to a characteristic morphological lesion in the glomerulus, and there may be increased vascular permeability leading to albumin loss from the intravascular space. Uteroplacental perfusion is often compromised, which may lead to fetal growth retardation.

Preeclampsia can lead to two life-threatening complications. The first is a rapidly developing syndrome characterized by microangiopathic hemolytic anemia and marked signs of liver dysfunction as well as coagulation changes. This variant, termed HELLP (hemolysis elevated liver enzymes low platelet count), constitutes an emergency requiring prompt pregnancy termination. The second complication is progression of preeclampsia to a convulsive phase termed eclampsia, at one time the major cause of cerebral bleeding and maternal mortality in this disorder. Pending or frank eclampsia also requires immediate termination of gestation.

Therapy for preeclampsia when gestation is advanced is delivery. Severe intrapartum hypertension is controlled with intravenous hydralazine, which is successful in most instances. Favorable results have been recorded with parenteral diazoxide, labetalol, and clonidine as well as oral nifedipine. Nitroprusside should be avoided unless maternal jeopardy is extreme. Magnesium sulfate remains the drug of choice to prevent or treat eclamptic convulsions.

Women with essential hypertension often experience reductions in blood pressure during the first two trimesters; failure for this to occur is an unfavorable prognostic sign. When pharmacological intervention is required, alpha methyldopa, because of its long history of safe use and a trial including a 7-year followup of the neonate, remains the drug of choice to treat chronic hypertension in pregnancy. Data relevant to beta blocking agents and combined beta and alpha adrenergic receptor antagonists demonstrate their usefulness with little or no evidence of fetal jeopardy. Thiazide diuretics, which have been used safely in normotensive gravidas, may be used in hypertensive pregnant women—especially those who are salt sensitive. Preliminary information concerning calcium channel antagonists is also encouraging, but angiotensin converting enzyme inhibitors are contraindicated in pregnant women.

Finally, like all pregnant women, those with hypertension should refrain from alcohol and tobacco. The roles of calcium supplementation and low-dose aspirin (which decreases thromboxane synthesis while sparing prostacyclin production) to prevent preeclampsia and/or chronic and transient hypertension are under investigation.

Certain Hypertension Drugs Dangerous for Pregnant Women

Pregnant women who take angiotensin-converting enzyme (ACE) inhibitors, drugs used to treat high blood pressure, should consult their doctors about switching treatment. Using the drugs past the first three months of pregnancy could result in significant harm and even death to the fetus.

At FDA's request, the six U.S. companies that manufacture the drugs sent a letter in March to doctors emphasizing the risks when women in the second and third trimesters of pregnancy take ACE inhibitors. In addition, FDA announced that all ACE inhibitors would be required to carry a boxed warning on the label.

The companies that manufacture ACE inhibitors are Bristol-Myers Squibb (Capoten, Capozide, Monopril), Ciba-Geigy (Lotensin), Hoechst-Roussel Pharmaceuticals (Altace), ICI Pharmaceuticals Group (Zestril, Zestoretic), Merck-Sharp & Dohme (Vasotec, Vasotec I.V., Vaseretic, Prinivil, Prinzide), and Parke-Davis (Accupril).

FDA's actions were prompted by continuing reports of fetal damage, including kidney failure and face or skull deformities, caused by these hypertension drugs. Although labeling for the products has for several years warned of the risks, more than 50 cases of fetal harm have been reported over the past several years.

In addition, very limited epidemiological evidence from Tennessee and Michigan Medicaid data bases indicates that fetal injury from exposure to ACE inhibitors in the second and third trimesters may be as high as 10 to 20 percent. FDA Commissioner David A. Kessler, M.D., noted, "The additional warnings will allow the safe use of ACE inhibitors by women who need them while helping to assure that women who become pregnant while taking these drugs promptly seek alternative treatment."

Pharmacists are being asked to counsel women of childbearing age who are taking ACE inhibitors about the risks and are being provided with warning stickers to place directly on the prescription bottles. Women taking ACE inhibitors who become pregnant should continue to take the medication because uncontrolled hypertension is dangerous to both mother and fetus, but they should consult their doctors immediately. There appears to be no risk to fetuses when the drugs are taken during the first trimester.

Chapter 54

Ambulatory Blood Pressure Monitoring

Introduction

Casual blood pressure measurements taken in a doctor's office or clinic or by patients themselves are not necessarily representative of blood pressure readings throughout the 24-hour day. Ambulatory blood pressure monitoring (ABPM) overcomes this problem by providing multiple readings over time with minimal intrusion into the patient's daily activities.

Techniques for ambulatory blood pressure measurement have evolved over the past 30 years as a means of obtaining multiple observations over time. Studies using direct, intraarterial equipment have been carried out primarily in Europe with Oxford equipment. While this technique measures beat-to-beat blood pressure and is less susceptible to environmental artifacts, it does require indwelling arterial catheters and does not lend itself to repeated studies on large numbers of subjects.

The development of techniques for indirect measurement of ambulatory blood pressure began with the introduction of the semiautomatic Remler device (no longer available). By the mid-1970's, fully automatic devices were available that were able to record approximately 200 blood pressures over a 24-hour period. These ambulatory devices measure blood pressure in the arm, either by auscultation of

Taken from NIH Pub. No. 92-3028.

503

Korotkoff sounds or oscillometry or both. Recently, finger cuff techniques have been developed, although they are not generally available.

Many reports have addressed the use of ambulatory devices in evaluating blood pressure changes with different antihypertensive drugs; correlating target organ damage and hypertension; and assisting with diagnostic problems such as "office" ("white-coat") hypertension, borderline hypertension, resistant hypertension, and special clinical situations such as orthostatic hypotension and pheochromocytoma. Researchers also have used ABPM coupled with electrocardiogram (ECG) monitoring to study such problems as syncope and "spells." This report addresses the current state of ABPM methodology, normal blood pressure profiles, the clinical and research uses of ABPM, cost considerations, and recommendations for use of this technique in selected circumstances.

Executive Summary

Ambulatory blood pressure monitoring (ABPM) is a technique by which multiple indirect blood pressure readings may be taken automatically over a period of 1 or more days with minimal intrusion into the daily activities of the patient. Although ABPM is not necessary for the diagnosis and management of most patients with hypertension, this technique appears to have certain benefits in selected research and clinical situations.

ABPM devices, which are now automatic, lightweight, and quiet, use either auscultatory or oscillometric methods to determine blood pressure. Before use, each device must be calibrated to the patient, who also may keep a diary of activities, medications, and emotions for the period in question. The data obtained through the devices are then analyzed with computer software and interpreted, often with the help of diary entries. The frequency of blood pressure readings and methods of analysis are not standardized and may depend on the biologic questions asked. Research needs with regard to ABPM methods include a rigorous comparison of auscultatory and oscillometric methods to determine if one method is more reliable. Also needed is a nonbiased assessment of all equipment to evaluate accuracy, reliability, and utility in the field.

Researchers have used ABPM to study 1) normal blood pressure patterns; 2) target organ complications of hypertension; 3) the prognosis of cardiovascular events and mortality; and 4) the effects of antihypertensive drugs.

Studies of normotensives show that blood pressure, which is characterized by a clear circadian rhythm, peaks during the daytime hours. Blood pressure also varies with work, activity, emotion, and possibly by race and age. Few studies of normative ABPM profiles are under way; normative data are needed for populations by age, race, gender, body habitus, and conditions such as pregnancy.

Research also has demonstrated that ABPM correlates with the target organ complications of hypertension better than casual office or home blood pressure readings. Thus, the correlation of blood pressure load with the development of target organ complications can be addressed with ABPM. In addition, the limited number of studies concerning prognosis indicate that, for patients with similar office blood pressures, the incidence of future cardiovascular events and mortality correlates best with mean ambulatory blood pressures.

ABPM also has proven useful in clinical trials of antihypertensive drug efficacy and in the investigation of drug dosage and effects. By excluding placebo responders, ABPM has reduced the number of mild hypertensives that researchers need to demonstrate drug efficacy. Longitudinal studies are needed to determine which ABPM profiles are associated with low and which with elevated cardiovascular risk and what changes in these profiles, induced by antihypertensive therapy, are associated with reduced risk.

Several clinical problems are better elucidated by ABPM than by casual readings. These are borderline hypertension with target organ involvement; "resistant" hypertension; episodic hypertension; "office" or "white coat" hypertension; and evaluation of episodic hypotensive symptoms.

On the other hand, ABPM is not appropriate for the diagnosis and management of a large majority of patients with hypertension, particularly in the presence of target organ damage and other risk factors. Unless there is a significant new problem in a well-managed patient such as syncope or new target organ damage, there is seldom an indication to obtain or repeat ABPM (aside from research purposes). Intermittent measurements by the patient at work and at home suffice to monitor the treatment response over a prolonged period of time between visits to the physician.

While indiscriminate use of ABPM on all hypertensive patients probably would increase costs out of proportion to any benefits gained, two economic models have demonstrated that ABPM, appropriately used, could be highly cost-effective for persons initially classified as having mild hypertension. Comprehensive cost-benefit models are still needed for the use of ABPM in the management and treatment of hypertension, and any such models will have to be evaluated in clinical trials.

In summary, various technical problems concerning ABPM need to be addressed and better normative and longitudinal data on its use must be obtained. Nonetheless, there are selected circumstances in which this technique has certain clinical uses as well as a number of research benefits.

Part Seven

Lifestyle Choices
For a Healthier
Cardiovascular System

Chapter 55

Obesity and Cardiovascular Disease

Overview

Obesity is one of the most prevalent diet-related problems in the United States, affecting more than a quarter of the U.S. population—nearly 44 million people. Obesity is associated with an increased risk for high blood pressure, high blood cholesterol, and diabetes, and is an independent risk factor for coronary heart disease (CHD). Studies reveal that reduction in body weight can lower blood pressure and improve blood cholesterol levels in overweight individuals and in individuals who have high blood pressure or high blood cholesterol. Obesity contributes to the development of sleep apnea, and weight loss is thought to improve this condition.

Obesity refers to an excess of body fat. Obesity is correlated with the degree of overweight, and these terms are often used interchangeably. Being overweight is also associated · ·+h an increased risk for Canaan diseases and conditions. Use of the term obesity or overweight in this data fact sheet does not imply extreme amounts of body fat in all cases.

In January 1991, the National Heart, Lung, and Blood Institute (NHLBI) launched the Obesity Education Initiative (OEI). The purpose of the initiative is to educate professionals and the public on the relationship of overweight and heart disease and impaired lung func-

An unnumbered publication of the National Heart, Lung, and Blood Institute.

tion. The OEI will address the determinants, consequences, and treatment issues related to obesity, and will integrate and enhance obesity education activities across NHLBI's other education programs, including the National High Blood Pressure Education Program, the National Cholesterol Education Program, and the NHLBI Smoking Education Program.

This data fact sheet examines the prevalence of obesity according to age, sex, race, and Hispanic origin, as well as the prevalence of obesity among persons with other cardiovascular risk factors (e.g., high blood pressure and high blood cholesterol). These data are derived from the second National Health and Nutrition Examination Survey 1976-80 (NHANES II), and the Hispanic Health and Nutrition Examination Survey 1982-84 (HHANES), both conducted by the National Center for Health Statistics (NCHS). The risk of high blood pressure and high blood cholesterol and the independent risk of cardiovascular disease (CVD) associated with obesity are described as reported in large NHLBI-funded cohort studies such as the Framingham Heart Study and the Nurses' Health Study. The benefits of weight loss in terms of reduction in blood pressure and improved lipid profiles are reported based on findings of research sponsored by NHLBI, including two multicenter clinical trials, Phase I of the Trials of Hypertension Prevention (TOHP) and the Trials of Antihypertensive Intervention and Management (TAIM).

Definition

Obesity and overweight are often used interchangeably. This is not precisely correct. Obesity really means an excess of body fat, regardless of weight. Overweight is defined as an excess of weight, generally in comparison to height.

The methods for estimating body fat vary in approach and in complexity—from estimates based on weight to height ratios or skinfold thickness—to more direct but difficult measures, such as hydrostatic weighing. The degree of excess body fat is highly correlated with the degree of overweight. The most common measure of relative weight is body mass index (BMI), which is calculated as weight in kilograms (kg) divided by the square of the height in meters [$BMI=weight(kg)/height(m)^2$].

The National Center for Health Statistics defines overweight as a BMI greater than or equal to 27.8 for men and 27.3 for women. This is approximately 20 percent above what many experts call the "desirable weight." Unless otherwise noted, this is the definition of overweight used in this data fact sheet. In addition, some scientific reports cited here compare the experience of various equal segments of their population—e.g., the heaviest and lightest fifths (or "quintiles"). Although the issues of measurement and definition are complex, the risks associated with obesity or overweight have been consistently shown regardless of the measurement.

Prevalence of Overweight

Data from the National Center for Health Statistics report that the prevalence of overweight is greater among women than men (27.1 vs. 24.2 percent), and the major differences appear in the older age groups [Figure 55.1]). More than 37 percent of older women (over 55 years of age) are overweight.

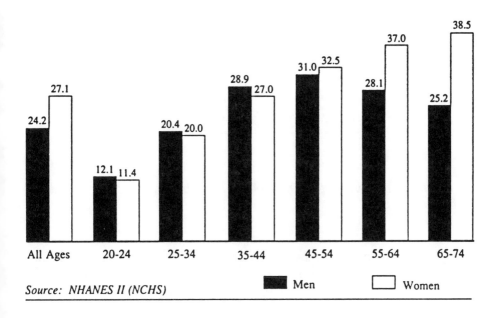

Figure 55.1. Prevalence of Overweight According to Sex and Age

Obesity is more common in minority populations, particularly women. [Figure 55.2] presents the percent of black, white, and Mexican-American men and women who are overweight. The prevalence of overweight among blacks and Mexican-Americans is greater than among whites, and the percent of black and Mexican-American women who are overweight is especially high.

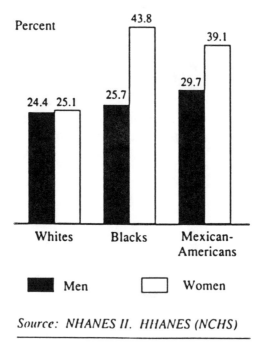

Source: NHANES II. HHANES (NCHS)

Figure 55.2. *Prevalence of Overweight Among blacks, Whites, and Mexican-Americans by Sex*

Obesity is associated with other cardiovascular disease risk factors. [Figure 55.3] presents the percent of persons with high blood pressure and high blood cholesterol who are also overweight. Fifty percent of women and 39 percent of men with high blood pressure are also overweight. Thirty-six percent of women and 31 percent of men with high blood cholesterol are also overweight.

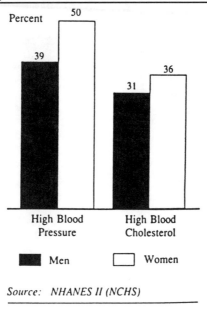

Source: NHANES II (NCHS)

Figure 55.3. Prevalence of Overseight Among Persons with HBP or HBCi

Obesity and High Blood Pressure

The prevalence of other risk factors for cardiovascular disease is greater in obese populations than nonobese populations. [Figure 55.4] shows that the prevalence of high blood pressure is at least twice as great in overweight populations as in nonoverweight populations. Persons with high blood pressure are defined here as those with a systolic and diastolic pressure of greater than or equal to 140/90 mmHg or those on antihypertensive medications. Fifty-five percent of overweight men have high blood pressure, compared to 27 percent of nonoverweight men. Similarly, 52 percent of overweight women have high blood pressure, compared to 19 percent of nonoverweight women.

Based on the Framingham cohort there appears to be a linear increase in blood pressures, both systolic and diastolic. associated with an increase in weight as defined by BMI [Figure 55.5]. The differences between the leanest one fifth of the population (or quintile) and the most obese quintile are 16-17 mmHg for systolic and 11 mmHg for diastolic, in both men and women.

A number of studies have shown that weight reduction in obese patients is an effective method for lowering blood pressure, not only in

513

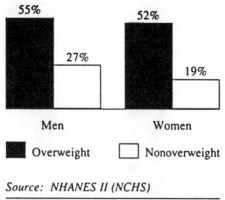

Source: NHANES II (NCHS)

Figure 55.4. Prevalence of High Blood Pressure in Overweight and Nonoverweight Men and Women

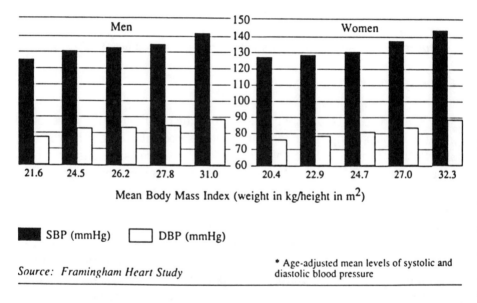

Source: Framingham Heart Study

* Age-adjusted mean levels of systolic and diastolic blood pressure

Figure 55.5. Mean Level of Systolic and Diastolic Blood Pressure* According to Body Mass Index

patients who have hypertension but also in individuals who are not diagnosed as hypertensive but who have blood pressure in the high normal range. In a recent clinical study, obese hypertensive patients lost a mean of 10.4 kg during treatment and decreased their systolic and diastolic blood pressure by 10.8 and 8.0 mmHg, respectively. [Figure 55.6] shows that the degree of reduction in blood pressure was greatest among unmedicated hypertensives (15.8/13.8 mmHg), followed by medicated hypertensives (14.9/7.2 mmHg), and normotensive patients (7.1/4.8 mmHg).

	Systolic Change (mmHg)	Diastolic Change (mmHg)
Unmedicated Hypertensive	15.8	13.8
Medicated Hypertensive	14.9	7.2
Normotensive	7.1	4.8

Source: Schotte and Stunkard

Figure 55.6. Reduction in systolic and Diastolic Blood Pressure With Weight Loss Among Obese Patients According to Hyptertension Status

Among mild hypertensives, data from the Trial of Antihypertensive Intervention and Management, a randomized controlled clinical trial, showed that when controlling for all other variables, weight loss of 4.7 kg yields a decrease of 23 mmHg diastolic blood pressure. This study concluded that weight loss is beneficial in the treatment of mild hypertension.

Finally, data from Phase I of the Trials of Hypertension Prevention, also a randomized controlled clinical trial, show that in obese individuals who are normotensive, a 3.9-kg weight loss produces a decrease of 2.3 mmHg in their diastolic blood pressure and 2.9 mmHg in their systolic blood pressure.

Results of these studies and others show that blood pressure and body weight are related and that the prevalence of hypertension is greater among obese individuals than among nonobese individuals. Furthermore, a reduction in weight, in both obese and nonobese individuals, whether or not they have hypertension, is associated with a reduction in blood pressure.

Obesity and High Blood Cholesterol

[Figure 55.7] presents the prevalence of high blood cholesterol among overweight men and women as compared to nonoverweight men and women. High blood cholesterol here is defined as cholesterol levels greater than 240 mg/dL. Among overweight men, 32 percent have high blood cholesterol as compared to 22 percent of nonoverweight men. Among overweight women, 38 percent have high blood cholesterol as compared to 25 percent of nonoverweight women.

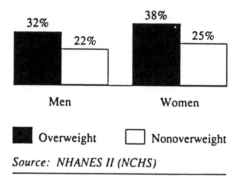

Men   Women

■ Overweight   □ Nonoverweight

Source: NHANES II (NCHS)

Figure 55.7. *Prevalence of High Blood Cholesterol in Overweight and Nonoverweight Men and Women*

Data from the Framingham cohort show that as weight increases there is an increase in the blood cholesterol level. Differences in cholesterol levels between the leanest group (the first quintile) as compared to the most obese group are 13 mg/dL for men and 9 mg/dL for women [Figure 55.8]. In addition, the Framingham study revealed that a change in weight was associated with a change in cholesterol level. In men, a 10-pound change in weight over 2 years was associated with a 7.5-mg/dL change in serum cholesterol, and in women this weight change was associated with a 5.8-mg/dL change in serum cholesterol.

A recent paper from investigators at Stanford University reported that when exercise is added to a diet reduced in total fat, saturated fat, and cholesterol, the blood lipid profile improves among

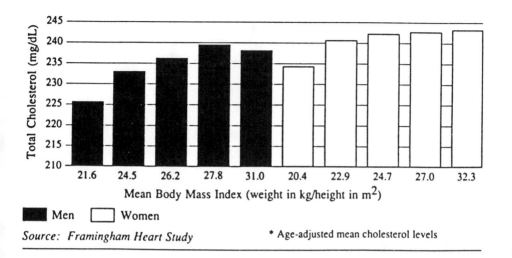

Figure 55.8. *Mean Cholesterol Level* According to Body Mass Index*

overweight men and women. After 1 year of followup in this random-ized controlled clinical trial, the two intervention groups—diet and diet plus exercise—resulted in a loss of weight and body fat as com-pared to the control group. The diet and exercise group lost signifi-cantly more body fat than the diet alone group. As a result of the two interventions both men and women had a drop in their total and LDL-cholesterol levels. This was significant among the women. The men in the diet plus exercise group had the advantage of increasing the level of protective HDL-cholesterol compared to the diet and control groups. In women, diet plus exercise prevented the decrease in HDL-choles-terol levels that occurred in the women who followed the diet only [Figure 55.9].

The effect of weight loss on serum cholesterol levels of obese in-dividuals has been shown to depend on the composition of the diet as well as the individual's initial blood cholesterol level. Both the Mul-tiple Risk Factor Intervention Trial and the National Diet and Heart Study reported that weight reduction combined with a diet low in saturated fat and cholesterol results in twice the reduction in serum cholesterol than a change in diet composition alone.

A recent meta analysis, which pooled the data from 70 studies, indicated that weight reduction was associated with significant de-

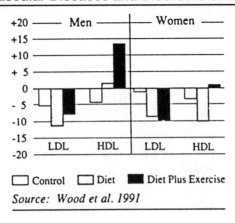

Figure 55.9. *Percent Change in Lipoprotein Cholesterol Concentration in the Study Groups After 1 Year*

creases in total cholesterol, LDL-cholesterol, and triglycerides. These results indicate that weight reduction through dieting can be a viable approach to help reduce lipid levels in overweight individuals with high blood cholesterol.

Obesity and Smoking

In general cigarette smokers weigh less and are leaner than non-smokers. Reviews of the relationship between weight gain and smoking cessation have estimated the average weight gain following smoking cessation to be between 4.5 and 7.5 pounds. Recent studies, however, have suggested that certain groups of individuals may be at risk for large amounts of weight gain.

Obesity and Coronary Heart Disease

In addition to increasing the risk of high blood pressure and high blood cholesterol, obesity is an independent risk factor for coronary heart disease. [Figure 55.10] presents the results of 28 years of followup of Framingham data. Age-adjusted rates per 100 persons are presented for incidence of coronary heart disease by BMI and smoking status among men and women. Rates are higher in smokers than in nonsmokers and increase with increasing BMI in both groups of men. Among women the rates are approximately the same for the three leanest groups and higher for the two heavier groups.

Event and smoking status		Mean BMI				
Men		21.6	24.5	26.2	27.8	31.0
CHD:	Nonsmokers	25.3	33.0	34.8	37.3	37.1
	Smokers	27.3	34.4	36.0	44.9	47.3
CHD-AP:	Nonsmokers	21.6	26.5	27.2	31.0	29.7
	Smokers	22.5	28.5	30.1	41.3	39.3
Total mortality:	Nonsmokers	47.3	45.3	47.7	47.1	50.5
	Smokers	52.7	52.3	59.7	58.5	64.1

		Mean BMI				
Women		20.4	22.9	24.7	27.0	32.3
CHD:	Nonsmokers	19.4	19.4	21.0	22.3	26.6
	Smokers	19.5	20.9	19.9	29.0	31.6
CHD-AP:	Nonsmokers	10.3	11.3	12.7	13.0	16.2
	Smokers	16.3	12.6	16.7	23.7	25.6
Total mortality:	Nonsmokers	33.5	32.4	33.7	34.2	39.4
	Smokers	39.4	38.8	38.2	45.0	51.6

Source: Framingham Heart Study, followup

Figure 55.10. *Age-Adjusted Rates per 100 of Coronary Heart Disease With and Without Angina Pectoris and Total mortality According to BMI and Smoking Status Among Men and Women*

The Nurses' Health Study examined the incidence of nonfatal and fatal coronary heart disease in relation to obesity in middle-aged women and concluded that obesity is a strong risk factor for coronary heart disease. Even mild to moderate overweight is associated with a substantial elevation in coronary risk [Figure 55.11].

The Framingham Heart Study and the Nurses' Health Study found that weight gain during adulthood further increases the risk of coronary heart disease. The Nurses Health Study found that a weight gain of 22-44 extra pounds (10-19.9 kg) during adulthood increases the risk of coronary heart disease by 60 percent. The Framingham data reflect the same conclusions regarding weight gain, but weight loss and obesity were found to be associated with mortality from all causes and cardiovascular disease.

Data that demonstrate a U- or J-shaped curve associated with body weight and all-cause mortality indicate that the leanest level is associated with a greater mortality. Although weight loss is associated

519

with improvements in blood pressure and blood cholesterol levels, leanness and weight loss is also associated with cigarette smoking. This is further complicated by studies that show decreases in weight associated with increased all-cause mortality. It is not clear if these data report the effect of illness on weight and mortality or the effect of weight on illness and mortality.

Interpretation of these data requires consideration of age, sex, level of BMI, presence of other risk factors, including cigarette smoking and high blood pressure or high blood cholesterol, and reasons for weight loss.

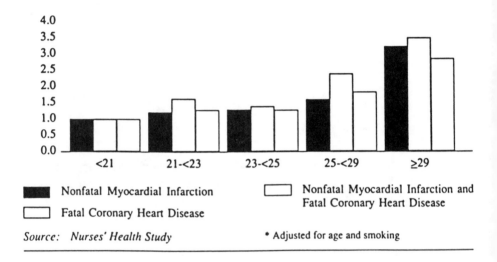

Figure 55.11. *Relative Risks of Nonfatal Myocardial Infarction, Fatal Coronary Heart Disease, and Nonfatal Myocardial Infarction and Fatal Coronary Heart Disease, Conbined, According to Body Mass Index**

Chapter 56

Eating to Lower
Your High Blood Cholesterol

High blood cholesterol is a serious problem. Along with high blood pressure and cigarette smoking, it is one of the three major modifiable risk factors for coronary heart disease. Approximately 25 percent of the adult population 20 years of age and older has "high" blood cholesterol levels—levels that are high enough to need intensive medical attention. More than half of all adult Americans have a blood cholesterol level that is higher than "desirable."

Because high blood cholesterol is a risk to your health, you need to take steps to lower your blood cholesterol level. The best way to do this is to make sure you eat foods that are low in saturated fat and cholesterol. The purpose of this brochure is to help you learn how to choose these foods...[Further information on cholesterol may be found in other chapters. Chapter 10 contains important basic facts about cholesterol. Chapter 26 contains information about cholesterol in children. Chapter 50 offers suggestions for improving your cholesterol levels using other strategies in addition to dietary modification. In this chapter] specific instructions are given for modifying eating patterns to lower your blood cholesterol, choosing low-saturated fat and low-cholesterol foods, and preparing low-fat dishes...

Taken from NIH Pub. No. 92-2920.

The Recommended Treatment:
A Blood Cholesterol-Lowering Diet

Whatever the reasons may be for your high blood cholesterol level—diet, heredity, or both—the treatment your doctor will prescribe first is a diet. If your blood cholesterol level has not decreased sufficiently after carefully following the diet for 6 months, your doctor may consider adding cholesterol-lowering medication to your dietary treatment. Remember, diet is a very essential step in the treatment of high blood cholesterol. Cholesterol-lowering medications are more effective when combined with diet. Thus they are meant to supplement, not replace, a low-saturated fat, low-cholesterol diet.

What Changes Should You Make in Your Diet?

The following [list] illustrates some guidelines for dietary changes to help you lower your blood cholesterol level. Your new diet is low in saturated fat and low in cholesterol and is adequate in all nutrients, including protein, carbohydrate, fat, vitamins, and minerals.

- Eat less high-fat food (especially those high in saturated fat).

- Replace part of the saturated fat in your diet with unsaturated fat.
- Eat less high-cholesterol food.
- Choose foods high in complex carbohydrates (starch and fiber).
- Reduce your weight, if you are overweight.

How Should You Change Your Daily Menu?

So far we have discussed the basic dietary trends for reducing your blood cholesterol level. Now, we will focus on how to make specific changes in the foods you choose to eat. The following [guidelines describe] these dietary changes in terms of percentages of daily calories.

Guidelines for Lowering Your High Blood Cholesterol Level

Specific Changes

- Eat less than 30% of your total daily calories from fat.

- Less than 10% of your calories should come from saturated fat.
- No more than 10% of your calories should come from polyunsaturated fat.
- 10-15% of your calories should come from monounsaturated fat.
- Eat less than 300 mg of cholesterol each day.
- Eat 50-60% of your daily calories from carbohydrates.
- Adjust your caloric intake to achieve or maintain a desirable weight.

You can calculate the percent of your total daily calories from fat with the following equations (use the numbers from the [published calorie and fat content guides] or from food labels):

$$\% \text{ calories from fat} = (\text{total fat calories/total calories}) \times 100$$

$$\text{total fat calories} = \text{total fat (grams)} \times 9$$

In other words, if your daily calorie need is 2,000 calories, 30% of your total daily calories from fat would equal 600 calories, or 67 grams of fat.

Remember, when you are using these equations, that not **everything** you eat must have fewer than 30% calories from fat, but that you should **balance** foods with a slightly higher fat content with foods that have a much lower fat content.

Since fat, carbohydrate, and protein are the three major sources of calories, the amounts that you eat of each of them makes up your daily calorie intake. For example, as shown below, the average diet of an adult American provides about 35-40 percent of calories from fat, and about 47 percent from carbohydrate and 16 percent from protein. On a cholesterol-lowering diet, the percentage of calories from total fat decreases, while the percentage of calories from carbohydrate increases and protein may stay the same.

Average American and Cholesterol-Lowering Diets

[The average American diet consists of:]

- 35-40% Fat (15-20% saturated; 14-16% monounsaturated; 7% polyunsaturated)

- About 47% carbohydrate
- About 16% protein
- 350-450 mg cholesterol a day

[A cholesterol-lowering diet consists of:]

- Less than 30% fat (less than 10% saturated; 10-15% monounsaturated; up to 10% polyunsaturated)
- 50-60% carbohydrate
- Up to 20% protein
- Less than 300 mg cholesterol a day

The differences between these two diets are subtle and appear to be small, but they are very important for lowering your blood cholesterol level. All of these small changes add up to big improvements in your blood cholesterol level. Take a look at the [following] sample menus. Although the new low-fat diet has the same number of calories as the average American diet, it has much less fat. And, the sample menus show that because the fat you were eating was so calorie-rich, the new diet actually allows you to eat more food!

Sample Menus

Average American Diet
(37% fat)

Breakfast
1 fried egg
2 slices white toast with 1 teaspoon butter
1 cup orange juice black coffee or tea

Snack
1 doughnut

Lunch
1 grilled cheese (2 ounces) sandwich on white bread
2 oatmeal cookies
black coffee or tea

Snack
20 cheese cracker squares

Dinner
3 ounces fried hamburger with ketchup
1 baked potato with sour cream
3/4 cup steamed broccoli with 1 teaspoon butter
1 cup whole milk
1 piece frosted marble cake

Nutrient Analysis
Calories 2,000
Total fat (percent of calories) 37
Saturated fat (percent of calories) 19
Cholesterol 505 mg

A New Low-Fat Diet
(30% fat)

Breakfast
1 cup corn flakes with blueberries
1 cup 1% milk
1 slice rye toast with 1 teaspoon margarine
1 cup orange juice
black coffee or tea

Snack
1 toasted pumpernickel bagel with 1 teaspoon margarine

Lunch
1 tuna salad (3 ounces) sandwich on whole wheat bread with lettuce
and tomato
1 graham cracker
tea with lemon

Snack
1 crisp apple

Dinner
3 ounces broiled lean ground beef with ketchup
1 baked potato with low-fat plain yogurt and chives
3/4 Cup steamed broccoli with 1 teaspoon margarine
tossed garden salad with 1 tablespoon oil and vinegar dressing
1 cup 1% milk

1 small piece homemade gingerbread* with a maraschino cherry and sprig of mint

Nutrient Analysis
Calories 2,000
Total fat (percent of calories) 30
Saturated fat (percent of calories) 10
Cholesterol 186 mg

A New Low-Fat Diet
(30% fat)

Breakfast
1 cup shredded wheat with peach slices
1 cup 1% milk
1 slice whole wheat toast with 1 teaspoon margarine
1 cup pink grapefruit juice
black coffee

Snack
1 toasted English muffin with
1 teaspoon margarine

Lunch
3 ounces turkey salad on lettuce with tomato wedges
1 thick slice of French bread
10 animal crackers
tea with lemon

Snack
1 banana

Dinner
3 ounces broiled halibut with lemon and herb seasoning
1/2 cup brown rice with mushrooms
1 dinner roll with 1 teaspoon margarine
3/4 cup carrot strips with 1 teaspoon margarine
spinach salad with 1 tablespoon oil and vinegar dressing
1 cup 1% milk
1 small piece homemade yellow cake*

Nutrient Analysis
Total calories 2,000
Total fat (percent of calories) 30
Saturated fat (percent of calories) 10
Cholesterol 172 mg

*Homemade desserts should be made with unsaturated fats instead of saturated fats. Two egg whites may be substituted for one egg yolk.

What Kind of Success Can You Expect?

Generally your blood cholesterol level should begin to drop 2 to 3 weeks after you start on a cholesterol-lowering diet. Over time, you may reduce your level 30-55 mg/dl. The reduction in your blood cholesterol level depends on several factors:

- The amount of saturated fat in your diet. If your diet is very high in saturated fats, you will probably see a greater reduction in your cholesterol level once you start to change your eating pattern than if your initial diet was only moderately high in saturated fat.

- Your blood cholesterol level prior to starting your new diet. In general, the higher your blood cholesterol level is, the greater reduction you can expect from your new diet. If your level is very high, you might be able to lower your cholesterol level even more than 55 mg/dl.

- How responsive your body is to your new diet—Genetic factors play a role in determining your blood cholesterol level and, to some extent, can determine your ability to lower your level by diet.

How to Change Your Eating Patterns

Look at your overall eating pattern and begin to plan. If you are eating few foods high in saturated fat, an occasional high-saturated fat food won't raise your blood cholesterol level. If you anticipate a high-saturated fat, high-cholesterol day, eat an especially low-saturated fat, low-cholesterol diet the day before and the day after. With a little planning, you can change your eating patterns and reduce your high blood cholesterol level.

Remember, the goal is to limit the saturated fat and cholesterol in your diet each day. You don't have to cut out all the high-saturated fat and high-cholesterol foods in your diet. Try to substitute one or two low-saturated fat or low-cholesterol foods each day, and soon you will reach your goal of a low-saturated fat, low-cholesterol diet.

Changing your eating patterns takes time. In fact, it may take you 6 months or longer to incorporate all the changes you'll want to make in your diet. Most likely you will be shopping for some different foods, preparing some food differently, even modifying your choices at restaurants and parties.

Remember: Eat foods high in unsaturated fats and high in complex carbohydrates in place of foods high in saturated fat and cholesterol. Make substitutions gradually and plan your meals ahead to adjust your diet and reduce your blood cholesterol level.

Shop for Foods That Are Low in Saturated Fat and Cholesterol

If you stock your kitchen shelves with foods that are low in saturated fat and cholesterol, it will be much easier to adjust your eating habits. With a little direction you can learn to shop for these foods.

This part of the brochure is divided into categories that will be helpful when you make out your grocery lists. The categories, or food groups, are listed below.

Food Groups. You must eat a variety of foods each day to get the nutrients you need. One way to do this is to choose foods from different food groups, which are categorized by the nutrients they provide. The number and size of portions should be adjusted to reach and maintain your desirable weight. Use the information in the following sections to identify specific foods in each of the food groups that are low in saturated fat and cholesterol.

- Meat, Poultry, Fish, and Shellfish (up to 6 ounces a day)
- Dairy Products (2 servings a day; 3 servings for women who are pregnant or breastfeeding)
- Eggs (no more than 3 yolks a week)
- Fats and Oils (up to 6-8 teaspoons a day)
- Breads, Cereals, Pasta, Rice, and Dried Peas and Beans (6 or more servings a day).

- Fruits and Vegetables (2-4 servings of fruit, 3-5 servings of vegetables a day)
- Sweets and Snacks (avoid too many sweets)

Meat, Poultry, Fish, and Shellfish. Meat, poultry, fish, and shellfish are important sources of protein and other nutrients in your diet. However, they also contain saturated fat and cholesterol. The following chart shows the differences between lean and fatty examples of each. As you can see, lean beef is lower in saturated fat than beef short ribs. Chicken without skin has less saturated fat than chicken with skin. Haddock has less saturated fat and cholesterol than either chicken or meat. And, of course, foods with less fat contain fewer calories as well.

Meat, Poultry, and Fish: A Comparison

Product (3 ounces, cooked*)	Saturated Fat (grams**)	Dietary Cholesterol (milligrams**)	Total Fat (grams**)
Beef, top round, broiled	2	84	6
Beef, short ribs, braised	8	93	18
Chicken, broiler/fryer, without skin, light meat, roasted	1	85	5
Chicken, broiler/fryer, with skin, light meat, roasted	3	85	11
Haddock, baked	0.1	63	1
Mackerel, baked	4	64	15

*About the size of a deck of cards, or ¼ pound when raw.
**The terms grams and milligrams are defined in the glossary.

Figure 56.1.

To lower your blood cholesterol level, choose the leanest meats and poultry, fish, and shellfish. Remember, all of these foods contain some saturated fat and cholesterol. Therefore the amount you eat is also important. The recommended amount of meat, poultry, fish, or shellfish is up to 6 ounces each day. For variety, consider dried beans or legumes as a main dish. If larger, more filling main dishes are desired, extend meat with pasta or vegetables for hearty dishes. Eating a diet that includes a variety of foods is important because a food lowest in fat may not have the same vitamins and minerals as one a little higher in fat.

Some people think well-marbled meat (meat with white fat running through it) tastes better than less well-marbled meat. However, the tasty cuts are not all high in fat. For example, well-trimmed cuts from the "round" cuts of the animal are tender if prepared appropriately and they are lower in saturated fat than well-marbled meat. The list below gives you other examples of trimmed, lean meats.

- Beef: Round; Sirloin; Chuck; Loin
- Veal: All trimmed cuts except commercially ground
- Pork: Tenderloin; Leg (fresh); Shoulder (arm or picnic)
- Lamb: Leg; Arm; Loin

Beef, veal, and lamb can be graded as "prime," "choice," or "good." The grade is determined by the amount of marbling (fat) in the meat. "Prime," which is the top grade, has the most fat, while "choice" has less marbling. Even though the difference in marbling between "good" and "choice" is small, **"good" grades of meat are lower in fat.** Keep in mind that it is not necessary to completely remove red meat from your diet. Lean meat is high in protein and iron. Women in particular should avoid severe reductions in lean meat that would increase their risk of iron-deficiency anemia.

Some producers now are using "lean" and "lite" and other similar labels to designate beef, lamb, and pork that have been produced with less trimmable fat (fat surrounding the meat) and, in some instances, less marbling. These labels frequently appear on processed meat products but may appear on fresh meats as well. "Light," "lite," "leaner," and "lower fat" generally refer to foods containing less fat. They can be, but are not necessarily low in fat. Read the label for information on grams of fat per serving.

High-fat processed meats should be eaten infrequently because 60-80 percent of their calories come from fat much of which is saturated. Some examples of these processed meats are bacon, bologna, salami, hot dogs, and sausage.

Organ meats, like liver, sweetbreads, and kidneys are relatively low in fat. However, these meats are high in cholesterol.

In general, poultry is low in saturated fat, especially when the skin is removed. Poultry is, therefore, an excellent choice for your new diet. When choosing poultry, keep these points in mind:

- Eat chicken and turkey pieces without skin to reduce the saturated fat.
- Limit goose, duck, and many processed poultry products like bologna and hot dogs, which are very high in saturated fat.

Most fish is lower in saturated fat and cholesterol than meat and poultry. Therefore, usually a good substitute for meats and poultry.

Shellfish varies in cholesterol content—some is relatively high and some is low—but all has less fat than meat, poultry, and most fish.

Dairy Products. Although many people believe that meats have the highest cholesterol and saturated fat content, dairy products that contain fat are also high in saturated fat and cholesterol. Since dairy products are often added to foods like casseroles, cakes, or pies, you might eat a significant amount of them without knowing it.

Milk provides many essential nutrients. And both 1% and skim milk provide the same nutrients as whole milk (3.3%) or 2% milk, while providing much less saturated fat and cholesterol and fewer calories.

Ease your way from whole milk to skim milk. Make the change gradually. Drink 2% milk for a few weeks, then 1%, and finally skim. With each step, you will decrease your intake of saturated fat cholesterol, and calories.

Often, when people cut back on meat, they replace it with cheese, thinking they are cutting back on their saturated fat and dietary cholesterol. They couldn't be more wrong. Because they are prepared from whole milk or cream, **most cheeses, while high in calcium, are also high in saturated fat and cholesterol**. Ounce for ounce, meat, poultry, and most cheeses have about the same amount of cholesterol. But cheeses for the most part have much more saturated fat. Also, cheese is not as good a source of some vitamins and minerals, especially iron, as meats. [Figure 56.2] compares the saturated fat and cholesterol content in chicken, a relatively lean cut of meat, and some cheeses.

Determining which cheeses are high and low in saturated fat and cholesterol can be confusing because there are so many different kinds on the market: part-skim milk, low-fat, imitation, processed, natural,

531

Poultry, Meat, and Cheese: A Comparison

Product (3 ounce serving)		Saturated Fat (grams)	Dietary Cholesterol (milligrams)	Total Fat (grams)
Beef, top round, lean only, broiled	♥	2	84	6
Chicken, broiler/fryer, without skin, light meat roasted	♥	1	85	5
Low-fat cottage cheese	♥	1	4	1
Part-skim mozzarella	♥	9	48	14
Mozzarella		11	66	18
American processed		17	81	26
Natural cheddar		18	90	28
Cream cheese		19	93	30

Figure 56.2.

hard, and soft. Imitation cheeses made with vegetable oil, part-skim-milk cheeses, and cheeses advertised as "low-fat" are usually lower in saturated fat and cholesterol than are natural and processed cheeses, which are made with whole milk. However, even part-skim-milk cheeses and "low-fat" cheeses are not necessarily lower in fat than many meats. Remember it this way:

• Natural and processed hard cheeses are highest in saturated fat.
• Low-fat and imitation cheeses may have less saturated fat.
• Meats have less saturated fat than many of these cheeses.

Therefore, substitute low-fat and imitation cheeses whenever possible for natural, processed, and hard cheeses. Read the label and choose low-fat cheeses that have between 2 and 6 grams of fat per ounce. When you get the urge for cheese, the following should be eaten instead of hard cheese, or low-fat imitation cheese:

532

- Cottage cheese (low-fat)
- Farmer cheese (made with skim milk)
- Pot cheese

Americans love ice cream. But, ice cream is made from whole milk and cream and therefore contains a considerable amount of saturated fat and dietary cholesterol. You do not need to eliminate ice cream, but do eat it in small amounts and less often. Try frozen desserts like ice milk, yogurt, sorbets, and popsicles which are low in saturated fat.

Eggs. Egg **yolks** are high in cholesterol: each contains about 270 mg. Eat no more than three egg yolks a week including those in processed foods and many baked goods. Egg **whites** contain no cholesterol and can be substituted for whole eggs in recipes. For cakes or cookies, this substitution will be acceptable for 1-2 eggs in most recipes and up to 3-4 whole eggs in some.

Fats and Oils. In your cooking, limit the amounts you use of these saturated fats:

- Butter
- Lard
- Fatback
- Solid Shortenings

Instead of using butter as a spread or in recipes, substitute margarine. Choose liquid vegetable oils that are highest in unsaturated fats like safflower, sunflower, corn, olive, sesame, and soybean oils for your cooking and in your salad dressings. Peanut oil and peanut butter may be eaten in small amounts. Choose margarines and oils that have more polyunsaturated fat than saturated fat.

Saturated fats often are found in commercially prepared products. Remember, some vegetable oils (like coconut, palm, and palm kernel oil) are saturated, and other vegetable oils can become saturated by hydrogenation—a process that solidifies them. They are called hydrogenated vegetable oils. Read the labels before deciding which products to buy.

Since avocados, olives, nuts, and seeds are high in fat, they are often grouped with fats and oils. Although the fat in nuts and seeds is mostly unsaturated fat, they are very high in calories.

Fruits and Vegetables. Fruits and vegetables contain no cholesterol and are very low in fat and low in calories (except for avocados and olives, which are high in fat and calories). By eating fruits as a snack or dessert and vegetables as snacks and side dishes, you can increase your intake of vitamins, minerals, and fiber and lower your intake of saturated fat and dietary cholesterol.

Breads, Cereals, Pasta, Rice, and Dried Peas and Beans. Breads, cereals, pasta, rice, and dried peas and beans are all high in complex carbohydrates and low in saturated fat. By substituting more foods from this group for high-saturated fat foods, you will:

• Decrease your saturated fat, dietary cholesterol, and calorie intake and
• Increase your complex carbohydrate consumption.

Try pasta, rice, and dried peas and beans (like split peas, lentils, kidney beans, and navy beans) as main dishes, casseroles, soups, or other one-dish meals without high-fat sauces. Also, try recipes that use small quantities of meat, poultry, fish, or shellfish as flavoring or seasoning in casseroles rather than as the main ingredient.

Cereal products, both cooked and dry, are usually low in saturated fat—with the exception of those that contain coconut or coconut oil, like many types of granola. (Most granolas are high in fat.)

Breads and most rolls also are low in fat (for more fiber, choose the whole-grain types). However, many other types of commercially baked goods are made with large amounts of saturated fats. Read the labels on these products to determine their fat content. The ones listed below (as well as many others) are high in saturated fat:

• Croissants
• Biscuits
• Doughnuts
• Muffins
• Butter rolls

Remember, you can make your own muffins and quick breads using unsaturated vegetable oils and egg whites. Two egg whites may be substituted for one egg yolk.

Sweets and Snacks. Sweets and snacks often are high in saturated fat, cholesterol, and calories. Examples of these foods are commercial cakes, pies, cookies, cheese crackers, and some types of chips. Once again, the key is to read labels carefully since some of these products may contain unsaturated fats and be low in total fat and calories.

If you are accustomed to eating commercially prepared pies, cakes, or cookies, there are some very tasty alternatives to these high-saturated fat and high-cholesterol items. A few examples of commercially prepared desserts that are acceptable include angel food cake, fig bars, and ginger snaps. Keep in mind that most desserts can be made at home substituting polyunsaturated oil or margarine for butter and lard, skim milk for whole milk, and egg whites for egg yolks (see "Low-Fat Cooking Tips"). Although this reduces their saturated fat and cholesterol content, these baked products remain a rich source of fat (and therefore calories) and should be eaten only occasionally if you are trying to lose weight. As an alternative, try fruit for dessert. And for your next snack, try a piece of fruit, some vegetables, or a low-fat snack like unbuttered popcorn or breadsticks.

Read the Labels

When you are shopping, compare labels. Some premixed, frozen, or prepared foods have a lower saturated fat or cholesterol content than others. Now that many products list their fat and cholesterol content, shopping for low-saturated fat, low-cholesterol foods is much easier. With a little guidance, you can learn how to use these labels when you shop.

Look at the Ingredients. All food labels list the product's ingredients in order by weight. The ingredient in the greatest amount is listed first. The ingredient in the least amount is listed last. To avoid too much total or saturated fat, limit your use of products that list a fat or oil first or that list many fat and oil ingredients. The checklist below helps you identify the names of common saturated fat and cholesterol sources in foods.

- Animal Fat
- Bacon Fat
- Beef Fat
- Butter
- Chicken Fat
- Cocoa Butter
- Coconut
- Coconut Oil
- Cream
- Egg and Egg-Yolk Solids
- Ham Fat
- Hardened Fat or Oil
- Hydrogenated Vegetable Oil
- Lamb Fat
- Lard
- Meat Fat
- Palm Kernel Oil
- Palm Oil
- Pork Fat
- Turkey Fat
- Vegetable Oil (could be coconut or palm oil)
- Vegetable Shortening
- Whole-Milk Solids

Read the Nutrition Information. Look for the amount of fat, polyunsaturated, and saturated fats and cholesterol. [Figure 56.3 shows] you how to identify products with lower saturated fat and cholesterol. The labels give the amount of fat in grams (g) and cholesterol in milligrams (mg) per serving. You can see that skim milk has less fat and cholesterol than whole milk. Tub margarine has less saturated fat and cholesterol than butter.

Low-Fat Cooking Tips

Your kitchen is now stocked with great tasting, low-saturated fat, low-cholesterol foods. But you may still be faced with the temptation to fix your favorite higher fat meats, rich soups, and baked breads and cookies. The suggestions below will help you to reduce the amount of total and saturated fats in these foods.

Nutrition Information Per Serving	Whole Milk	2% Milk	Skim Milk
Serving Size	1 cup	1 cup	1 cup
Calories	150	121	86
Protein	8 g	8 g	8 g
Carbohydrates	11 g	12 g	12 g
Fat	8 g	5 g	less than 1 g
Polyunsaturates	less than 1 g	less than 1 g	0 g
Saturates	5 g	3 g	less than 1 g
Cholesterol	33 mg	18 mg	4 mg

Nutrition Information Per Serving	Butter, Stick	Margarine, Tub
Serving Size	1 T	1 T
Calories	101	101
Protein	0.1 g	0.1 g
Carbohydrates	0.1 g	0 1 g
Fat (100% calories from fat)	11.4 g	11.4 g
Polyunsaturates	0.4 g	3.9 g
Saturates	7.1 g	1.8 g
Cholesterol	31 mg	0 mg

Note: The amount of monounsaturated fat is not listed.

Figure 56.3.

New Ways To Prepare Meat, Poultry, Fish, and Shellfish.
When you prepare meats, poultry, and fish, remove as much saturated fat as possible. Trim the visible fat from meat. Remove the skin and fat from the chicken, turkey, and other poultry. And, if you buy tuna or other fish that is packed in oil, rinse it in a strainer before making tuna salad or a casserole, or buy it packed in water.

Changes in your cooking style can also help you remove fat. Rather than frying meats, poultry, fish, and shellfish, try broiling, roasting, poaching, or baking. Broiling browns meats without adding fat. When you roast, place the meat on a rack so that the fat can drip away.

Finally, if you baste your roast, use fat-free ingredients such as wine, tomato juice, or lemon juice instead of the fatty drippings. If you baste turkeys and chickens with fat use vegetable oil or margarine instead of the traditional butter or lard. Self-basting turkeys can be high in saturated fat—read the label!

537

New Ways To Make Sauces and Soups. Sauces, including gravies and homemade pasta sauces, and many soups often can be prepared with much less fat. Before thickening a sauce or serving soup, let the stock or liquid cool—preferably in the refrigerator. The fat will rise to the top and it can easily be skimmed off. Treat canned broth-type soups the same way.

For sauces that call for sour cream, substitute plain low-fat yogurt. To prevent the yogurt from separating, mix 1 tablespoon of cornstarch with 1 tablespoon of yogurt and mix that into the rest of the yogurt. Stir over medium heat just until the yogurt thickens. Serve immediately. Also, whenever you make creamed soup or white sauces, use skim or 1% milk instead of 2% or whole milk.

New Ways To Use Old Recipes. There are dozens of cookbooks and recipe booklets that will help you with low-fat cooking. But there is no reason to stop using your own favorite cookbook. The following list summarizes many of the tips. Using them, you can change tried and true recipes to low-saturated fat, low-cholesterol recipes. In some cases, especially with baked products, the quality or texture may change. For example, using vegetable oil instead of shortening in cakes that require creaming will affect the result. Use margarine instead; oil is best used only in recipes calling for melted butter. Substituting yogurt for sour cream sometimes affects the taste of the product. Experiment! Find the recipes that work best with these substitutions:

- Instead of 1 tablespoon butter, use 1 tablespoon margarine or 2/3 tablespoon oil
- Instead of 1 cup shortening, use 2.3 cup vegetable oil
- Instead of 1 whole egg, use 2 egg whites
- Instead of 1 cup sour cream, use 1 cup yogurt (plus 1 tablespoon cornstarch for some recipes)
- Instead of 1 cup whole milk, use 1 cup skim milk

Where Can You Go for Help?

If you want additional help in planning an approach to low-saturated fat, low-cholesterol eating, make an appointment with a registered dietitian or qualified nutritionist. They can help you design an eating plan particular to your own needs and preferences. Dietitians may be identified through a local hospital as well as through state and district affiliates of the American Dietetic Association. The American Dietetic Association maintains a roster of registered dietitians. By calling the Division of Practice [(312) 899-0040] you can request names of qualified dietitians in your area. Others can be found in public health departments, health maintenance organizations, cooperative extension services, and colleges.

These health professionals can assist you in making dietary changes by providing additional advice on shopping and preparing foods, eating away from home, and changing your eating behaviors to help you maintain your new eating pattern. Their expertise will help you set short-term goals for dietary change so that you can success-fully lower your high blood cholesterol levels without drastically changing your eating pattern or overall lifestyle.

If you would like more information to help you start your new ap-proach to healthy eating, contact the National Cholesterol Education Program (NCEP) of the National Heart, Lung, and Blood Institute. NCEP has developed a *Community Guide to Cholesterol Resources*, which includes the names and addresses of other organizations that can provide additional information. *So You Have High Blood Choles-terol* provides more specific information on the significance of high blood cholesterol and how it affects your health. To request additional information, write:

National Cholesterol Education Program
National Heart, Lung, and Blood Institute
National Institutes of Health
C-200
Bethesda, MD 20892

Chapter 57

The Healthy Heart Handbook for Women

The Healthy Heart

You owe it to yourself to take this handbook to heart. For coronary heart disease is a woman's concern. Every woman's concern. It is not something that only affects your husband, your father, your brother, your son. This handbook tells you why you should be concerned about your own heart health, and what you can do to prevent coronary disease. A little prevention can have a big payoff—a longer, healthier, more active life.

Each year, 245,000 women die of coronary heart disease, making it the number one killer of American women. Another 90,000 women die each year of stroke. Although death rates from coronary heart disease and stroke have declined in recent years, these conditions still rank first and third, respectively, as causes of death for women.

Overall, about 10 million American women of all ages suffer from heart disease. One in ten women 45 to 64 years of age has some form of heart disease, and this increases to one in four women over 65. Each year, one-half million women suffer heart attacks. Cardiovascular diseases and their prevention, therefore, are pressing personal concerns for every woman.

Taken from NIH Pub. No. 92-2720.

541

What Are Cardiovascular Diseases?

Cardiovascular diseases are diseases of the heart and blood vessel system, such as coronary heart disease, heart attack, high blood pressure, stroke, angina (chest pain), and rheumatic heart disease. Coronary heart disease—the primary subject of this handbook—is a disease of the blood vessels of the heart that causes heart attacks. A heart attack happens when an artery becomes blocked, preventing oxygen and nutrients from getting to the heart. A stroke results from a lack of blood to the brain, or in some cases, bleeding in the brain.

Who Gets Cardiovascular Diseases?

Some women have more "risk factors" for cardiovascular diseases than others. Risk factors are traits or habits that make a person more likely to develop a disease. Some risk factors for heart-related problems cannot be changed, but others can be. The three major risk factors for cardiovascular disease that you can do something about are cigarette smoking, high blood pressure, and high blood cholesterol. Other risk factors, such as overweight, diabetes, and physical inactivity, also are conditions you have some control over. Although growing older is a risk factor that cannot be changed, it is important to realize that other risks can be reduced at any age. This handbook identifies some key risk factors that you can control, and suggests changes in living habits to lessen your chances of developing cardiovascular diseases.

Some groups of women are more likely to develop cardiovascular diseases than other groups. Black women are 24 percent more likely to die of coronary heart disease than white women, and their death rate for stroke is 83 percent higher. Older women have a greater chance of developing cardiovascular diseases than younger women, partly because the tendency to have heart-related problems increases with age. Older women, for example, are more likely to develop high blood pressure and high blood cholesterol levels, to be diabetic, to be overweight, and to exercise less than younger women. Also, after menopause, women are more apt to get cardiovascular diseases, in part because their bodies produce less estrogen. Women who have had early menopause, either naturally or by means of a hysterectomy, are twice as likely to develop coronary heart disease as women of the same age who have not begun menopause.

While any one risk factor will raise your chances of developing heart-related problems, the more risk factors you have, the more concerned you should be about prevention. If you smoke cigarettes and have high blood pressure, for example, your chance of developing coronary heart disease goes up dramatically. Having all three major changeable risk factors—smoking, high blood pressure, and high blood cholesterol—can boost your risk to eight times that of women who have no risk factors.

We're Making Progress

Changing habits isn't easy—but experience shows that it works. As Americans have learned to control blood pressure and make healthful changes in their eating, smoking, and exercise habits, death rates for heart attack and stroke have dropped dramatically. Between 1970 and 1988 the death rate for women from coronary heart disease was cut in half. During the same period, the death rate for stroke went down 55 percent.

Cardiovascular diseases remain the leading cause of death for American women. But the message is clear: by taking an active role in your own heart health, you can make a difference. Beginning with the chapter on "Self-Help Strategies for a Healthy Heart," this handbook supplies a number of practical tips to help you get started. Also, for information about other organizations and materials available to help you, see [the section titled] "Resources for a Healthy Heart."

Major Risk Factors

Smoking

Cigarette smoking has been described as "the most important individual health risk in this country." Approximately 26 million American women smoke. Although the smoking rate for women dropped 8 percent between 1965 and 1988, women who smoke today are apt to smoke more heavily than they did in the past.

Surprising as it may seem, smoking by women in the United States causes almost as many deaths from heart disease as from lung cancer. Women who smoke are two to six times as likely to suffer a heart attack as nonsmoking women, and the risk increases with the number of cigarettes smoked per day. Smoking also boosts the risk of stroke.

543

Cardiovascular diseases are not the only health risks for women who smoke. Cigarette smoking greatly increases the chances that a woman will develop lung cancer. In fact, the lung cancer death rate for women is now higher than the death rate for breast cancer, the chief cause of cancer deaths in women for many years. Cigarette smoking is also linked with cancers of the mouth, larynx, esophagus, urinary tract, kidney, pancreas, and cervix. Smoking also causes 80 percent of cases of chronic obstructive lung disease, which includes bronchitis and emphysema.

Smoking is also linked to a number of reproductive problems. Women who smoke are more apt to have problems getting pregnant and to begin menopause at a slightly younger age. Further, cigarette use during pregnancy poses serious risks for the unborn. Babies of women who smoked during pregnancy tend to weigh less at birth than babies of nonsmokers. Smoking while pregnant also increases risks of bleeding, miscarriage, premature delivery, stillbirth, and sudden infant death syndrome, or "crib death." Moreover, young children who are exposed to a parent's cigarette smoke have more lung and ear infections.

There is simply no "safe way" to smoke. Although low-tar and low-nicotine cigarettes may reduce the lung cancer risk to some extent, they do not lessen the risks of heart diseases or other smoking-related diseases. The only safe and healthful course is not to smoke at all.

High Blood Pressure

High blood pressure, also known as hypertension, is another major risk factor for coronary heart diseases and the most important risk factor for stroke. Even slightly high levels double the risk. High blood pressure also boosts the chances of developing kidney disease.

Nearly 58 million Americans have high blood pressure, and about half of them are women. Older women have a higher risk, with more than half of all women over the age of 55 suffering from this condition. High blood pressure is more common and more severe in black women than it is in white women. Use of birth control pills can contribute to high blood pressure in some women.

Blood pressure is the amount of force exerted by the blood against the walls of the arteries. Everyone has to have some blood pressure, so that blood can get to the body's organs and muscles. Usually, blood pressure is expressed as two numbers, such as 120/80, and is measured in millimeters of mercury (mmHg). The first number is the systolic blood pressure, the force used when the heart beats. The second number, or diastolic blood pressure, is the pressure that exists in the arteries between heartbeats. Depending on your activities, blood pressure may move up or down in the course of a day. Blood pressure is considered high when it stays above normal levels over a period of time.

High blood pressure is sometimes called the "silent killer" because most people have it without feeling sick. Therefore, it is important to have it checked each time you see your doctor or other health professional. Blood pressure can be easily measured by means of the familiar stethoscope and inflatable cuff placed around one arm. However, since blood pressure changes so often and is affected by many factors, your health professional should check it on several different days before deciding if your blood pressure is too high. If your blood pressure stays at 140/90 mmHg or above, you have high blood pressure.

Although high blood pressure can rarely be cured, it can be controlled with proper treatment. If your blood pressure is not too high, you may be able to control it entirely through weight loss if you are overweight, regular exercise, and cutting down on alcohol, table salt, and sodium. (Sodium is an ingredient in salt that is found in many packaged foods, baking soda, and some antacids.)

However, if your blood pressure remains high, your doctor will probably prescribe medicine in addition to the above changes. The amount you take may be gradually reduced, especially if you are successful with the changes you make in your lifestyle. While few people like the idea of taking any medicine for a long time, the treatment benefits are real and will reduce the risk of stroke, heart attack, and kidney disease. If you are prescribed a drug to control high blood pressure and find you have any uncomfortable side effects, ask your doctor about changing the dosage or possibly switching to another type of medicine.

During pregnancy, some women develop high blood pressure for the first time. Between 10 and 20 percent of first-time mothers develop a high blood pressure problem during pregnancy called preeclampsia. Other women who already have high blood pressure may find that it worsens during pregnancy. If untreated, these conditions can be life-threatening to both mother and baby. Since a woman can feel perfectly normal and still have one of these conditions, it is important to get regular prenatal checkups so that your doctor can discover and treat a possible high blood pressure problem.

Small Dose, Big Benefit

If you are one of the 3 million older Americans with a type of high blood pressure called isolated systolic hypertension (ISH), there is good news. A recent study shows that treating ISH with a low dose of a common blood pressure-lowering drug, a diuretic called cholorthalidone, cut the risk of stroke by more than one-third, and reduced the risk of coronary heart disease by 27 percent. The dose of the diuretic used in the study was only half of the smallest dose usually given to patients, One in five patients also took a low dose of a second drug, a beta-blocker, to help lower their blood pressure.

If you have ISH and are already doing well on another type of blood pressure-lowering drug, you should not necessarily switch medicines. But you may want to discuss with your doctor whether the treatment used successfully in this study might work for you.

High Blood Cholesterol

High blood cholesterol is a third important risk factor for coronary heart diseases that you can do something about. Although young women tend to have lower cholesterol levels than young men, between the ages of 45 and 55, women's cholesterol levels begin to rise higher than men's. After age 55, the gap between women and men becomes still wider. Today, about one-third of American women have blood cholesterol levels high enough to pose a serious risk for coronary heart diseases. The higher your blood cholesterol level, the higher your heart disease risk. For all adults, a desirable blood cholesterol level is less than 200 mg/dL. A level of 240 mg/dL or above is considered "high" blood cholesterol. But even levels in the "borderline-high" category (200-239 mg/dL) boost the risk of heart disease.

The body needs cholesterol to function normally. It is found in all foods that come from animals—that is all meats and dairy products. However, the body can make all of the cholesterol that it needs. Over a period of years, extra cholesterol and fat circulating in the blood settle on the inner walls of the arteries that supply blood to the heart. These deposits make the arteries narrower and narrower. As a result, less blood gets to the heart and the risk of coronary heart disease increases.

Ask your health professional to check your blood cholesterol level once every 5 years. This simple test involves taking a small blood sample and measuring the amount of cholesterol. The cholesterol level is expressed as, for example, "215 mg/dL" or 215 milligrams of cholesterol per deciliter of blood. Be sure to ask what your cholesterol number is and whether you should take steps to lower it. Before age 45, the total blood cholesterol level of women averages below 220 mg/dL. But between the ages of 45 and 55, women's average cholesterol levels soar to between 240 and 260 mg/dL. Women between 45 and 74 years of age who have a cholesterol level over 240 mg/dL are more than twice as likely to develop coronary heart disease as women with levels below 200 mg/dL.

Total blood cholesterol is the first measurement used to identify persons with high blood cholesterol. As you read above, a blood cholesterol level of 240 or more means you have "high" blood cholesterol. But even "borderline-high" levels (200-239) boost your risk of coronary heart disease. If your total blood cholesterol is in the high or borderline-high category and you have other risk factors for coronary heart disease, your doctor will want a more complete "cholesterol profile" before making a decision about treatment. Specifically, your doctor will measure your LDL and HDL levels after an overnight fast.

Cholesterol travels in the blood in packages called lipoproteins. Cholesterol packaged in low density lipoprotein (LDL) is often called "bad cholesterol" because LDL carries most of the cholesterol in the blood and if not removed, cholesterol and fat can build up in the arteries. Another type of cholesterol, which is packaged in high density lipoprotein (HDL), is known as "good cholesterol." That is because HDL helps remove cholesterol from the blood, preventing it from piling up in the arteries.

A "cholesterol profile" includes measurements of both HDL and LDL levels. An LDL level below 130 mg/dL is desirable. LDL levels of 130-159 mg/dL are "borderline-high." Levels of 160 mg/dL or above mean you have a high risk of developing coronary heart disease. As with total cholesterol, the higher the LDL number, the higher the risk. On the other hand, the lower your HDL number is, the greater your risk for coronary heart disease. Any HDL level below 35 mg/dL is considered too low. After studying your LDL- and HDL-cholesterol levels and other risk factors for coronary heart disease, your doctor may recommend a specific treatment program for you.

For many people, a change in eating habits is the only step needed to lower blood cholesterol levels. Cutting back on foods rich in fat, especially saturated fat, and in cholesterol, can lower both total and LDL-cholesterol. Weight loss for overweight persons also will lower blood cholesterol levels. Losing extra weight, as well as quitting smoking and becoming more active, also may help boost your HDL-cholesterol levels. Although we don't know for sure that raising HDL levels in this way will reduce the risk of coronary heart disease, these measures are likely to be good for your heart in any case.

While changing the way you eat is the first and most important action you can take to improve your blood cholesterol levels, your doctor may also suggest that you take cholesterol-lowering medications. This recommendation will depend on how much your new diet lowers your blood cholesterol and whether you have any other risk factors for coronary heart disease. If your doctor does prescribe medicines, you must also continue your cholesterol-lowering diet because the combination may allow you to take less medicine. Also, because diet is still the safest treatment, you should always try to lower your cholesterol levels with diet changes before adding medication.

Triglycerides are another type of fat found in the blood and in food. Triglycerides in food are made up of saturated, polyunsaturated, and monounsaturated fats. The liver also produces triglycerides. When alcohol is consumed or when excess calories are taken in, the liver produces more triglycerides. A number of studies have found that some people with coronary heart disease have high triglyceride levels. However, more research is needed to determine whether high triglycerides cause narrowing of the arteries or are just associated with other risk factors like low levels of HDL-cholesterol and being overweight.

Extremely high levels of triglycerides can cause a dangerous inflammation of the pancreas called pancreatitis.

To reduce blood triglyceride levels, doctors recommend a low-fat, low-calorie diet, weight control, increased exercise, and no alcohol. Occasionally drugs are needed.

Other Risk Factors

Overweight (obesity) is a proven risk factor for cardiovascular diseases. People who are obese—more than 30 percent overweight—are more likely to develop heart-related problems even if they have no other risk factors. According to an important study of cardiovascular diseases called the Framingham Heart Study, overweight in women is linked with coronary heart disease, stroke, congestive heart failure, and death from heart-related causes.

The Framingham Heart Study found that the more overweight a woman was, the higher her risk for heart disease. This was true for women of all ages, but especially for women under age 50. Among women younger than 50, the heaviest group was two and a half times more likely to develop coronary heart disease than the group with desirable weight. Overweight women under age 50 had more than four times the stroke rate of the group with desirable weight.

Overweight contributes not only to cardiovascular diseases, but to other risk factors as well. For example, overweight women under age 50 are three times as likely to develop high blood pressure as women of desirable weight. Overweight women also are more apt to have high blood cholesterol levels and diabetes. Fortunately, these conditions often can be controlled with weight loss and regular exercise.

What is a healthy weight for you? Currently, there is no exact answer. Researchers are trying to develop better ways to measure healthy weight. In the meantime, [if you have questions about you the proper weight for you, check published tables or consult with your doctor].

Research also suggests that body shape as well as weight affects heart health. "Apple-shaped" individuals with extra fat at the waistline may have a higher risk than "pear-shaped" people with heavy hips and thighs. If your waist is larger than the size of your hips, you may have a higher risk for coronary heart disease.

Diabetes

Diabetes, or high blood sugar, is a serious disorder that raises the risk of coronary heart disease. More than 80 percent of people who have diabetes die of some type of cardiovascular disease, usually heart attack. The risk of death from coronary heart disease is doubled in women with diabetes. Compared with nondiabetic women, diabetic women are also more apt to suffer from high blood pressure and high blood cholesterol. Besides helping to cause coronary heart disease, untreated diabetes can contribute to the development of kidney disease, blindness, problems in pregnancy and childbirth, nerve and blood vessel damage, and difficulties in fighting infection.

Diabetes is often called a "woman's disease" because after age 45, about twice as many women as men develop diabetes. The type of diabetes that develops in adulthood is usually "noninsulin-dependent diabetes mellitus," or NIDDM. This type of diabetes, in which the pancreas makes insulin but the body is unable to use it well, is the most common form of the disease. For unknown reasons, the risks of heart disease and heart-related death are higher for diabetic women than for diabetic men.

While there is no cure for diabetes, there are steps one can take to control it. Eighty-five percent of all NIDDM diabetics are at least 20 percent overweight. It appears that overweight and growing older promote the development of diabetes in certain people. Losing excess weight and boosting physical activity may help postpone or prevent the disease. For lasting weight loss, get regular, brisk exercise and eat a diet that is limited in calories and fat, especially saturated fat.

Stress

In recent years, we have read and heard much about the connection between stress and coronary heart disease. In particular, we have heard that "type A" behavior—aggressiveness, a need to compete, a constant concern about time—is linked to the development of heart disease. Some studies have shown such a relationship in men. But recent research on type A behavior in women shows no link between this kind of behavior and coronary heart disease.

Another factor that has often been connected to women's heart disease is employment outside the home. The "price of liberation" for working women, according to many media reports, is a high level of stress leading to soaring rates of coronary heart disease. But research from the Framingham Heart Study shows no difference in rates of coronary heart disease between housewives and employed women.

But it is too early to rule out stress as a risk factor for women. Certainly, some common ways of coping with stress, such as overeating and heavy drinking, are bad for your heart. On the other hand, stress-relieving activities such as exercise can lower your risk of heart disease. Researchers will need to study larger groups of women over time to find out whether certain behaviors, personality types, or stressful situations are linked to the development of coronary heart disease in women.

Birth Control Pills

Studies show that women who use high-dose birth control pills (oral contraceptives) are more likely to have a heart attack or a stroke because blood clots are more likely to form in the blood vessels. These risks are lessened once the birth control pill is stopped: Using birth control pills also may worsen the effects of other risk factors, such as smoking, high blood pressure, diabetes, high blood cholesterol, and overweight.

Much of this information comes from studies of birth control pills containing higher doses of hormones than those commonly used today. Still, the risks of using low-dose birth control pills are not fully known. Therefore, if you are now taking any kind of birth control pill or are considering using one, keep these guidelines in mind:

Smoking and "the pill" don't mix. If you smoke cigarettes, stop smoking or choose a different form of birth control. Cigarette smoking boosts the risks of serious cardiovascular problems from birth control pill use, especially the risk of blood clots. This risk increases with age and with the amount smoked. For women over 35, the risk is particularly high. Women who use oral contraceptives should not smoke.

Pay attention to diabetes. Glucose metabolism, or blood sugar, sometimes changes dramatically in women who take birth control pills. Any woman who is diabetic, or has a close relative who is, should have regular blood sugar tests if she takes birth control pills.

Talk with your doctor. If you have a heart defect, if you have suffered a stroke, or if you have any other kind of cardiovascular disease, oral contraceptives may not be a safe choice. Be sure your doctor knows about your condition before prescribing birth control pills for you.

Alcohol

Over the last several years, a number of studies have reported that moderate drinkers—those who have one or two drinks per day-are less likely to develop heart disease than people who don't drink any alcohol. Alcohol may help protect against heart disease by raising levels of "good" HDL cholesterol. On the other hand, it may also raise blood pressure which could lead to stroke.

If you are a nondrinker, this is not a recommendation to start using alcohol. And certainly, if you are pregnant or have another health condition that could make alcohol use harmful, you should not drink. But if you're already a moderate drinker, evidence suggests that you may be at a lower risk for heart attack.

But remember, moderation is the key. Heavy drinking can definitely cause heart-related problems. More than two drinks per day can raise blood pressure, and recent research shows that binge drinking can lead to stroke. It is well-known that people who drink heavily on a regular basis have higher rates of heart disease than either moderate drinkers or nondrinkers.

Keep in mind, too, that alcohol provides no nutrients—only extra calories. Most drinks contain 100-200 calories each. Women who are trying to control their weight may want to cut down on alcohol and substitute calorie-free iced tea, mineral water, or seltzer with a squeeze of lemon or lime.

What is moderate drinking? For women, "moderate drinking" is no more than one drink per day according to the U.S. Dietary Guidelines for Americans.

Count as one drink:

- 12 ounces of beer
- 5 ounces of wine
- 1 1/2 ounces of hard liquor (80 proof)

Source: *Dietary Guidelines for Americans*, U.S. Department of Agriculture/U.S. Department of health and Human Services, 1990.

Prevention: A Personal Project

Preventing heart disease, by and large, means making changes in the way we live. For each individual a healthy heart requires a personal action plan. But where does one begin? A complete medical checkup is a sensible first step. With the help of your doctor or other health professional, you can find out if you have any cardiovascular disease risk factors, and if so, work out a practical treatment plan. Even if you don't have any risk factors now, you can discuss ways to lessen your chances of developing them. Good communication with your health professional is very important. Choose someone you trust who will listen to your questions, answer them fully, and take your concerns seriously.

But while advice from a health professional is important, the final responsibility for heart health lies with each woman. Only you can make the kinds of lifestyle changes—changes in eating, drinking, smoking, and exercise habits—that will help protect against cardiovascular diseases. To learn about the many organizations and reading materials available to help you, see [the section titled] "Resources for a Healthy Heart." In the meantime, keep reading. The self-help suggestions that follow can help you get started on a personal program for a healthy heart.

To Do!

The *Healthy Heart Action Plan:*

* Quit smoking
* Cut back on foods high in fat, saturated fat, and cholesterol
* Check blood pressure and blood cholesterol levels
* Get more exercise
* Lose weight if you are overweight

Self Help Strategies for a Healthy Heart

Kicking the Smoking Habit

There is nothing easy about giving up cigarettes. But as hard as quitting may be, the results are well worth it. In the first year after stopping smoking, the risk of coronary heart disease drops sharply. It then gradually returns to "normal"—that is, the same risk as someone who never smoked. This means that no matter what your age, quitting will lessen your chances of developing heart disease.

Quitting will also save you money. Over 10 years, a two-pack-a-day smoker can spend more than $7,500 on cigarettes. And that price tag doesn't take into account the extra costs of smoking-related illness, such as doctors' bills, medicines, and lost wages.

Take some time to think about other benefits of being an ex-smoker. Check the reasons that apply to you in the [list] that follows. Add any others you think are important. This is an important first step in kicking the smoking habit—figuring out for yourself what you have to gain.

- I will greatly lessen my chances of having a heart attack or stroke.
- I will greatly lessen my chances of getting lung cancer, emphysema, and other lung diseases.
- I will have fewer colds or flu each year.
- I will have better smelling clothes, hair, breath, home, and car.
- I will climb stairs and walk without getting out of breath.
- I will have fewer wrinkles.
- I will be free of my morning cough.
- I will reduce the number of coughs, colds, and earaches my children will have.
- I will have more energy to pursue physical activities I enjoy.
- I will have more control over my life.

Many women fear that if they stop smoking they will gain unwanted weight. But you do not have to gain a lot of weight. Here are the facts:

- The average weight gain for ex-smokers is only about 5 pounds.
- Only about 3 percent of women gain a lot of weight (more than 20 pounds) after quitting.

Weight gain may be partly due to changes in the way the body uses calories after smoking stops. Also, some people eat more when quitting because they substitute high-calorie food for cigarettes. Choosing more foods lower in calories and boosting your exercise level will help guard against weight gain. And if you do gain some weight, you can work on losing it after you have become comfortable as a nonsmoker. When you think about the enormous health risks of smoking, the possibility of putting on a few pounds is not a reason to continue.

Getting Ready to Quit

Once you decide to stop smoking, a few preparations are in order. Set a target date for quitting—perhaps the first day of a month. Don't choose a time when you know you will be under a lot of stress. To help you stick to your quit date, write [and date a contract like the one] that follows and have someone sign it with you. And don't forget to list how you'll reward yourself for becoming an ex-smoker.

Consider asking your contract cosigner—or another friend or family member—to give you special support in your efforts to quit. Plan to get in touch with your supporter regularly to share your progress and to ask for encouragement. Give your "cheerleader" a copy of your list of "Why I Want to Quit" so that he or she can remind you of your goals. If possible, quit with a spouse or a friend.

Ex-Smoker's Contract

I WILL QUIT SMOKING ON: (date)

I WILL REWARD MYSELF FOR NOT SMOKING AS FOLLOWS:

First 3 days of not smoking:

Each week of not smoking:

Each month of not smoking:

Signed by:

Cosigned by:

Breaking the Habit

Surviving "Day One." On the evening before your quit day, "clean house." Throw away all cigarettes, matches, and lighters and give away your ashtrays. Plan some special activities for the next day to keep you busy, such as a long walk, a bike ride, a movie, or an outing with a good friend. Ask family members and friends not to offer you cigarettes or to smoke in front of you. Your goal is to get through that first important day smoke-free. If you succeed on the first day, it will help give you the confidence to succeed on the second-and on each day after that.

Know yourself. To quit successfully, you need to know your personal smoking "triggers." These are the situations and feelings that typically bring on the urge to light up. Some common triggers include drinking coffee, finishing a good meal, watching television, having an alcoholic drink, talking on the phone, or watching someone else smoke. Stress can also be a trigger. Make a list of the situations and feelings that particularly tempt you to smoke. Especially during the first weeks after quitting, try to avoid as many triggers as you can.

Find new habits. Replace "triggers" with new activities that you don't associate with smoking. For example, if you always had a cigarette with a cup of coffee, switch to tea for awhile. If you always smoked at the table after dinner, get up as soon as the meal is over and go out for a walk. If you're feeling tense or angry, try a relaxation exercise such as deep breathing to calm yourself. (Take a slow, deep breath, count to five, and release it. Repeat 10 times.)

Keep busy. Get involved in projects that require you to use your hands: needlework, gardening, jigsaw puzzles. Try out new physical activities that make smoking impossible, such as swimming, jogging, tennis, or aerobic dancing. When you feel the need to put something in your mouth, have low-calorie substitutes on hand, such as vegetable sticks, apple slices, or sugarless gum. Some people find it helpful to inhale on a straw or chew on a toothpick until the urge passes.

Know what to expect. During the first few weeks after quitting, you may experience some temporary withdrawal symptoms, such as headaches, irritability, tiredness, constipation, and trouble concentrating. These symptoms may come and go, and be stronger or weaker on different days. While these feelings are not pleasant, it is important to know that they are signs that your body is recovering from smoking. Most symptoms end within 2 to 4 weeks.

Two things to help you. Nicotine chewing gum and a nicotine patch are both available by prescription. The gum and the patch can help you stay off cigarettes by lessening your withdrawal symptoms. They give you nicotine at a lower, more even dose than your cigarettes did. Gradually, you should chew fewer pieces of the gum each day until you stop using it altogether. Similarly, you gradually use patches with a lower dose of nicotine. Nicotine gum and the nicotine patch are not for everyone—talk to your health professional about using them. Pregnant women, nursing mothers, and people with serious heart problems cannot use them safely. But for those who can, both the gum and the patch can help one "over the hump" and on the road to smoke-free living.

More help is available. There are a number of free or low-cost programs available to help you stop smoking. They include programs offered by local chapters of the American Lung Association and the American Cancer Society (see "Resources for a Healthy Heart"). Other low-cost programs can be found through hospitals, health maintenance organizations (HMOs), workplaces, and community groups. Some programs offer special support groups for women.

Be good to yourself. Get plenty of rest, drink lots of fluids, and eat three balanced, healthful meals per day. If you are not as productive or cheerful as usual during the first several weeks after quitting, don't feel guilty. Give yourself a chance to adjust to your new non-smoking lifestyle. Ask your friends and family to give you lots of praise for kicking the habit—and don't forget to pat yourself on the back. You are making a major change in your life, and you deserve a lot of credit.

If You "Slip"

A "slip" means that you have had a small setback and smoked a cigarette after your quit date. Don't worry. It doesn't mean that you've become a smoker again. Most smokers "slip" three to five times before they quit for good. But to get right back on the nonsmoker track, here are some tips:

Don't get discouraged. Having a cigarette or two doesn't mean you have failed. It doesn't mean you can't quit smoking. A slip happens to many, many people who successfully quit. Keep thinking of yourself as a nonsmoker. You are one.

Learn from experience. What was the trigger that made you light up? Were you driving home from work, having a glass of wine at a party, feeling angry at your boss? Think back on the day's events until you remember what the specific trigger was.

Take charge. Make a list of things you will do the next time you are in that particular situation—and other tempting situations as well. Sign a new contract with your support person to show yourself how determined you are to kick the habit. Reread your list of all the reasons you want to quit. You're on your way.

Getting Physical

Regular exercise can help you reduce your risk of coronary heart disease. Exercise helps women take off extra pounds, helps to control blood pressure, lessens a diabetic's need for insulin, and boosts the level of "good" HDL-cholesterol.

Some studies also show that being inactive boosts the risk of heart attack.

Exercise has many other benefits. It strengthens the lungs, tones the muscles, keeps the joints in good condition, and helps many people cope better with stress.

While many physical activities are fun, only regular, brisk exercise will improve heart health. This is called "aerobic" exercise and includes jogging, swimming, jumping rope, and cross-country skiing. Walking, biking, and dancing can also strengthen your heart, if you do them fast enough and long enough. Choose an activity that you think you will enjoy and that will fit most easily into your schedule.

Most people do not need to see a doctor before they start a gradual, sensible exercise program. Some people, however, should get medical advice. For example, if you have heart trouble or have had a heart attack, if you are over 50 years old and are not used to energetic activity, or if you have a family history of developing heart disease at a young age, check with your doctor before you start.

[For more information on exercising for a healthy heart see Chapter 58 "Exercise and Your Heart."]

Eating for Health

The health of your heart has a lot to do with the food you eat. Changing your eating habits according to the Dietary Guidelines for Americans lessens your risk of heart disease in three ways:

• It helps reduce high blood cholesterol levels.
• It helps control high blood pressure.
• It helps take off extra pounds.

As a bonus, the kinds of eating habits that are good for your heart may also help prevent certain types of cancer and a number of other health problems.

Dietary Guidelines for Americans

- Eat a variety of foods
- Maintain a healthy weight
- Choose a diet low in fat, saturated fat, and cholesterol
- Choose a diet with plenty of vegetables, fruits, and grain products
- Use sugars only in moderation
- Use salt and sodium only in moderation
- If you drink alcoholic beverages, do so in moderation

Use these seven guidelines together as you choose a healthful and enjoyable diet.

[For more information on lowering your blood cholesterol through dietary changes see Chapter 56 "Eating to Lower Your High Blood Cholesterol."]

Controlling Blood Pressure

More than half of American women will develop high blood pressure at some point in their lives. Women who have the highest risk include those who are black, have a family history of high blood pressure, are overweight, or have "high-normal" blood pressure. To help keep blood pressure under control, take these steps:

- Lose weight, if you are overweight.

- If you drink alcohol, have no more than one drink per day- that means no more than 12 ounces of beer, 5 ounces of wine, or 1 1/2 ounces of hard liquor.

- Exercise regularly. A regular aerobic exercise program-for example, brisk walking, bicycling, jogging, or swimming-helps weight control and is good for your entire cardiovascular system.

- Use salt in small amounts, if at all, in cooking and at the table. Try seasoning foods instead with pepper, garlic, ginger, minced onion or green pepper, and lemon juice. Keep in mind that sodium, an ingredient in salt, is "hidden" in many foods such as cured meats, cheese, canned vegetables and soups, frozen dinners, prepared snacks, and condiments such as catsup, soy sauce, pickles, and olives. Check product labels for the amount of sodium in each serving, or buy products labeled "no sodium," or "reduced in sodium."

• While salt substitutes containing potassium chloride may be useful for some individuals, they can be harmful to people with certain medical conditions. Ask your doctor before trying salt substitutes.

• If your doctor prescribes medication, take it regularly as directed.

Losing Weight: Four Ways to Win

If you are overweight, taking off pounds can lower the chances of developing cardiovascular disease in several ways. First, since being overweight raises the risk of heart disease, losing weight will directly lower your risk. Secondly, weight loss will also help reduce the risk of developing diabetes and help control it. Third and fourth, shedding pounds can lower both high blood pressure and cholesterol. In fact, if your blood pressure or blood cholesterol count is not too high, weight loss along with other changes in your diet may be the only treatment you will need. But even if medication is required, the more healthful your weight, the less medication you may need.

In a society so concerned about thinness, it may be hard to listen to yet more advice about the need to take off pounds. But too often, women are pressured to lose too much weight and for the wrong reasons: to look better in trendy clothes, to attract male attention, to have today's super-slim athletic look. The aim here is not to promote the false and discouraging idea that "thin is beautiful," but to show the link between reasonable weight and good health—especially the health of your heart.

Weight loss is advised only to reach a healthy weight, not to drop to an extreme level.

Taking off pounds—and especially keeping them off—can be quite a challenge. Here are some suggestions for making weight loss an easier, safer, and more successful process:

Eat for health. Choose a wide variety of low-calorie, nutritious foods in moderate amounts from each food group. Make sure that these foods are low in fat, since fat is the richest source of calories. To make every calorie count cut out snack foods that are high in calories but provide few other nutrients. If you have a lot of weight to lose, ask your doctor, a nutritionist, or registered dietitian to help you develop a sensible, well-balanced plan for gradual weight loss. To lose weight you will need to take in fewer calories than you burn. That means that you must either choose food with fewer calories or boost your physical activity—and preferably, do both.

Keep milk on the menu. Don't cut out dairy products in trying to reduce calories and fat. Dairy products are rich in calcium, a nutrient that is particularly important for women. Instead, choose low-fat, lower calorie dairy products. For instance, if you are used to drinking whole milk, gradually cut back to 2 percent milk, move to 1 percent, and then perhaps to skim milk. This way the calories are reduced while the amount of calcium remains the same.

Beyond dieting. To keep the pounds off, change your basic eating habits rather than simply "go on a diet." Keep a food diary of what, how much, when, and why you eat to help you understand your eating patterns and what affects them. Learn to recognize social and emotional situations that trigger overeating and figure out ways to cope with them. Set short-term goals at first.

Forget the fads. Tempting as their promises are, fad diets are not the answer. Most provide poor nutrition and cause a number of side effects, especially those with less than 800 calories. Although fad diets can give quick and dramatic results, much of the weight loss is due to water loss. The weight returns quickly once you stop dieting.

Steer clear of diet pills. Studies show that most diet medicines have troublesome side effects and don't work for long-term weight loss.

Get a move on. Although physical activity alone won't take off many pounds, exercise can help burn calories, tone muscles, and control appetite. (It will also give you something to do when you feel that familiar urge for a slice of chocolate fudge cake.) Even moderate activity, such as brisk walking, will burn up calories and help control weight.

Ask for support. Tell your family and friends about your weight-loss plans and let them know how they can be most helpful to you. You might also want to join a self-help group devoted to weight control. These groups provide companionship, support, and practical suggestions on changing eating habits and long-term weight loss.

Other Prevention Issues

Hormones and Menopause

Should menopausal women use "hormone replacement therapy"? There is no simple answer to this question.

Menopause is caused by a decrease in estrogen and other hormones produced by a woman's ovaries. It happens naturally in most women between the ages of 45 and 55, and it also occurs in any woman whose ovaries are removed by an operation. As estrogen levels begin to drop, some women develop uncomfortable symptoms such as "hot flashes" and mood changes. Hormone replacement therapy—a term for prescription hormone pills that are taken daily—can be used to relieve these symptoms. Some women are prescribed pills that contain only estrogen. Others take estrogen combined with a second hormone called progestin.

Estrogen pills have several important benefits. They can help you feel more comfortable as your body adjusts to lower estrogen levels. They also help to prevent osteoporosis, a thinning of the bones that makes them more likely to break in later life. Many studies also have found that estrogen pills help protect women from developing coronary heart disease, but more research is needed before we will know this for sure.

Estrogen therapy also has risks. It may increase the chances of developing gallbladder disease, and it may worsen migraine headaches. It may also increase the risk of breast cancer. But by far, the biggest risk of taking estrogen pills is cancer of the uterus. Women on estrogen therapy after menopause are up to six times more likely to develop uterine cancer than women not on this treatment. It is important to point out that women are much more likely to die of coronary heart disease than from uterine cancer. Still, the cancer risk exists and must be taken seriously and discussed with your doctor.

Because of the risk of uterine cancer, some doctors now prescribe estrogen in combination with the hormone progestin. When progestin is taken along with estrogen, the risk of cancer of the uterus is reduced. While this is good news, we don't yet know how this newer "combo" treatment affects other aspects of women's health. We don't know, for example, whether the progestin-estrogen combination is a safe and effective way to prevent heart disease. We don't know whether the combined hormones are as successful as estrogen alone in protecting women from osteoporosis. Finally, we don't yet know whether this combination will boost the risk of breast cancer. Studies are now under way to find answers to these important questions.

In the meantime, a woman and her doctor must decide whether the benefits of hormone therapy are worth the risks. If you are considering this treatment, you will need to consider your overall health and your personal and family history of heart disease, uterine and breast cancer, and osteoporosis.

If you are now on hormone therapy, check with your doctor to be sure you are taking the lowest possible effective dose. At least every 6 months, you and your doctor should discuss whether you need to continue treatment. Be alert for signs of trouble—abnormal bleeding, breast lumps, shortness of breath, dizziness, severe headaches, pain in your calves or chest-and report them immediately. See your doctor at least once a year for a physical examination.

The Aspirin Question

You may have heard that taking aspirin regularly can help prevent heart attacks. Is this a good idea for you? Maybe.

A recent study of more than 87,000 women found that those who took a low dose of aspirin regularly were less likely to suffer a first heart attack than women who took no aspirin. Older women appeared to benefit most: those over age 50 had a 32 percent lower risk of heart attack, while women overall had a 25 percent lower risk. While earlier research has shown that aspirin can help prevent heart attacks in men, this was the first study to suggest a similar benefit for women. Other recent research suggests that only a tiny daily dose of aspirin may be needed to protect against heart attacks. One study found that for both women and men, taking only 30 mg of aspirin daily—one-tenth the strength of a regular aspirin—helped prevent heart attacks as effectively as the usual 300 mg dose. The smaller dose also caused less stomach irritation.

While these recent reports are encouraging, more study is needed before we can be sure that aspirin is safe and effective in preventing heart attacks in women. What is known for sure is that you should not take aspirin to prevent a heart attack without first discussing it with your doctor. Aspirin is a powerful drug with many side effects. It can increase your chances of getting ulcers and stroke from a hemorrhage. Only a doctor who knows your complete medical history and current health can judge whether the benefit you may gain from aspirin outweighs the risks.

Research: New Focus on Women

As you have read through this handbook, you may have noticed the recurring words: "more research is needed." This is true. Until very recently, men were the main subjects of heart disease research. We now know, however, that coronary heart disease is indeed a woman's concern. We know that we need to understand more about women's heart problems if we are to prevent and treat these problems successfully. As a result, several major research projects are now under way. They include studies on:

- The effects of hormone replacement therapy on cardiovascular diseases, uterine cancer, breast cancer, and osteoporosis. Both estrogen pills and estrogen-progestin combinations are being studied.

- Whether low doses of aspirin can safely and successfully protect women from heart attacks.

- The effect of a low-saturated-fat diet on preventing coronary heart disease in women.

- Whether commonly used programs to encourage exercise, weight control, and quitting smoking are successful for women.

- Possible links between stress, hormonal changes, and risk for coronary heart disease in women.

These and other important research projects will give us new information and tools to better protect ourselves from coronary heart disease. They will also help doctors identify and treat women's heart problems more successfully. Where women's hearts are concerned,

564

knowledge is power—the power to improve our health and enrich our lives.

The Heart of the Matter

Getting serious about heart health may seem like a huge project. Because it means making basic changes in health and living habits, for many it is a major effort. But it doesn't have to be an overwhelming one. Some people find it easier to tackle only one habit at a time. If you smoke cigarettes and also eat a high-fat diet, for example, work on kicking the smoking habit first. Then, once you have gotten used to life without cigarettes, begin skimming the fat from your diet.

And remember: nobody's perfect. Nobody always eats the ideal diet or gets just the right amount of exercise. Few smokers are able to swear off cigarettes without a slip or two along the way. The important thing is to want to make healthful changes, and then to follow a sensible, realistic plan that will gradually lessen your chances of developing cardiovascular diseases.

Women are taking a more active role in their own health care. We are asking more questions and we are seeking more self-help solutions. We are concerned not only about treatment, but about the prevention of a wide range of health problems. Taking steps to prevent cardiovascular diseases is part of this growing movement to promote and protect personal health. The rewards of a healthy heart are well worth the effort.

[For more information on low-cholesterol meal planning, see Chapter 56, "Eating to Lower Your High Blood Cholesterol."]

Recipies for a Healthy Heart

Corn Chowder

Add a mixed green salad, whole grain bread, plus a fruit for a satisfying supper...

NUTRIENTS PER SERVING
Calories/cup: 182
Total fat: 4 gms
Saturated fat: 1 gm

565

Corn Chowder (continued)
Polyunsaturated fat: 1 gm
Cholesterol: 5 mgs
Sodium: 236 mgs

[INGREDIENTS]
1 Tbsp margarine
2 Tbsp finely chopped celery
2 Tbsp finely chopped onion
2 Tbsp finely chopped green pepper
1 10-oz pkg frozen whole kernel corn
1 C peeled, diced, raw potatoes
2 Tbsp chopped fresh parsley
1 C water
1/4 tsp salt
Freshly ground black pepper
1/4 tsp paprika
2 Tbsp flour
2 C low-fat (1%) milk

Melt margarine in medium saucepan. Add celery, onion, and green pepper and sauté for 2 minutes. Add corn, potatoes, water, salt, pepper, and paprika. Bring to a boil; reduce heat to medium; and cook, covered, about 10 minutes or until potatoes are tender. Place 1/2 cup milk in a jar with tight fitting lid. Add flour and shake vigorously. Add gradually to cooked vegetables and add remaining milk. Cook, stirring constantly, until mixture comes to a boil and thickens. Serve garnished with chopped fresh parsley.
4 servings, 1 cup each

Homemade Turkey Soup

A good recipe to make ahead and refrigerate or freeze until needed...

NUTRIENTS PER SERVING
Calories: 226
Total fat: 5 gms
Saturated fat: 1 gm
Polyunsaturated fat: 1 gm
Cholesterol: 93 mgs
Sodium 217 mgs

Homemade Turkey Soup (continued)

[INGREDIENTS]
6 lb turkey breast
2 medium onions
3 stalks celery
1 tsp dried thyme
1/2 tsp dried rosemary
1/2 tsp dried sage
1 tsp dried basil
1/2 tsp dried marjoram
1/2 tsp dried tarragon

1/2 lb Italian pastina
1/2 tsp salt
Pepper to taste

Place turkey breast in a large 6-qt pot. Cover with water (at least 3/4 full). Add peeled onions, cut in large pieces. Wash celery stalks, slice, and add. Simmer covered for about 2 1/2 hours. Remove carcass from pot and cool soup in refrigerator. After cooling, skim off fat. While soup is cooling, remove remaining meat from carcass. Cut into pieces. Add meat to skimmed soup along with herbs and spices. Bring to boil. Add pastina. Continue cooking, low boil, 20 minutes until pastina is done. Serve at once or refrigerate and reheat later. **16 servings, 1 cup each.**

Very Lemony Chicken

Serve with wild rice and barley casserole, a curly endive salad, peas, and sorbet...

NUTRIENTS PER SERVING
Calories: 154
Total fat: 5 gms
Saturated fat: 2 gms
Polyunsaturated fat: 1 gm
Cholesterol: 63 mgs
Sodium: 202 mgs

Very Lemony Chicken (continued)

[INGREDIENTS]
1 1/2 lb chicken parts (breast, leg, and thigh), skinned and fat removed
1/2 C fresh lemon juice
2 Tbsp white wine vinegar
1/2 C fresh sliced lemon peel
3 tsp chopped fresh oregano or 1 tsp dried oregano, crushed
1 medium onion, sliced
1/4 tsp salt
Freshly ground black pepper
1/2 tsp paprika

Place chicken in a 13x9x2 glass baking dish. Mix lemon juice, vinegar, lemon peel, oregano, and onion. Pour over chicken, cover, and marinate in refrigerator several hours or overnight, turning occasionally. Sprinkle with salt, pepper, and paprika. Cover and bake at 300 degrees for 30 minutes. Uncover and bake 30 minutes more or until done.
4 servings

Barbeque Chicken

Make this your specialty—serve with cornbread and a salad of distinctive greens...

NUTRIENTS PER SERVING
Calories: 180
Total fat: 6 gms
Saturated fat: 2 gms
Polyunsaturated fat: 1 gm
Cholesterol: 68 mgs
Sodium: 242 mgs

[INGREDIENTS]
3 lb chicken parts (breast, leg, and thigh) skinned and fat removed
1 large onion, thinly sliced
3 Tbsp vinegar
3 Tbsp Worcestershire sauce
2 Tbsp brown sugar
Dash of pepper

Barbeque Chicken (continued)

1 Tbsp hot pepper flakes
1 Tbsp chili powder
1 C chicken stock or broth, fat removed

Place chicken in a 13x9x2 pan. Arrange onion over the top. Mix together vinegar, Worcestershire sauce, brown sugar, pepper, hot pepper flakes, chili powder, and stock. Pour over the chicken and bake at 350 degrees 1 hour or until done. Baste occasionally.
8 servings

Fish Veronique

A classic preparation of delicate white fillets of sole with green grapes in a creamy sauce...

NUTRIENTS PER SERVING
Calories: 148
Total fat: 4 gms
Saturated fat: 1 gm
Polyunsaturated fat: 1 gm
Cholesterol: 53 mgs
Sodium: 316 mgs

[INGREDIENTS]
1 lb white fish (sole, turbot, etc.)
1/4 tsp salt
1/8 tsp freshly ground pepper
1/4 C dry white wine
1/4 C chicken stock or broth, fat removed
1 Tbsp lemon juice
1 Tbsp margarine
2 Tbsp flour
3/4 C low-fat (1%) milk
1/2 C seedless green grapes

Place fish in a lightly oiled 10x6 flameproof baking dish. Sprinkle with salt and pepper. Mix wine, stock, and lemon juice in small bowl and pour over fish. Cover and bake at 350 degrees for 15 minutes. Melt margarine in small saucepan. Remove from heat and blend in

Fish Veronique (continued)

flour. Gradually add milk and cook over moderately low heat, stirring constantly until thickened. Remove fish from oven and pour liquid from baking dish into cream sauce, stirring until blended. Pour sauce over fish and sprinkle with grapes. Broil about 4 inches from heat 5 minutes or until sauce starts to brown.
4 servings

Stir-Fried Beef and Vegetables

This Japanese-style dish is savory and delicious...

NUTRIENTS PER SERVING
Calories: 187
Total fat: 8 gms
Saturated fat: 2 gms
Polyunsaturated fat: 3 gms
Cholesterol: 38 mgs
Sodium: 218 mgs

2 Tbsp dry red wine
1 Tbsp soy sauce
1/2 tsp sugar
1 1/2 tsp grated, peeled ginger root
1 lb boneless round steak, fat trimmed, and cut across grain
        into 1 1/2" strips, raw
1 Tbsp corn oil
2 medium onions, each cut into 8 wedges
1/2 lb fresh mushrooms, rinsed, trimmed, and sliced
2 stalks celery, bias cut into 1/4" slices (about 1/2 cup)
2 small green peppers, cut into thin lengthwise strips
1 C water chestnuts, drained and sliced
2 Tbsp cornstarch
1/4 C water
1 Tbsp corn oil

Prepare marinade mixing together wine, soy sauce, sugar, and ginger. Marinate meat in mixture while preparing vegetables. Heat 1 Tbsp oil in large skillet or wok. Stir-fry onions and mushrooms 3 minutes over medium-high heat. Add celery and cook 1 more minute. Add

Stir-Fried Beef and Vegetables (continued)

remaining vegetables and cook 2 minutes or until green pepper is tender crisp. Transfer vegetables to warm bowl. Add remaining 1 Tbsp oil to skillet. Stir-fry meat in oil about 2 minutes or until meat loses its pink color. Blend cornstarch and water. Stir into meat. Cook and stir until thickened. Return vegetables to skillet; stir gently and serve.
6 servings

Picnic Potato Salad

Excellent new low-fat version of an old favorite and very good with barbecue chicken...

NUTRIENTS PER SERVING
Calories: 92
Total fat: 4 gms
Saturated fat: .6 gms
Polyunsaturated fat: 2 gms
Cholesterol: 3 gms
Sodium: 199 mgs

[INGREDIENTS]
1/2 C plain low-fat (1%) yogurt
1/2 C mayonnaise-type salad dressing
1 Tbsp vinegar
1 tsp salt
1 tsp fresh chopped parsley
2 tsp prepared mustard
1 clove garlic, minced
freshly ground black pepper
6 C peeled, cooked potatoes, diced (about 4 large)
1 C coarsely chopped celery
1/2 C sliced radishes
1/4 C sliced scallions with tops

Combine yogurt, salad dressing, vinegar, salt, parsley, mustard, garlic, and pepper in large mixing bowl. Add vegetables; mix well. Refrigerate until serving time. Variation: cauliflower salad—omit rad-

571

Picnic Potato Salad (continued)

ishes and potatoes and substitute 6 cups diced, cooked cauliflower (about 1 lg head).
16 servings, 1/2 cup

Italian Vegetable Bake

Enough colorful vegetables baked together deliciously to feed a crowd...

NUTRIENTS PER SERVING
Calories: 36
Total fat .5 gms
Saturated fat: .2 gms
Polyunsaturated fat: .1 gm
Cholesterol .4 mgs
Sodium: 86 gms

[INGREDIENTS]
1 28-oz can whole tomatoes
1/2 lb fresh green beans, sliced
1/2 lb fresh okra, cut into 1/2" pieces or 1/2 10-oz pkg frozen okra
1 medium eggplant, pared and cut into 1" cubes
3/4 C finely chopped green pepper
1 Tbsp chopped fresh oregano leaves, or 1/2 tsp dried oregano, crushed
1 Tbsp chopped fresh basil, or 1 tsp dried basil, crushed
3 7"-long zucchini, cut into 1" cubes
2 Tbsp grated parmesan cheese
1 medium onion, sliced
2 Tbsp lemon juice

Drain and coarsely chop tomatoes. Reserve liquid. Mix together tomatoes and reserved liquid, onion, green beans, okra, green pepper, lemon juice, and herbs. Cover and bake at 325 degrees for 15 minutes. Mix in zucchini and eggplant and continue baking, covered, 60-70 more minutes or until vegetables are tender. Stir occasionally. Sprinkle top with parmesan cheese just before serving.
18 servings, 1/2 cup

Apricot-Orange Bread

A moist, rich-tasting bread to round out a light meal...

NUTRIENTS PER SERVING
Calories: 97
Total fat: 2 gms
Saturated fat: <1 gm
Polyunsaturated fat: <1 gm
Cholesterol: 6 mgs
Sodium: 113 mgs

[INGREDIENTS]
6-oz pkg dried apricots cut into small pieces
2 C water
2 Tbsp margarine
1 C sugar
1 egg, slightly beaten
1 Tbsp freshly grated orange peel
3 1/2 C sifted all-purpose flour
1/2 C nonfat dry milk powder
2 tsp baking powder
1 tsp baking soda
1 tsp salt
1/2 C orange juice
1/2 C chopped pecans

Preheat oven to 350 degrees. Lightly oil two 9x5x3 pans. Cook apricots in water in a covered medium-size saucepan 10 to 15 minutes or until tender but not mushy. Drain; reserve 3/4 cup liquid. Set apricots aside to cool. Cream together margarine and sugar. By hand, beat in egg and orange peel. Sift together flour, dry milk, baking powder, soda, and salt. Add to creamed mixture alternately with reserved apricot liquid and orange juice. Stir apricot pieces and pecans into batter. Turn batter into prepared pans. Bake 40-45 minutes or until bread springs back when lightly touched in center. Cool 5 minutes in pans. Remove from pans and completely cool on wire rack before slicing.
2 loaves, 36 1/2-inch slices

Rainbow Fruit Salad

A new twist to a back-to-basics favorite...either a side dish or dessert...

NUTRIENTS PER SERVING
Calories: 96
Total fat: 1 gm
Saturated fat: <1 gm
Polyunsaturated fat: <1 gm
Cholesterol: O mgs
Sodium: 4 mgs

[INGREDIENTS]
1 large mango, peeled and diced
2 C fresh blueberries
2 bananas, sliced
2 C fresh strawberries, halved
2 C seedless grapes
2 nectarines, unpeeled and sliced
1 kiwi fruit, peeled and sliced

HONEY ORANGE SAUCE
1/3 C unsweetened orange juice
2 Tbsp lemon juice
1 1/2Tbsp honey
1/4 tsp ground ginger
dash of nutmeg

Prepare the fruit. Combine all ingredients for sauce and mix. Just before serving, pour Honey Orange Sauce over fruit.
12 servings

Resources for a Healthy Heart

If you would like more information on the topics discussed in this booklet, the following organizations may be able to help you.

Federal Government

National Heart, Lung, and Blood Institute (NHLBI)
Information Center
P.O. Box 30105
Bethesda, MD 20824-0105
(301) 951-3260

The NHLBI Information Center is a service of the National Heart, Lung, and Blood Institute (NHLBI). It provides public and patient education materials on high blood pressure, cholesterol, smoking, obesity, and heart disease. Publications include: *Facts About High Blood Pressure; Eating to Lower Your High Blood Cholesterol; Check Your Weight and Heart Disease I.Q.*; and *Check Your Smoking I.Q.: An Important Quiz for Older Smokers.* The NHLBI also offers a number of fact sheets on heart disease-related topics such as *Facts About Coronary Heart Disease.*
A directory of publications is available.

Consumer Information Center (CIC)
Pueblo, CO 81009

The Consumer Information Catalog from the CIC lists over 200 free or low-cost booklets on consumer topics. Many are health-related and include booklets on nutrition, foods, exercise, women's health, and smoking. Write for a free copy.

Food and Drug Administration (FDA)
Office of Consumer Affairs, HFE-88
5600 Fishers Lane
Rockville, MD 20857
(301) 443-3170

The FDA offers publications on topics such as general drug information, medical devices, and food-related subjects including fiber, fats, sodium, and cholesterol. The FDA also publishes a monthly journal, *FDA Consumer,* which reports on recent developments in the regulation of foods, drugs, and cosmetics. Recent articles have covered topics such as heart bypass surgery, balloon angioplasty, dieting, and nutrition for women. Subscriptions can be ordered through the Consumer Information Catalog listed above. To order materials, contact the FDA at the address above or contact the consumer affairs office nearest you. Copies are available free of charge.

Food and Nutrition Information Center (FNIC)
National Agricultural Library
10301 Baltimore Avenue, Room 304
Beltsville, MD 20705-2351
(301) 504-5917

The FNIC answers questions concerning food and nutrition and provides database searches, bibliographies, and resource guides on a wide variety of food and nutrition topics.

Human Nutrition Information Service (HNIS)
Department of Agriculture
6505 Belcrest Road
Room 328A
Hyattsville, MD 20782
(301) 436-8617

HNIS reports results of research on food consumption, food composition, and dietary guidance in both technical and popular publications. A list of Department of Agriculture publications is available.

National Cancer Institute (NCI)
Office of Cancer Communications
Bldg. 31, Room 10A24
9000 Rockville Pike
Bethesda, MD 20892
(800) 4-CANCER
(301) 496-5583

The NCI provides information on how to stop smoking. Publications include: *Why Do You Smoke?* (a self-test); *Clearing the Air: A Guide to Quitting Smoking*; and *Guia Para Dejar de Fumar*. Publications are available free of charge.

National Clearinghouse for Alcohol and Drug Abuse Information (NCADI)
P.O. Box 2345
Rockville, MD 20852
(800) 729-6686
(301) 468-2600

NCADI is the central point within the Federal Government for current print and audiovisual information about alcohol and other drugs. Publications for women include: *Alcohol Alert #10; Alcohol and Women; Alcohol, Tobacco, and Other Drugs May Harm the Unborn*; and *Women and Alcohol*. A publications catalog is available.

National Diabetes Information Clearinghouse (NDIC)
Box NDIC
9000 Rockville Pike
Bethesda, MD 20892
(301) 468-2162

The NDIC provides information to diabetic patients and provides materials on topics such as diabetes management and treatment, nutrition, dental care, insulin, and self-blood glucose monitoring. Topical bibliographies are produced on subjects such as diet and nutrition, sports and exercise, and pregnancy. A bimonthly newsletter, *Diabetes Dateline*, is also available. Some mailing fees may apply.

Office of Disease Prevention and Health Promotion
National Health Information Center (ONHIC)
P.O. Box 1133
Washington, DC 20013-1133
(800) 336-4797
(301) 565-4167

The ONHIC helps the public and health professionals locate health information through identification of health information resources, an information and referral system, and publications. The ONHIC provides resource guides on a variety of health-related topics. A publications list is available.

Office on Smoking and Health (OSH)
Center for Chronic Disease Prevention and Health Promotion
Mail Stop K-50
Centers for Disease Control
1600 Clifton Road, N.E.
Atlanta, GA 30333
(404) 488-5705

The Office on Smoking and Health provides information on smoking cessation. Current titles include: *Out of the Ashes: Choosing a Method to Quit Smoking; At A Glance—The Health Benefits of Smoking Cessation: A Report of the Surgeon General; Is Your Baby Smoking?*; and a poster, *Pregnant? That's Two Good Reasons to Quit*. Single copies are available free of charge.

Superintendent of Documents
U.S. Government Printing Office
Washington, DC 20402-9352
(202) 783-3238

The Superintendent of Documents makes available many health-related publications from Government agencies. There are charges for publications. Write for a free copy of *U.S. Government Books and New Books* to receive information on what is available.

Voluntary Health Agencies

American Cancer Society (ACS)
1599 Clifton Road, N.E.
Atlanta, GA 30329
(404) 320-3333
(800) ACS-2345

Contact the local chapters or the national office for information. The ACS provides materials, individual and group support, self-help groups, and a speakers bureau. Publications include: *How Can We Reach You?*, which describes risks specific to women who smoke and tips for quitting without weight gain; *Why Start Life Under a Cloud; Eating Smart*; and *Nutrition, Common Sense, and Cancer*. The Taking Control program provides an introduction to a healthful, enjoyable lifestyle that may reduce one's risk of developing cancer. All publications and services are free.

American Diabetes Association
1660 Duke Street
Alexandria, VA 22314
(800) 232-3472
(703) 549-1500

Contact the local chapters or the national office. The group offers patient and family education activities such as educational meetings, weekend retreats, counseling and discussion, self-help, and support groups. Patient education publications include: *Diabetes in the Family; Diabetes: A to Z*; and the *Family Cookbook* series. *Diabetes Forecast*, a monthly magazine, and *Diabetes*, a quarterly newsletter, are available. There are membership fees and costs for some publications.

American Heart Association (AHA)
National Center
7320 Greenville Avenue
Dallas, TX 75231
(214) 373-6300

The AHA provides fact sheets, brochures, and audiovisuals on topics such as general cardiovascular disease risk reduction, exercise, high blood pressure, smoking, and nutrition. Publications include: *What Every Woman Should Know About High Blood Pressure; About Your Heart and Blood Pressure; American Heart Association Diet: An Eating Plan for Healthy Americans; Now You're Cookin': Healthful Recipes to Help Control High Blood Pressure; Eat Well, But Eat Wisely—To Reduce Your Risk of Heart Attack; Exercise and Your Heart*; and more. Write to the national office or the local AHA affiliate nearest to you. Single copies of most publications are free.

American Lung Association (ALA)
1740 Broadway
New York, NY 10019
(212) 315-8700

The ALA and its local affiliates conduct smoking cessation programs and offer a catalog of publications, including many on smoking. *The Stop Smoking, Stay Trim* booklet explains how stopping smoking affects weight and what you can do to prevent weight gain. *Freedom*

From Smoking in 20 Days is a self-help quit smoking program. Other publications include: *Q and A of Smoking and Health; Because You Love Your Baby*; and *Facts About Nicotine, Addiction, and Cigarettes.* Contact your local ALA affiliate or write to the above address. Some fees may apply.

Professional Association

American Dietetic Association (ADA)
216 W. Jackson Blvd., Suite 800
Chicago, IL 60606
(312) 899-0040

The ADA offers cookbooks and other materials for consumers designed to educate about food and nutrition. These include: *Lowfat Living: A Guide to Enjoying a Healthful Diet; Food Facts: What You Should Know About Nutrition and Health*; and *Food 3: Eating the Moderate Fat and Cholesteral Way.* Write or call for price information.

The National Center for Nutrition and Dietetics is the public education initiative of the ADA. It sponsors a consumer nutrition hotline that can be reached at (800) 366-1655 (9:00-4:00, central time). Callers can listen to recorded messages on current issues in nutrition or speak to a registered dietitian.

—by Marian Sandmaier

Chapter 58

Exercise and Your Heart: A Guide to Physical Activity

Foreword

Coronary heart disease remains the No. 1 cause of death and disability in the United States for both men and women. Almost half a million Americans die of coronary heart disease each year, and approximately half of these deaths are women. Preventing coronary heart disease remains the leading challenge to biomedical researchers and public health workers today. On the average, almost three Americans will suffer a heart attack every minute of the day, adding up to almost one and a half million attacks each year.

At the National Heart, Lung, and Blood Institute (NHLBI) and the American Heart Association (AHA), we are committed to addressing this challenge by encouraging fundamental research on the causes and treatment of coronary heart disease and by strengthening our disease prevention and health promotion programs. We have seen a dramatic decline in coronary heart disease mortality during the past two decades. This has been accompanied by a growing interest in making lifestyle changes which can reduce the risks for coronary heart disease.

With prevention as our ultimate goal, the communication of health information to the public will continue to be an important part of our activities. We have long provided the public with educational

NIH Pub. No. 93-1677.

materials to help reduce three primary risk factors: high blood pressure, cigarette smoking and high blood cholesterol. In recent years, the NHLBI and the AHA have addressed another major risk factor—sedentary lifestyle, or physical inactivity. The results of various studies now show that regular physical activity can help reduce the risk of heart disease. It also can help control other contributing risk factors, including obesity and diabetes. We hope that this booklet will help to stimulate a sensible exercise program as one way of keeping a healthy heart.

We are delighted to join together to provide this message about physical activity. We believe that collaboration is one improtant way of performin common public health missions. Revising and distributing this publication is only one example of this ongoing partnership.

Edward S. Cooper, M.D.
President American Heart Association

Claude M. Lenfant M.D.
Director
National Heart, Lung, and Blood Institute

Do We Get Enough Exercise from Our Daily Activities?

Most Americans get little vigorous exercise at work or during leisure hours. Today, only a few jobs require vigorous physical activity. People usually ride in cars or buses and watch TV during their free time rather than be physically active. Activities like golfing and bowling provide people with some benefit. But they do not provide the same benefits as regular, more vigorous exercise.

Evidence suggests that even low- to moderate-intensity activities can have both short- and long-term benefits. If done daily, they help lower your risk of heart disease. Such activities include pleasure walking, stair climbing, gardening, yardwork, moderate to heavy housework, dancing and home exercise. More vigorous exercise can help improve fitness of the heart and lungs, which can provide even more consistent benefits for lowering heart disease risk.

Today, many people are rediscovering the benefits of regular, vigorous exercise—activities like swimming, brisk walking, running, or jumping rope. These kinds of activities are sometimes called "aerobic"—meaning the body uses oxygen to produce the energy needed for the activity. Aerobic exercises can condition your heart and lungs if performed at the proper intensity for at least 30 minutes, 3-4 times a week.

But you don't have to train like a marathon runner to become more physically fit! Any activity that gets you moving around, even it it's done for just a few minutes each day, is better than none at all. For inactive people, the trick is to get started. One great way is to take a walk for 10-15 minutes during your lunch break. Other ideas in this pamphlet will help you get moving and living a more active life.

What Are the Benefits of Regular Physical Activity?

These are the benefits often experienced by people who get regular physical activity.

Feeling Better

Regular physical activity:

- gives you more energy
- helps in coping with stress
- improves your self-image
- increases resistance to fatigue
- helps counter anxiety and depression
- helps you to relax and feel less tense
- improves the ability to fall asleep quickly and sleep well
- provides an easy way to share an activity with friends or family and an opportunity to meet new friends

Looking Better

Regular physical activity:

- tones your muscles
- burns off calories to help lose extra pounds or helps you stay at your desirable weight
- helps control your appetite

You need to burn off 3,500 calories more than you take in to lose 1 pound. If you want to lose weight, regular physical activity can help you in either of two ways.

583

First, you can eat your usual amount of calories, but be more active. For example: A 200-pound person who keeps on eating the same amount of calories, but decides to walk briskly each day for 1 1/2 miles will lose about 14 pounds in 1 year. Or second, you can eat fewer calories and be more active. This is an even better way to lose weight.

About three-fourths of the energy you burn every day comes from what your body uses for its basic needs, such as sleeping, breathing, digesting food and reclining. A person burns up only a small amount of calories with daily activities such as sitting. Any physical activity in addition to what you normally do will burn up extra calories.

The average calories spent per hour by a 150-pound person are listed below. (A lighter person burns fewer calories; a heavier person burns more.) Since exact calorie figures are not available for most activities, the figures below are averaged from several sources and show the relative vigor of the activities.

- Bicycling 6 mph burns 240 cals./hr.
- Bicycling 12 mph burns 410 cals./hr.
- Cross-country skiing burns 700 cals./hr.
- Jogging 5 1/2 mph burns 740 cals./hr.
- Jogging 7 mph burns 920 cals./hr.
- Jumping rope burns 750 cals./hr.
- Running in place burns 650 cals./hr.
- Running 10 mph burns 1280 cals./hr.
- Swimming 25 yds/min. burns 275 cals./hr.
- Swimming 50 yds/min. burns 500 cals./hr.
- Tennis-singles burns 400 cals./hr.
- Walking 2 mph burns 240 cals./hr.
- Walking 3 mph burns 320 cals./hr.
- Walking 4 1/2 burns mph 440 cals./hr.

The calories spent in a particular activity vary in proportion to one's body weight. For example, a 100-pound person burns 1/3 fewer calories, so you would multiply the number of calories by 0.7. For a 200-pound person, multiply by 1.3.

Working harder or faster for a given activity will only slightly increase the calories spent. A better way to burn up more calories is to increase the time spent on your activity.

Working Better

Regular physical activity:

• helps you to be more productive at work
• increases your capacity for physical work
• builds stamina for other physical activities
• increases muscle strength
• helps your heart and lungs work more efficiently

Consider the benefits of a well-conditioned heart:
In 1 minute with 45 to 50 beats, the heart of a well-conditioned person pumps the same amount of blood as an inactive person's heart pumps in 70 to 75 beats. Compared to the well-conditioned heart, the average heart pumps up to 36,000 *more* times per day, 13 million *more* times per year.

Feeling, looking, and working better—all these benefits from regular physical activity can help you enjoy your life more fully.

Can Physical Activity Reduce My Chances of Getting a Heart Attack?

Yes! Various studies have shown that physical inactivity is a risk factor for heart disease. Overall, the results show heart disease is almost twice as likely to develop in inactive people than in those who are more active. Regular physical activity (even mild to moderate exercise) can help reduce your risk of heart disease. In fact, burning calories through physical activity may help you lose weight or stay at your desirable weight—which also helps lower your risk of heart disease. The best exercises to strengthen your heart and lungs are the *aerobic* ones like brisk walking, jogging, cycling and swimming.

Coronary artery disease is the major cause of heart disease and heart attack in America. It develops when fatty deposits build up on the inner walls of the blood vessels feeding the heart (*coronary arteries*). Eventually one or more of the major coronary arteries may become blocked—either by the buildup of deposits or by a blood clot forming in the artery's narrowed passageway. The result is a heart attack.

We know that there are several factors that can increase your risk for developing coronary artery disease—and thus the chances for a heart attack. Fortunately, many of these risk factors can be reduced or eliminated.

The Risk Factors for Heart Disease That You Can Do Something about Are:

- Cigarette Smoking
- High Blood Pressure
- High Blood Cholesterol
- Physical Inactivity and
- Obesity.

The more risk factors you have, the greater your risk for heart disease and heart attack.

Cigarette Smoking. Heavy smokers are two to four times more likely to have a heart attack than nonsmokers. The heart attack death rate among all smokers is 70 percent greater than among nonsmokers. People who are active regularly are more likely to cut down or stop cigarette smoking.

High Blood Pressure. The higher your blood pressure, the greater your risk of developing heart disease or stroke. A blood pressure of 140/90 mmHg (millimeters of mercury) or greater is generally classified as high blood pressure. Regular physical activity, even of moderate intensity, can help reduce high blood pressure in some people. This type of activity may also help *prevent* high blood pressure.

High Blood Cholesterol. A blood cholesterol level of 240 mg/dl (milligrams per deciliter) or above is high and increases your risk of heart disease. A total blood cholesterol of under 200 mg/dl is desirable and usually puts you at a lower risk of heart disease. Cholesterol in the blood is transported by different types of particles. One of these particles is a protein called *high density lipoprotein* or HDL. HDL has been called "good" cholesterol because research has shown that high levels of HDL are linked with a lower risk of coronary artery disease. Regular moderate-to-vigorous physical activity is linked with increased HDL levels.

Physical Inactivity. The lack of physical activity increases your risk for developing heart disease. Even persons who have had a heart attack can increase their chances of survival if they change their habits to include regular physical activity. It can help control blood lipids, diabetes and obesity as well as help to lower blood pressure. Also, physical activity of the right intensity, frequency and duration can increase the fitness of your heart and lungs—which may help protect you against heart disease even if you have other risk factors.

Obesity. Excess weight may increase your risk of developing high blood pressure, high blood cholesterol and diabetes. Regular physical activity can help you maintain your desirable body weight. People at their desirable weight are less likely to develop diabetes. And, exercise may also decrease a diabetic person's need for insulin.

Remember that even if you are active, you should not ignore other risk factors. Reduce or eliminate any risk factors you can to lower your chances of having a heart attack.

Tips for your heart's health:

- Stay physically active
- Stop smoking and avoid other people's smoke if possible
- Control high blood pressure and high blood cholesterol
- Cut down on total fats, saturated fats, cholesterol and salt in your diet.
- Reduce weight if overweight

Are There Any Risks in Exercising?

Muscles and Joints

The most common risk in exercising is injury to the muscles and joints. This usually happens from exercising too hard or for too long—particularly if a person has been inactive for some time. However, most of these injuries can be prevented or easily treated as explained in [the section below titled] "Effective ways to avoid injuries."

Heat Exhaustion and Heat Stroke

If precautions are not taken during hot, humid days, heat exhaustion or heat stroke can occur—although they are fairly rare. Heat stroke is the more serious of the two. Their symptoms are similar:

587

- Heat exhaustion: dizziness, headache, nausea, confusion, body temperature below normal
- Heat stroke: dizziness, headache, nausea, thirst, muscle cramps, sweating stops, high body temperature

The last two symptoms of heat stroke are important to know. If the body temperature becomes dangerously high, it can be a serious problem.

Both heat exhaustion and heat stroke can be avoided if you drink enough liquids to replace those lost during exercise. And be sure to take the other important precautions listed in the section on avoiding injuries.

Heart Problems

In some cases, people have died while exercising. Most of these deaths are caused by overexertion in people who already had heart conditions. In people under age 30, these heart conditions are usually *congenital heart defects* (heart defects present at birth). In people over age 40, the heart condition is usually *coronary artery disease* (the buildup of deposits of fats in the heart's blood vessels). Many of these deaths have been preceded by warning signs such as chest pain, lightheadedness, fainting and extreme breathlessness. These are symptoms that should not be ignored and should be brought to the attention of a doctor immediately.

Some of the deaths that occur during exercise are not caused by the physical effort itself. Death can occur at any time and during any kind of activity—eating, sleeping, sitting. This does not necessarily mean that a particular activity caused the death—only that the two events happened at the same time.

No research studies have shown that physically active people are more likely to have sudden, fatal heart attacks than inactive people. In fact, a number of studies have shown a reduced risk of sudden death for people who are physically active.

Exercising too hard is not beneficial for anyone, however, and is especially strenuous for out-of-shape, middle-aged and older persons. It is very important for these people to follow a gradual and sound exercise program.

If you consider the time your body may have been out of shape, it is only natural that it will take time to get it back into good condition.

A gradual approach will help you maximize your benefits and minimize your risks.

Comparing the Benefits and the Risks

Should you begin a regular exercise program? Consider the ways physical activity can benefit you and weigh them against the possible risks.

Potential benefits:

- more energy and capacity for work and leisure activities
- greater resistance to stress, anxiety and fatigue, and a better outlook on life
- increased stamina, strength and flexibility
- improved efficiency of the heart and lungs
- loss of extra pounds or body fat
- help in staying at desirable weight
- reduced risk of heart attack

Potential risks:

- muscle or joint injuries
- heat exhaustion or heat stroke on hot days (rare)
- aggravation of existing or hidden heart problems

Should I Consult a Doctor Before I Start an Exercise Program?

Most people do not need to see a doctor before they start since a gradual, sensible exercise program will have minimal health risks. However, some people should seek medical advice. Use the following checklist to find out if you should consult a doctor before you start or significantly increase your physical activity. (This checklist has been developed from several sources, particularly the Physical Activity Readiness Questionnaire, British Columbia Ministry of Health, Department of National Health and Welfare, Canada (revised 1992).)

Mark those items that apply to you:

- Your doctor said you have a heart condition and recommended only medically supervised physical activity.

- During or right after you exercise, you frequently have pains or pressure in the left or mid-chest area, left neck, shoulder or arm.

- You have developed chest pain within the last month.

- You tend to lose consciousness or fall over due to dizziness.

- You feel extremely breathless after mild exertion.

- Your doctor recommended you take medicine for your blood pressure or a heart condition.

- Your doctor said you have bone or joint problems that could be made worse by the proposed physical activity.

- You have a medical condition or other physical reason not mentioned here which might need special attention in an exercise program. (For example, insulin-dependent diabetes.)

- You are middle-aged or older, have not been physically active, and plan a relatively vigorous exercise program.

If you've checked one or more items, see your doctor before you start. If you've checked no items, you can start on a gradual, sensible program of increased activity tailored to your needs. If you feel any of the physical symptoms listed above when you start your exercise program, contact your doctor right away.

What If I've Had a Heart Attack?

Regular, brisk physical activity can help reduce your risk of having another heart attack. People who include regular physical activity in their lives after a heart attack improve their chances of survival. Regular exercise can also improve the quality of your life—how you feel and look. It can help you do more than before without pain (angina) or shortness of breath.

If you've had a heart attack, consult your doctor to be sure you are following a safe and effective exercise program. Your doctor's guidance is very important because it could help prevent heart pain and/or further damage from overexertion.

Five Common Myths about Exercise

Myth 1: Exercising Makes You Tired

As they become more physically fit, most people feel physical activity gives them even more energy than before. Regular, moderate-to-brisk exercise can also help you reduce fatigue and manage stress.

Myth 2: Exercising Takes Too Much Time

It only takes a few minutes a day to become more physically active. To *condition* your heart and lungs, regular exercise does not have to take more than about 30 to 60 minutes, three or four times a week. If you don't have 30 minutes in your schedule for an exercise break, try to find two 15-minute periods or even three 10-minute periods. Once you discover how much you enjoy these exercise breaks, you may want to make them a habit! Then physical activity becomes a natural part of your life.

Myth 3: All Exercises Give You the Same Benefits

All physical activities can give you enjoyment. Low-intensity activities—if performed daily—also can have some long-term health benefits and lower your risk of heart disease. But only regular, brisk and sustained exercises such as brisk walking, jogging or swimming improve the efficiency of your heart and lungs and burn off substantial extra calories. Other activities may give you other benefits such as increased flexibility or muscle strength, depending on the type of activity.

Myth 4: The Older You Are, the Less Exercise You Need

We tend to become less active with age, and therefore need to make sure we are getting enough physical activity. In general, middle-aged and older people benefit from regular physical activity just as young people do. Age need not be a limitation. In fact, regular physi-

591

cal activity in older persons increases their capacity to perform activities of daily living. What is important, no matter what your age, is tailoring the activity program to your own fitness level.

Myth 5: You Have to Be Athletic to Exercise

Most physical activities do not require any special athletic skills. In fact, many people who found school sports difficult have discovered that these other activities are easy to do and enjoy. A perfect example is walking—an activity that requires no special talent, athletic ability or equipment.

How Do Different Activities Help My Heart and Lungs?

Some types of activity will improve the condition of your heart and lungs if they are brisk, sustained and regular. Low-intensity activities do not condition the heart and lungs much. But they can have other long-term health benefits.

The [list below describes] three types of activities and how they affect your heart.

[No. 1: Activities that do condition heart and lungs.] These vigorous exercises are especially helpful when done regularly. To condition your heart and lungs, the AHA recommends that you do them for at least 30 minutes, three or four times a week, at more than 50 percent of your exercise capacity. (See [chart in section titled "How Do I Pace Myself?"] on target heart rate zone.) Other health experts suggest a shorter period for higher-intensity activities. These exercises can also burn up more calories than those that are not so vigorous.

[No. 2: Activities that can condition heart and lungs.] These activities are moderately vigorous but still excellent choices. When done briskly for 30 minutes or longer, three or four times a week, they can also condition your heart and lungs.

[No. 3: Activities that do not condition much.] These activities are not vigorous or sustained. They still have benefits—they can be enjoyable, improve coordination and muscle tone, relieve tension, and also help burn up some calories.

These and other low-intensity activities—like gardening, yardwork, housework, dancing and home exercise—can help lower your risk of heart disease if done daily.

1. [Activities that] do condition heart and lungs: Aerobic Dancing; Bicycling; Cross-Country Skiing; Hiking (uphill); Ice Hockey; Jogging; Jumping Rope; Rowing; Running in Place; Stair-climbing; Stationary Cycling; Swimming; Walking Briskly

2. [Activities that] can condition heart and lungs: Downhill Skiing; Basketball; Field Hockey; Calisthenics; Handball; Racquetball; Soccer; Squash; Tennis (singles); Volleyball; Walking Moderately

3. [Activities that] do not condition much: Badminton; Baseball; Bowling; Croquet; Football; Gardening; Golf (on foot or by cart); Housework; Ping-pong; Shuffleboard; Social Dancing; Softball; Walking Leisurely

The Key to Success

How Do I Begin?

The key to a successful program is choosing an activity (or activities) that you will enjoy. Even moderate levels of activity have important health benefits. Here are some questions that can help you choose the right kind of activity for you:

How physically fit are you? If you've been inactive for a while, you may want to start with walking or swimming at a comfortable pace. Beginning with less strenuous activities will allow you to become more fit without straining your body. Once you are in better shape, you can gradually change to a more vigorous activity if you wish.

How old are you? If you are over 40 and have not been active, avoid very strenuous programs such as jogging when you're first starting out. For the first few months, build up the length and intensity of your activity gradually. Walking and swimming are especially good forms of exercise for all ages.

What benefits do you want from exercising? If you want the benefits of exercise that condition your heart and lungs, check the activities [listed under No. 1 and No. 2 above]. These activities—as well as those listed in [No. 2]—also give you other benefits as described in this booklet.

Do you like to exercise alone or with other people? Do you like individual activities such as swimming, team sports such as soccer, or two-person activities such as racquetball? How about an aerobics class or ballroom dancing? Companionship can help you get started and keep going. If you would like to exercise with someone else, can you find a partner easily and quickly? If not, choose another activity until you can find a partner.

Do you prefer to exercise outdoors or in your home? Outdoor activities offer variety in scenery and weather. Indoor activities offer shelter from the weather and can offer the convenience of exercising at home as with stationary cycling. Some activities such as bench stepping, running in place or jumping rope can be done indoors or outdoors. If your activity can be seriously affected by weather, consider choosing a second, alternate activity. Then you can switch activities and still stay on your regular schedule.

How much money are you willing to spend for sports equipment or facilities? Many activities require little or no equipment. For example, brisk walking only requires a comfortable pair of walking shoes. Also, many communities offer free or inexpensive recreation facilities and physical activity classes.

When can you best fit the activity into your schedule? Do you feel more like being active in the morning, afternoon, or evening? Consider moving other activities around. Schedule your activity as a regular part of your routine. Remember that exercise sessions are spread out over the week and needn't take more than about 10 to 15 minutes at a time.

By choosing activities you like, you will be more likely to keep doing them regularly and enjoying the many benefits of physical activity.

How Do I Pace Myself?

Build up *slowly*. If you've been inactive for a long while, remember it will take time to get into shape. Start with low- to moderate-level activities for at least several minutes each day. See the sample walking program [in the section titled "Two Sample Activity Programs"], for example. You can slowly increase your time or pace as you become more fit. And you will feel more fit after a few weeks than when you first started.

How Hard Should I Exercise?

It's important to exercise at a comfortable pace. For example, when jogging or walking briskly you should be able to keep up a conversation comfortably. If you do not feel normal again within 10 minutes of stopping exercise, you are pushing yourself too much.

Also, if you have difficulty breathing, experience faintness or prolonged weakness during or after exercising, you are exercising too hard. Simply cut back.

If your goal is to improve the fitness of your heart and lungs, you can find out how hard to exercise by keeping track of your heart rate. Your maximum heart rate is the fastest your heart can beat. Exercise above 75 percent of your maximum heart rate may be too strenuous unless you are in excellent physical condition. Exercise below 50 percent gives your heart and lungs little conditioning.

Therefore, the best activity level is 50 to 75 percent of this maximum rate. This 50-75 percent range is called your *target heart rate zone*.

When you begin your exercise program, aim for the lower part of your target zone (50 percent) during the first few months. As you get into better shape, gradually build up to the higher part of your target zone (75 percent). After 6 months or more of regular exercise, you can exercise at up to 85 percent of your maximum heart rate—if you wish. However, you do not have to exercise that hard to stay in good condition. To find your target zone, look for the age category closest to your age in the table below and read the line across. For example, if you are 30, your target zone is 95 to 142 beats per minute. If you are 43, the closest age on the chart is 45; the target zone is 88 to 131 beats per minute.

Age	Target HR Zone 50–75%	Average Maximum Heart Rate 100%
20 years	100–150 beats per min.	200
25 years	98–146 beats per min.	195
30 years	95–142 beats per min.	190
35 years	93–138 beats per min.	185
40 years	90–135 beats per min.	180
45 years	88–131 beats per min.	175
50 years	85–127 beats per min.	170
55 years	83–123 beats per min.	165
60 years	80–120 beats per min.	160
65 years	78–116 beats per min.	155
70 years	75–113 beats per min.	150

Figure 58.1.

Your maximum heart rate is approximately 220 minus your age. However, the above figures are averages and should be used as general guidelines.

Note: A few high blood pressure medicines lower the maximum heart rate and thus the target zone rate. If you are taking high blood pressure medications, call your physician to find out if your exercise program needs to be adjusted.

To see if you are within your target heart rate zone, take your pulse immediately after you stop exercising.

1. When you stop exercising, quickly place the tips of your first two fingers lightly over one of the blood vessels on your neck (carotid arteries) located to the left or right of your Adam's apple. Another convenient pulse spot is the inside of your wrist just below the base of your thumb.

2. Count your pulse for 10 seconds and multiply by six.

3. If your pulse falls within your target zone, you're doing fine. If it is below your target zone, exercise a little harder next

time. And if you're above your target zone, exercise a little easier. Don't try to exercise at your maximum heart rate—that's working too hard.

4. Once you're exercising within your target zone, you should check your pulse at least once each week during the first 3 months and periodically after that.

A Special Tip

Some people find that exercising within their target zone seems too strenuous. If you start out lower, that's okay, too. You will find that with time you'll become more comfortable exercising and can increase to your target zone at your own rate.

How Long Should I Exercise?

That depends on your age, your level of physical fitness, and the level of intensity of your exercise. If you are inactive now, you might begin slowly with a 10-15 minute walk or other short session, three times a week. As you become more fit, you can do longer sessions or short sessions more often. If you're active already and your goal is to condition your heart and lungs, try for a minimum of 30 minutes at your target heart rate zone. Each exercise session should include:

Warm up—5 minutes. Begin exercising slowly to give your body a chance to limber up and get ready for more vigorous exercise. Start at a medium pace and gradually increase it by the end of the 5-minute warm-up period.

Note: With especially vigorous activities such as jumping rope, jogging or stationary cycling, warm up for 9-10 minutes by jumping rope or jogging slowly, warming up to your target zone. It is often a good idea to do stretching exercises after your warm-up period and after your exercise period. Many of these stretching exercises can be found in books on sports medicine and running. Below are three stretches you can use in your warm-up period and after your cooldown period. Each of these exercises help stretch different parts of your body. Do stretching exercises slowly and steadily, and **don't bounce** when you stretch.

- Wall push: Stand about 1 1/2 feet away from the wall. Then lean forward pushing against the wall, keeping heels flat. Count to 10 (or 20 for a longer stretch), then rest. Repeat one to two times.

- Palm touch: Stand with your knees slightly bent. Then bend from the waist and try to touch your palms to the floor. Count to 10 or 20, then rest. Repeat one to two times. If you have lower back problems, do this exercise with your legs crossed.

- Toe touch: Place your right leg level on a stair, chair, or other object. With your other leg slightly bent, lean forward and slowly try to touch your right toe with right hand. Hold and count to 10 or 20, then repeat with left hand. Do not bounce. Then switch legs and repeat with each hand. Repeat entire exercise one to two times.

Exercising within your target zone—30-60 minutes. Build up your exercising time gradually over the weeks ahead until you reach your goal of 30-60 minutes. Once you get in shape, your exercising will last from 30 to 60 minutes depending on the type of exercise you are doing and how briskly you do it. For example—for a given amount of time, jogging requires more energy than a brisk walk. Jogging will thus take less time than walking to achieve the same conditioning effect. For two examples of how to build up to the goal of 30-60 minutes, see [the section titled] "Two Sample Exercise Programs."

Cool down—5 minutes. After exercising within your target zone, slow down gradually. For example, swim more slowly or change to a more leisurely stroke. You can also cool down by changing to a less vigorous exercise, such as changing from running to walking. This allows your body to relax gradually. Abrupt stopping can cause dizziness. If you have been running, walking briskly, or jumping rope, repeat your stretching and limbering exercises to loosen up your muscles.

How Often Should I Exercise?

If you are exercising in your target zone, exercise at least three or four times per week (every other day). If you are starting with less intense exercise, you should try to do at least something every day.

Exercising regularly is one of the most important aspects of your exercise program. If you don't exercise at least three times a week, you won't experience as many of the benefits of regular physical activity as you could or make as much progress. Try to spread your exercise sessions throughout the week to maximize the benefits. An every-other-day schedule is recommended and may work well for you.

What If I Miss a Few Sessions?

Whenever you miss a few sessions (more than a week), you may need to resume exercising at a lower level than before.

If you miss a few sessions because of a temporary, minor illness such as a cold, wait until you feel normal before you resume exercising. If you have a minor injury, wait until the pain disappears. When you resume exercising, start at one-half to two-thirds your normal level, depending on the number of days you missed and how you feel while exercising.

Whatever the reasons for missing sessions, don't worry about the missed days. Just get back into your routine and think about the progress you will be making toward your exercise goal.

Is There a Top Limit to Exercising?

That depends on the benefits you are seeking.

Anything beyond 60 minutes daily of a vigorous or moderately vigorous activity will result in little added conditioning of your heart and lungs. And it may increase your risk of injury.

If you want to lose extra pounds or control your present weight, there is no upper limit in that the longer you exercise, the more calories you burn off. But remember that the most effective weight loss program includes cutting down on calories in addition to exercise.

Remember: How you exercise is just as important as the kind of activity you do. Your activity should be brisk, sustained and regular—but you can do it in gradual steps. Common sense and your body will tell you when you are exercising too long or too hard. Don't push yourself to the point where exercise stops being enjoyable.

Effective Ways to Avoid Injuries

The most powerful medicine for injuries is prevention. Here are some effective ways to avoid injuries:

Build up Your Level of Activity Gradually over the Weeks to Come.

- Try not to set your goals too high—otherwise you will be tempted to push yourself too far too quickly.

- For activities such as jogging, walking briskly and jumping rope, limber up gently and slowly before and after exercising.

- For other activities, build up slowly to your target zone, and cool down slowly afterwards.

Listen to Your Body for Early Warning Pains

- Exercising too much can cause injuries to joints, feet, ankles and legs. So don't make the mistake of exercising beyond early warning pains in these areas or more serious injuries may result. Fortunately, minor muscle and joint injuries can be readily treated by rest and aspirin.

Be Aware of Possible Signs of Heart Problems Such As:

- Pain or pressure in the left or mid-chest area, left neck, shoulder or arm during or just after exercising. (Vigorous exercise may cause a side stitch while exercising—a pain below your bottom ribs—which is not the result of a heart problem.)

- Sudden lightheadedness, cold sweat, pallor or fainting.

Ignoring these signals and continuing to exercise may lead to serious heart problems. Should any of these signs occur, stop exercising and call your doctor.

For Outdoor Activities, Take Appropriate Precautions Under Special Weather Conditions

On hot, humid days:

- Exercise during the cooler and/or less humid parts of the day such as early morning or early evening after the sun has gone down.

- Exercise less than normal for a week until you become adapted to the heat.

- Drink lots of fluids, particularly water—before, during and after exercising. Usually, you do not need extra salt because you get enough salt in your diet. (And a well-conditioned body is better able to conserve salt so that most of the sweat is water.) However, if you exercise very vigorously for an extended time in the heat (for example, running a marathon), it's a good idea to increase your salt intake a little.

- Watch out for signs of heat stroke—feeling dizzy, weak, lightheaded, and/or excessively tired; sweating stops; or body temperature becomes dangerously high.

- Wear a minimum of light, loose-fitting clothing.

- Avoid rubberized or plastic suits, sweatshirts, and sweat pants. Such clothing will not actually help you lose weight any faster by making you sweat more. The weight you lose in fluids by sweating will be quickly replaced as soon as you begin drinking fluids again. This type of clothing can also cause dangerously high temperatures, possibly resulting in heat stroke.

On cold days:

- Wear one layer less of clothing than you would wear if you were outside but not exercising. It's also better to wear several layers of clothing rather than one heavy layer. You can always remove a layer if you get too warm.

- Use old mittens, gloves, or cotton socks to protect your hands.

- Wear a hat, since up to 40 percent of your body's heat is lost through your neck and head.

On rainy, icy or snowy days:

- Be aware of reduced visibility (for yourself and for drivers) and reduced traction on pathways.

Other Handy Tips Are:

- If you've eaten a meal, avoid strenuous exercise for at least 2 hours. If you exercise vigorously first, wait about 20 minutes before eating.

- Use proper equipment such as goggles to protect your eyes for handball or racquetball, or good shoes with adequate cushioning in the soles for running or walking.

- Hard or uneven surfaces such as cement or rough fields are more likely to cause injuries. Soft, even surfaces such as a level grass field, a dirt path, or a track for running are better for your feet and joints.

- If you run or jog, land on your heels rather than the balls of your feet. This will minimize the strain on your feet and lower legs.

- Joggers or walkers should also watch for cars and wear light-colored clothes with a reflecting band during darkness so that drivers can see you. Remember, drivers don't see you as well as you see their cars. Face oncoming traffic and do not assume that drivers will notice you on the roadway.

- If you bicycle, you can help prevent injuries by always wearing a helmet and using lights and wheel-mounted reflectors at night. Also, ride in the direction of traffic and try to avoid busy streets.

- Check your shopping malls. Many malls are open early and late for people who do not wish to exercise alone in the dark. They also make it possible to be active in bad weather and to avoid summer heat, winter cold or allergy seasons.

Two Sample Activity Programs

There are many ways to begin an activity program. [Figures 58.2 and 58.3 describe two sample programs]—a walking and a jogging program. These activities are easy ways for most people to get regular exercise because they do not require special facilities or equipment other than good, comfortable shoes.

If walking or jogging does not meet your needs, look for other exercise programs in pamphlets and books on aerobic exercise and sports medicine. Check out the programs and facilities of your local park and recreation department or community recreation centers. Many programs have adapted facilities for the disabled and for seniors.

If you find a particular week's pattern tiring, repeat it before going on to the next pattern. You do not have to complete the walking program in 12 weeks or the jogging program in 15 weeks.

A new AHA brochure called "Walking. . .Natural Fun, Natural Fitness" has a walking readiness questionnaire and a one-mile fitness test. You can ask your local American Heart Association for a copy.

If you are over 40 and have not been active, you should not begin with a program as strenuous as jogging. Begin with the walking program instead. After completing the walking program, you can start with week 3 of the jogging program [described in Figure 58.3].

The exercise patterns for both of the sample activity programs are suggested guidelines. Listen to your body and build up less quickly, if needed.

How Do I Keep Going?

Here are some tips to help you stay physically active:

1. Set your sights on short-term as well as long-term goals. For example, if your long-term goal is to walk 1 mile, then your short-term goal can be to walk the first quarter mile. Or if your long-term goal is to lose 10 pounds, then focus on the immediate goal of losing the first two or three pounds. With short-term goals you will be less likely to push yourself too hard or too long. Also, think back to where you started. When you compare it to where you are now, you will see the progress you've made.

2. Discuss your program and goals with your family or friends. Their encouragement and understanding are important sources of support that can help you keep going. Your friends and family might even join in.

	Warm up	Target zone exercising	Cool down	Total time
Week 1				
Session A	Walk 5 min.	Then walk briskly 5 min.	Then walk more slowly 5 min.	15 min.
Session B	Repeat above pattern			
Session C	Repeat above pattern			

Continue with at least three exercise sessions during each week of the program.

	Warm up	Target zone exercising	Cool down	Total time
Week 2	Walk 5 min.	Walk briskly 7 min.	Walk 5 min.	17 min.
Week 3	Walk 5 min.	Walk briskly 9 min.	Walk 5 min.	19 min.
Week 4	Walk 5 min.	Walk briskly 11 min.	Walk 5 min.	21 min.
Week 5	Walk 5 min.	Walk briskly 13 min.	Walk 5 min.	23 min.
Week 6	Walk 5 min.	Walk briskly 15 min.	Walk 5 min.	25 min.
Week 7	Walk 5 min.	Walk briskly 18 min.	Walk 5 min.	28 min.
Week 8	Walk 5 min.	Walk briskly 20 min.	Walk 5 min.	30 min.
Week 9	Walk 5 min.	Walk briskly 23 min.	Walk 5 min.	33 min.
Week 10	Walk 5 min.	Walk briskly 26 min.	Walk 5 min.	36 min.
Week 11	Walk 5 min.	Walk briskly 28 min.	Walk 5 min.	38 min.
Week 12	Walk 5 min.	Walk briskly 30 min.	Walk 5 min.	40 min.

Week 13 on:

Check your pulse periodically to see if you are exercising within your target zone. As you become more fit, try exercising within the upper range of your target zone. Gradually increase your brisk walking time to 30 to 60 minutes, three or four times a week. Remember that your goal is to get the benefits you are seeking and enjoy your activity.

Figure 58.2. A Sample Walking Program

	Warm up	Target zone exercising	Cool down	Total time
Week 1				
Session A	Walk 5 min., then stretch and limber up	Then walk 10 min. Try not to stop	Then walk more slowly 3 min. and stretch 2 min.	20 min.
Session B	Repeat above pattern			
Session C	Repeat above pattern			

Continue with at least three exercise sessions during each week of the program.

	Warm up	Target zone exercising	Cool down	Total time
Week 2	Walk 5 min., then stretch and limber up	Walk 5 min., jog 1 min., walk 5 min., jog 1 min.	Walk 3 min., stretch 2 min.	22 min.
Week 3	Walk 5 min., then stretch and limber up	Walk 5 min., jog 3 min., walk 5 min., jog 3 min.	Walk 3 min., stretch 2 min.	26 min.
Week 4	Walk 5 min., then stretch and limber up	Walk 4 min., jog 5 min., walk 4 min., jog 5 min.	Walk 3 min., stretch 2 min.	28 min.
Week 5	Walk 5 min., then stretch and limber up	Walk 4 min., jog 5 min., walk 4 min., jog 5 min.	Walk 3 min., stretch 2 min.	28 min.
Week 6	Walk 5 min., then stretch and limber up	Walk 4 min., jog 6 min., walk 4 min., jog 6 min.	Walk 3 min., stretch 2 min.	30 min.
Week 7	Walk 5 min., then stretch and limber up	Walk 4 min., jog 7 min., walk 4 min., jog 7 min.	Walk 3 min., stretch 2 min.	32 min.

Figure 58.3(a): A Sample Jogging Program

605

Week 8	Walk 5 min., then stretch and limber up	Walk 4 min., jog 8 min., walk 4 min., jog 8 min.	Walk 3 min., stretch 2 min.	34 min.
Week 9	Walk 5 min., then stretch and limber up	Walk 4 min., jog 9 min., walk 4 min., jog 9 min.	Walk 3 min., stretch 2 min.	36 min.
Week 10	Walk 5 min., then stretch and limber up	Walk 4 min., jog 13 min.	Walk 3 min., stretch 2 min.	27 min.
Week 11	Walk 5 min., then stretch and limber up	Walk 4 min., jog 15 min.	Walk 3 min., stretch 2 min.	29 min.
Week 12	Walk 5 min., then stretch and limber up	Walk 4 min., jog 17 min.	Walk 3 min., stretch 2 min.	31 min.
Week 13	Walk 5 min., then stretch and limber up	Walk 2 min., jog slowly 2 min., jog 17 min.	Walk 3 min., stretch 2 min.	31 min.
Week 14	Walk 5 min., then stretch and limber up	Walk 1 min., jog slowly 3 min., jog 17 min.	Walk 3 min., stretch 2 min.	31 min.
Week 15	Walk 5 min., then stretch and limber up	Jog slowly 3 min., jog 17 min.	Walk 3 min., stretch 2 min.	30 min.

Week 16 on:

Check your pulse periodically to see if you are exercising within your target zone. As you become more fit, try exercising within the upper range of your target zone. Gradually increase your jogging time from 20 to 30 minutes (or more, up to 60 minutes), three or four times a week. Remember that your goal is to get the benefits you are seeking and enjoy your activity.

Figure 58.3(b). A Sample Jogging Program (continued)

3. If you're having trouble sticking to your regular activity program, use the questions [listed in the above section titled "The Keys to Success"] to think through the kinds of things that can affect your exercise enjoyment.

4. What were your original reasons for starting an activity program? Do these reasons still apply or are others more important? If you are feeling bored or aren't enjoying a particular activity, consider trying another one.

By continuing to be active regularly, you'll be building a good health habit with benefits you can enjoy throughout your life.

How Can I Become More Active Throughout My Day?

To become more physically active throughout your day, take advantage of any opportunity to get up and move around. Here are some examples:

- Use the stairs—up and down—instead of the elevator. Start with one flight of stairs and gradually build up to more.
- Park a few blocks from the office or store and walk the rest of the way. Or if you ride on public transportation, get off a stop or two before and walk a few blocks.
- Take an activity break—get up and stretch, walk around and give your muscles and mind a chance to relax.
- Instead of eating that extra snack, take a brisk stroll around the neighborhood.
- Do housework, such as vacuuming, at a more brisk pace.
- Mow your own lawn.
- Carry your own groceries.
- Go dancing instead of seeing a movie.
- Take a walk after dinner instead of watching TV.

If you have a family, encourage them to take part in an exercise program and recreational activities they can either share with you or do on their own. It is best to build healthy habits when children are young. When parents are active, children are more likely to be active and stay active after they become adults.

Whatever your age, moderate physical activity can become a good health habit with lifelong benefits.

For more information about heart health, contact:

National Heart, Lung, and Blood Institute
Education Programs Information Center
P. O. Box 30105
Bethesda, Maryland 20824-0105

or

Your local American Heart Association

or

call 1-800-AHA-USA1 (1-800-242-8721)

Chapter 59

Aerobic Fitness
Affects Blood Pressure

Aerobic fitness affects the diurnal patterns of blood pressure in adolescents, particularly in blacks, according to investigators at the University of Tennessee General Clinical Research Center at LeBonheur Children's Medical Center in Memphis.

This finding is the result of a recent study of blood pressure in adolescents by Dr. Gregory A. Harshfield, Dr. Bruce S. Alpert, and their associates, who were extending previous research findings involving adults. The earlier studies determined that although black and white adults have similar blood pressure while awake, blacks have higher blood pressure during sleep. According to the investigators, whites show a decline in blood pressure during sleep, whereas nocturnal pressure remains constant or shows a much smaller drop in blacks. The investigators reasoned that this difference in nocturnal blood pressure may account in part for the increased prevalence of hypertension among blacks, which is nearly 1.5 times higher than that among whites.

"If blood pressure remains elevated at night, one is exposed to an additional 8 hours of cardiovascular load per night. Think about how that would impact a person over the course of 4 decades. The arteries, the heart, and the kidneys of that person would be exposed to much greater pressure over a 40-year period," Dr. Harshfield explains.

Research Resources Reporter, April 1992

"As part of a larger, ongoing study of hypertension risk factors in children, we have amassed data on a large number of possible factors that could influence blood pressure. They were evaluated by exercise tests, blood tests, 24-hour urine tests, family histories, and measures of psychological reactivity," he says. To examine the relationships among race, fitness, and blood pressure in this age group the researchers first analyzed ambulatory blood pressure measurements to determine whether black adolescents had higher pressures during sleep than did white adolescents, then evaluated how aerobic fitness influenced this 24-hour rhythm of blood pressure.

The subject group consisted of 175 normotensive blacks and whites (80 boys and 95 girls) 10 to 18 years old. The subjects underwent 24-hour ambulatory blood pressure monitoring while pursuing normal daily activities and kept diaries of their times of sleep and awakening. Blood pressure readings were taken automatically at 20-minute intervals from 6 a.m. to midnight and at 60-minute intervals from midnight until 6 a.m.

Dr. Harshfield's previous findings on nocturnal blood pressure differences between black and white adults held true in these adolescents. "All the children had comparable systolic pressure while awake, but while asleep, black males had higher levels than any other group. For diastolic blood pressure we had similar findings: while awake, all the children had similar pressures, but while asleep, black males and females had higher levels."

Dr. Harshfield describes his discovery of this difference in nocturnal blood pressures as somewhat serendipitous. "Ambulatory monitoring is my area of expertise. When I worked at Cornell University, it was very rare to find a white subject who didn't show a nocturnal drop in blood pressure, and that was among close to 2,000 subjects. Then I moved to Los Angeles in California where my institution was located near the Watts area [which is predominantly inhabited by blacks]. Subjects there almost never showed this blood pressure response. It was so striking. We were totally surprised," he says.

Researching the literature, Dr. Harshfield found that studies documenting the "universal" nocturnal decline in blood pressure had included extremely few black subjects. "Our finding worried us at first, because no one else had reported anything like it," he says, adding that the confirmation provided by this study of adolescents and additional studies by other investigators not yet reported in the literature has eased his mind.

610

Dr. Harshfield and his associates went on to examine factors that might be responsible for this racial difference in blood pressure patterns, analyzing the results of concurrent bicycle ergometer maximal exercise testing for the same group of black and white adolescents. Subjects were divided into "more-fit" and "less-fit" categories based on whether their maximal oxygen consumption during the exercise test fell above or below the median for their sex. The more-fit group of boys comprised 23 whites and 18 blacks who had a mean resting blood pressure of 111/60 mmHg. The less-fit group included 21 white and 18 black boys who had a mean resting blood pressure of 108/59 mmHg. The more-fit girls' group comprised 19 white and 27 black girls who had a mean resting blood pressure of 99/57 mmHg; the less-fit group included 18 white and 31 black girls who had a mean blood pressure of 102/65 mmHg.

For both boys and girls, the less-fit subjects were heavier than the more-fit subjects. Parental hypertension was similar in the groups.

"In white children, awake or asleep, there were no differences in the blood pressures of less-fit and more-fit boys or girls. However, less-fit black children, awake or asleep, had consistently elevated systolic blood pressure relative to that of more-fit black children and all white children," Dr. Harshfield says.

Further analysis showed that the differences in blood pressure between more-fit and less-fit children could not be accounted for by differences in body surface area, height, weight, and weight-to-height index, Dr. Harshfield notes.

"The obvious implication is that in the United States blacks have a much bigger problem with hypertension than do whites. One way to control the risk for developing hypertension is to stay fit. Staying fit to keep blood pressure in check therefore appears to be more important for blacks than for whites," he says.

The investigators have no immediate plans for a prospective study to determine whether improving aerobic fitness will indeed lower nocturnal blood pressure in blacks, and whether that will subsequently decrease the risk of developing hypertension. But they are pursuing other aspects of the relationship between race and hypertension.

"It all comes down to a racial difference in regulation of sodium metabolism, and it fits in with the accepted model of how sodium regulation affects blood pressure," Dr. Harshfield says.

In a study that has not yet been published, the researchers examined sodium excretion in a subgroup of 159 of the children. "We did find that black children with a sodium excretion of less than 150 milliequivalents (mEq) per 24 hours had nocturnal blood pressure that was similar to that of whites. Those with sodium excretion greater than 150 mEq had elevated nocturnal blood pressure," Dr. Harshfield says. He suggests that black children on a high salt diet (as reflected by sodium excretion) may have difficulty excreting the excessive sodium load during the day. As a result, blood pressure remains elevated into the night until the additional sodium load has been excreted and the children return to a state of sodium balance.

"So I don't think this is a black/white issue. I think it's an issue of how the kidney handles salt. If a person's kidneys retain salt, it doesn't make any difference if the person is black or white—he or she is going to have trouble with blood pressure," Dr. Harshfield says.

He and his associates currently are studying the relationship between blood pressure and plasma renin activity relative to sodium excretion. High sodium levels are known to suppress plasma renin activity, which increases blood pressure through its stimulation of angiotensin II production, Dr. Harshfield says.

The investigators also are examining the relationship between sodium regulation and stress. "Many colleagues assume that psychological stress doesn't impact sodium regulation, but it's our view that it does. We're looking at how the same subjects handle salt during and after a laboratory test that induces psychological stress. Preliminary results suggest that half the subjects retain salt both during the test and for some time afterward," he says.

—by Mary Ann Moon

Additional Reading:

1. Harshfield, G. A., Hwang, C., and Grim, C., Circadian variation of blood pressure in blacks: Influence of age, gender, and activity. *Journal of Human Hypertension* 4:43-47, 1990.

2. Harshfield, G. A., Dupaul, L. M., Alpert, B. S., et al., Aerobic fitness and the diurnal rhythm of blood pressure in adolescents. *Hypertension* 15:810-814, 1990.

3. Hoffman, A., Walter, H., Connelly, P., and Vaughan, R., Blood pressure and physical fitness in children. *Hypertension* 9:188-191, 1987.

The research described in this article was supported by the General Clinical Research Centers Program of the National Center for Research Resources and the National Heart, Lung, and Blood Institute.

Chapter 60

Older Athletes
Outrun Heart Disease

Regular intense exercise is safe for healthy older people and carries little risk of heart attack or other cardiovascular events, according to a recent study by University of Florida scientists. Perhaps more important, scientists found, the benefits can be dramatic: Intense exercise appeared to slow the aging process, maintaining fitness and muscle mass and attenuating the development of such age-related disorders as heart disease, hypertension, and diabetes.

The study began more than 20 years ago when a 70-year-old man, overweight and out of shape, was told by his physician that he was headed for a heart attack. He vowed to turn his life around and embarked on a program that combined aerobic exercise, strength and flexibility training, and a healthy diet. Remarkably, within 2 years, he had achieved the status of "elite" athlete and competed in national track events. But no one knew for sure whether the high-intensity training and competition were safe for a man his age, or whether it could strain his cardiovascular system and induce a serious or even fatal cardiac event.

When the man faced this dilemma in the early 1970's, concern about the safety of moderate- to high-intensity exercise in middle-aged and elderly people had peaked, along with the popularity of jogging. While vigorous exertion was known to increase the risk of acute car-

NCRR Reporter July/August 1994.

diac events, the cardioprotective effects of exercise were thought, but not known, to offset this risk.

To help settle this issue, and to evaluate the long-term effect of intense training on risk factors for cardiovascular disease, scientists enrolled this man and other older male track athletes in a study that evaluated their aerobic capacity and heart function at 10-year intervals. Recently, Dr. Michael L. Pollock, director of the University of Florida's Center for Exercise Science, Gainesville, and his associates completed a 20-year followup on 21 of the athletes, who are now 60 to 92 years old and have maintained regular aerobic training for 22 years or more.

Aerobic capacity—the body's ability to use oxygen in the blood—correlated with activity level and did not necessarily decline with age, as scientists had previously believed. Subjects who maintained the frequency, intensity, and duration of their training showed no reduction in aerobic capacity, while those who decreased their training because of medical problems showed the greatest decline in aerobic capacity.

Other researchers have postulated a nine-percent reduction in aerobic capacity with each decade of life. The reduction observed in those studies probably was due to subjects' increasingly sedentary lifestyle, not a natural effect of aging, Dr. Pollock notes.

His results also contradict another "given" in the medical literature. Currently, one calculates an individual's maximal heart rate using a formula that subtracts the individual's age from 220 beats per minute. As a result of this formula, the maximum rate drops 10 beats per minute for each decade a person ages. But the Florida researchers found that maximal heart rate declines only 5-7 beats per minute for each decade of life—a finding that was confirmed in a separate study of more than 200 healthy elderly subjects. Dr. Pollock suggests that the previous estimates of maximal heart rate were inaccurate because researchers have been reluctant to push elderly subjects to their true limit during treadmill testing.

Subjects in the study had few age-related heart problems, detected by electrocardiographic recordings. An age-related increase in minor abnormalities in the heart's normal rhythm was found, but it was not of medical concern. Over the entire study period, there were no acute cardiac events during exertion. And the overall incidence of cardiovascular disease was a fraction of what would be expected in an average population of this age, Dr. Pollock says. He emphasizes that his subjects are a select group of athletes, and caution should be used in extrapolating these findings to the average population.

His associate Dr. Larry Mengelkoch notes a similar pattern for other disorders. The incidence of hypertension in American males in this age group is estimated to be 59 to 67 percent; in contrast, only 19 percent of the subjects in the study developed hypertension, with only 1 of 21 subjects requiring antihypertensive medication. Also, Americans in this age range usually have 23 percent body fat, but the study group had only 17 percent body fat. And the incidence of diabetes, which reaches nearly 20 percent among older Americans, was 0 percent in the study group.

Using tolerance testing, which establishes whether a subject has diabetes mellitus and detects more subtle problems in glucose metabolism, scientists found that none of the subjects were diabetic, two had impaired glucose tolerance, and two had high blood levels of the hormone insulin. None of these four patients required treatment, Dr. Mengelkoch says.

The investigators also found that exercise appeared to prevent the decrease in bone density normally associated with aging, with the highest densities occurring in subjects who routinely ran longer distances and who kept a faster pace. "The bones in some of our 90-year-olds looked like those you would see in 60-year-olds, which may be due in part to the fact that these subjects had been active all their lives," Dr. Pollock says.

In a final—and surprising—study result, scientists found that achieving aerobic fitness does not prevent a natural drop in muscle mass of about 3 pounds per decade. At the 10-year followup, subjects who had not done any weight training had lost about 4 pounds of muscle mass, mostly from their upper bodies; those who had done weight training had maintained their muscle mass. At the recently completed 20-year followup, 16 of the 21 athletes were doing weight training and had maintained their muscle mass; the other five subjects had lost another 2 pounds of muscle mass in the intervening decade.

"Very clearly, you need to have a well-rounded fitness program. Aerobic fitness alone will keep the cardiovascular system healthy, but you must have strength and flexibility training as well to maintain whole-body health," Dr. Pollock says. He adds that both the American College of Sports Medicine and the Centers for Disease Control and

Prevention, relying in part on these data, added a weight training component to their recommendations on overall fitness.

Scientists plan to continue monitoring the athletes and to complete another followup study in 5 years. The man described at the beginning of this article plans to take part: Now 92, he continues to follow an intense exercise program, still qualifies as an elite athlete, and regularly competes in marathons.

—by Mary Ann Moon

Additional Reading

1. Pollock, M. L., Mengelkoch, L. J., Graves, J. E., et al., Twenty year follow-up of aerobic power of champion master track athletes (abstract). *Medicine and Science in Sports and Exercise* 25:S105, 1993.

2. Paffenbarger, R. S., Hyde, R. T., Wing, A. L., et al., The association of changes in physical activity level and other lifestyle characteristics with mortality among men. *New England Journal of Medicine* 328:538-545, 1993.

The research described in this article was supported by the General Clinical Research Centers Program of the National Center for Research Resources and by the American Heart Association.

Chapter 61

Finding Resources for Healthy Heart Programs at Work

How To Use This Guide

The National Heart, Lung, and Blood Institute (NHLBI) offers this book of resources to the many people who make wellness at the worksite a reality. [Inclusion in this resource guide does not indicate endorsement by the National Heart, Lung, and Blood Institute. This guide is also not intended to be comprehensive.]

What You Will Find in This Guide

Those of you who are new to health promotion at the worksite will find the first few sections especially helpful. They contain suggestions on how to get started and for finding resources at your own worksite and in your own community. For readers who are familiar with these health resources, there is updated information about organizations, and perhaps even about new ones with which you are unfamiliar.

This guide focuses on resources for worksite healthy heart programs—such as publications, prepackaged programs, videotapes, people, and organizations that can advise you on how to plan a pro-

Taken from NIH Pub. No. 92-737. To obtain a complete copy of this book of resources, contact the National Heart, Lung, and Blood Institute, NHLBI Information Center, P.O. Box 30105, Bethesda, MD 20824-0105; (301) 951-3260.

gram, and more. All the resources in this guide relate to cardiovascular health, which includes:

- High blood pressure
- High blood cholesterol
- Smoking
- Nutrition
- Weight control
- Exercise and physical activity.

Many of the resources are specifically for employers to use in worksite health promotion programs. And many are more general and can be used in the worksite as well as in other community settings, such as schools, hospitals, and health care settings. Many publications are free or low cost, especially those from government agencies. Some are also available in large quantities, and others may have a handling charge. Contact the supplier for the most current information.

How To Choose the Resources That Are Right for You

As you can see by the scope of this guide, there is a wide array of health promotion materials, programs, and services offered by the many agencies and organizations at the local, state, and national level. You may wonder how to choose the resources that are right for you and your worksite. We offer these suggestions:

- Ask the resource organization to provide you with information about the background and training of staff and the names of former clients. Follow up with these clients—with a visit, if possible.

- Ask your colleagues in professional organizations and other worksites about their experience with a group's publications or services.

- If you are not an expert in a topic area, ask an expert. Contact your local or state health department for advice from health educators, dietitians and nutritionists, nurses, fitness specialists, and other health professionals. [A list of state health department contacts is provided.]

Locating People and Organizations: From Coworkers to National Agencies

Find Resources at Your Own Worksite

Often the best place to start looking for resources for a health promotion program is right in your own worksite. The most active collaboration and cooperation usually come from individuals you already know. They can be valuable links to the network of organizations that are already active in your community. In addition, your worksite may already sponsor activities that can provide the starting point of a health promotion program. Talk with people in these jobs:

- Managers
- Labor union officials
- Human resource managers
- Occupational health nurses and physicians
- Industrial hygienists
- Employee assistance program staff
- Personnel administrators
- Employee benefits staff
- Safety and health staff
- Food service directors
- Fitness directors
- Health educators
- Interested volunteers from the employees at large.

Ask them to join an employee committee. The most successful worksite programs include an advisory or coordinating committee composed of employees from various levels and departments. This committee can offer advice to the professional staff and help plan wellness activities. They will feel ownership for the program from the start and help to keep it going.

Check with your health insurance carrier. Many health insurance carriers offer information on and assistance in establishing health promotion programs. They may be able to tell you where your health care dollars are being spent. Some companies, including many Blue Cross and Blue Shield plans, can actually help you set up a pro-

621

gram. Also, contact your health maintenance organization (HMO) for health promotion programs and services they offer to your employees.

Look Beyond Your Own Worksite: Start With the Basics in Your Community

After you have checked out the resources available at your own worksite, look for health promotion resources in your local community by starting with these basic sources of help.

Look in your telephone directory. Check the white pages of the telephone directory for addresses and telephone numbers of organizations listed in this guide. Also, look in the yellow pages under appropriate listings—such as hospitals, HMOs, dietitians, nutritionists, weight control services, health and fitness program consultants, health clubs, and libraries.

Call a local information and referral service. Local governments, the United Way, Health and Welfare Councils, or similar organizations often establish information and referral services in communities. Many produce directories for locating health and social services in addition to responding to telephone or written requests for information.

Visit your public library. The reference room, the information desk, or a special section on health or consumer resources may provide listings of local services, programs, and organizations for health promotion. In addition, find healthy heart cookbooks, health and nutrition magazines, and many [other] publications.

Locate the "Healthy" Organizations in Your Town

The following agencies and organizations may offer programs, materials, staff expertise, volunteers, facilities, or equipment to help you set up or expand a worksite program. Some offer help at no cost, while others charge fees. They may conduct wellness screenings, train your employees in blood pressure measurement, or offer followup counseling for employees with high blood pressure or cholesterol. Well-coordinated and efficient community resources will be especially helpful to smaller worksites. [Addresses and telephone numbers are listed at the end of this chapter.]

Wellness councils. Wellness councils are local groups of businesses and other employers interested in promoting worksite wellness. Ask your local Chamber of Commerce if there is a wellness council in your community. Or call or write the Wellness Councils of America (WELCOA), the national organization of wellness councils, to obtain a local contact. WELCOA is dedicated to providing direction and support services to community-based wellness councils. It also offers detailed reports on programs under way in local councils and a newsletter. WELCOA offers manuals and videotapes on health promotion topics. Contact WELCOA for an order form for current resources.

Business/health coalitions. Business/health coalitions are groups of businesses organized to find solutions to the rising cost of employer-paid health care. One of their interests is health promotion. Ask your local Chamber of Commerce whether there is a local coalition nearby. The National Business Coalition Forum on Health is a national association of more than 40 business/health coalitions in 28 States. They have published a survey of 64 coalitions, *Health Care Coalitions in the United States* ($35). The Washington Business Group on Health (WBGH) is a national employer organization dedicated to representing the purchaser's view of health care. Its members include more than 200 of the Nation's largest employers. Within WBGH, the Prevention Leadership Forum publishes the Worksite Wellness series of over 20 papers. Titles available include: *Reaching Families Through Worksite and Community Health Promotion Programs, Healthy Communities: A Growing Corporate Commitment*, and *Community-Based Health Promotion Programs for Employees and Their Families*. WBGH also publishes a national magazine, *Business and Health* and houses the National Resource Center on Worksite Health Promotion.

City and county public health departments. Check with these units of your local health department: chronic disease control, community health nursing, health promotion, nutrition, preventive health, disease prevention, or adult health. One or more of these units may offer materials, protocols, staff assistance, training, or suggestions about other resources. Some local health departments may have special initiatives to reach out into local businesses to promote health among the employees. See [the list provided later in this chapter] of individuals to contact in your state health department. Ask them for names of contacts in your local health department.

Local recreation departments. City and county departments of recreation often offer a wide range of exercise, fitness, and sports activities, including team sports and walking clubs.

Public school systems or education departments of counties and towns. For healthy heart cooking classes, weight control courses, and other health programs, contact the adult education or evening education departments in your local government. Consult the government blue pages in the telephone book under education or schools.

Community and county colleges and universities. Contact these departments: health education, recreation, physical education, adult education, home economics, nutrition, food sciences, dietetics, human ecology, and nursing and medical schools. Both faculty and students may offer training in cholesterol and blood pressure measurement, assistance in developing healthy heart courses and other education activities, protocols for screening and followup, and many other services.

Voluntary health agencies and professional associations. Contact your local units of voluntary health groups, professional associations, and other community organizations. They may offer services and assistance at the local level, such as materials, programs, training, professional advice, and technical assistance. Several major groups most likely to have local units are highlighted here:

American Association of Occupational Health Nurses (AAOHN). This national professional membership organization for occupational health nurses provides educational opportunities through traditional continuing education activities, self-instructional modular materials, an annual national conference with workshops on various risk factors for developing cardiovascular disease, and a comprehensive library. Publications include the monthly refereed *AAOHN Journal*, a monthly newsletter, and special manuals, brochures, and guides. Local and state AAOHN chapters can provide referrals to local occupational health nurse experts. They can also offer information on developing and maintaining wellness programs in local business and industry and resources for carrying out a program. Contact the AAOHN professional affairs department at the national office for a contact person at the 183 local and state AAOHN chapters.

The American Dietetic Association (ADA). The ADA offers publications on food and good nutrition for worksite program planners, health professionals, and employees and their families. The ADA sponsors National Nutrition Month in March and a Nutrition InfoCenter. Toll-free nutrition advice: Employees and their families can get answers to their nutrition questions by calling the ADA toll-free consumer hotline. To reach a registered dietitian in person, callers can dial (800) 366-1655 Monday through Friday from 10 a.m. to 5 p.m. (EST). Taped messages about nutrition are available 24 hours a day. Dietitians sometimes work as consultants in developing worksite nutrition programs. Contact the division of practice of The American Dietetic Association at (312) 899-0040, ext. 4815, for a list of consultant dietitians in your state. In addition, officers in state ADA affiliates can help identify local dietitians who will accept employees for nutrition counseling. Local nutrition councils may also offer classes or have nutrition hotlines staffed by dietitians. Through State and local dietetic associations, it also provides technical assistance and speakers to outside groups.

American Heart Association (AHA). The AHA provides materials, conducts programs and training, and offers support to individuals and groups. Materials include catalogs, fact sheets, brochures, and audiovisual materials on topics such as heart disease, exercise, high blood pressure, cholesterol, smoking, and nutrition. Contact the corporate health account executive at the national center to receive information on the American Heart Association nearest you or to conduct national worksite wellness programs. For information about the AHA film library, call (214) 747-8048 in Texas or (800) 527-3211 outside Texas.

American Lung Association (ALA). The ALA offers materials and programs on such topics as quitting smoking, occupational health, lung diseases, and air conservation. The ALA offers a catalog of all its publications, including *On the Air: A Guide to Promoting a Smoke-Free Workplace, Team Up for Freedom from Smoking, Freedom from Smoking for You and Your Family, Stop Smoking: Stay Trim*, and *Helping Smokers Get Ready to Quit*. Fees are determined by local affiliates. Contact your local ALA unit or the national office to find one near you.

Association for Fitness in Business (AFB). The AFB represents over 3,500 health and fitness professionals who are employed by corporations, hospitals, and other worksites that conduct fitness programs for employees. The AFB promotes employee health and fitness by publishing data and current information, offering continuing education programs, and encouraging professional networking. The AFB also serves as a clearinghouse on employee health and fitness. Members belong to one of 11 regional chapters to exchange ideas and information locally through publications and through state and regional conferences. The AFB publishes the bimonthly newsletter, *Action*, and the *AFB Annual Information Directory and Resource Guide*, which includes a list of members by state and profession. The AFB also developed the publication *Guidelines for Employee Health Promotion Programs*.

United Way. The United Way in many communities offers a worksite presence program that includes such activities as lunchtime seminars, health fairs, community service directories, and referral services. Contact your local United Way for more information on programs available in your area.

YMCA of the USA. The Corporate Health and Fitness Program provides services to worksites, ranging from YMCA membership as an employee benefit to full-scale health and fitness programs for employees. The YMCA also offers educational materials and seminars, fitness and health testing, health monitoring, and program management. Program topics include nutrition education, weight management, exercise, quitting smoking, and stress management, along with traditional sports such as swimming and aerobics. Participation is open to men and women. Fees are determined by local YMCAs. Contact your local YMCA or the associate director for health and fitness, program services division, at the national office for further information.

There are many other groups that may be able to help you establish your wellness program. You may want to contract for services with individuals who are members of these professional groups. Or staff people at voluntary health groups can sometimes offer their time and talents for a modest fee or for free. In addition, they may have established programs that can be used at the worksite. Look for local units of these organizations:

• American Cancer Society
• American Red Cross

- American College of Occupational and Environmental Medicine
- National Kidney Foundation
- Society for Nutrition Education
- Society for Public Health Education
- YWCA

Hospitals and HMOs. Contact local hospitals and HMOs for classes on healthy heart topics such as cholesterol control, high blood pressure education, stop-smoking programs, and weight control. Consider the health promotion offerings of local HMOs when choosing future health care providers for your employees.

Occupational health clinics and other health promotion providers. In industrial and well-populated areas, businesses have been established to provide traditional occupational health services and the newer health promotion services to local employers. Look in the yellow pages of your telephone book under health and fitness program consultants, health promotion programs, and occupational health services.

Nutritionists, including registered dietitians and other qualified nutrition professionals. Nutritionists sometimes work as consultants in developing worksite nutrition programs. In addition, employees may need individualized nutrition counseling, and you will want to refer them to qualified nutritionists. The American Dietetic Association (ADA) maintains a roster of dietitians and will respond to written requests for assistance in locating registered dietitians in your state. In addition, officers in state ADA affiliates could help identify local dietitians who will accept employees for nutrition counseling. The Society for Nutrition Education may sponsor a local nutrition council that offers classes or has a nutrition hotline staffed by nutritionists.

Visiting Nurse Associations. Visiting nurse associations (VNAs) offer a wide range of community-based health care services, including those associated with worksite wellness programs, such as nutrition counseling and blood pressure screening. The Visiting Nurse Associations of America maintain a toll-free telephone number, (800) 426-2547, for patient referral and other public information. Call to obtain the name, address, and telephone number of a local VNA.

Labor unions. Local community services committees—composed of labor union members with special training—help meet the health needs of their fellow union members and their families. Contact your shop steward, local president, or central labor council officers to find out how organized labor can help in your worksite.

USDA Cooperative Extension Service. The Extension Service has a network of professionals across the country ready to deliver food and nutrition education programs to the public. In cooperation with the land-grant universities, they share nutrition information with people in every state and 3,150 counties in the United States. To find a local office, consult the county or state government section of the white telephone pages under Cooperative Extension or Extension.

Check Out Your State Health Department

Publications, services, and other resources offered by state health departments vary. Check with these units of your state health department: chronic disease control, community health nursing, health promotion, nutrition, preventive health, disease prevention, family health, or adult health. One or more of these units may offer materials, screening procedures and standards, staff assistance, training, or suggestions about other resources. Check to see whether your state offers resources that are tailored to specific groups and reading levels.

A list of cardiovascular disease contacts in state health departments [is reproduced below]. Contact the person in your state health department to find out the resources available to you. These contacts may also be able to put you in touch with someone in your local health department or other agency.

Get Help From National Groups

Many national organizations offer health promotion materials, programs, and services to worksites. The following three national information centers are good places to start in your search for health promotion materials and other resources. [Address and telephone numbers are listed at the end of this chapter.]

NHLBI Information Center. The National Heart, Lung, and Blood Institute (NHLBI) Information Center is the source of a wide variety of information and materials on high blood pressure, high blood cholesterol, smoking, obesity, nutrition, and general heart health. The Information Center offers materials for planning wellness programs aimed at employees and their families. Materials for planning worksite wellness programs include *Make Workplace Wellness Programs Work for Your Company, Workplace Facts on Heart Disease and Stroke, Wellness Outreach at Work: A How-To Guide*, and this guide.

Other materials include those developed for health professionals, such as guidelines for the detection and evaluation of high blood pressure and cholesterol. NHLBI also has numerous brochures, booklets, and posters for employees and their families. A kit, designed to help carry out awareness activities in communities, includes many short reproducible handouts on high blood pressure, cholesterol, and smoking. The Information Center publishes the newsletter HEART*MEMO*, which contains information on NHLBI activities and resources. Most materials are available in limited quantities and are free. *Life in the Health Lane: A Directory of Resources From the National Heart, Lung, and Blood Institute* lists all the resources available from the NHLBI for health professionals, program planners, and consumers. NHLBI maintains the cholesterol, high blood pressure, and smoking education subfile of the Combined Health Information Database (CHID).

National Resource Center on Worksite Health Promotion. This resource center provides information for employers on worksite health promotion programs currently in place in U.S. corporations and other worksites. The information is contained in a database that includes information related to worksite health promotion programs, evaluation, research, and supporting organizations. The resource center also gathers experts to discuss emerging issues in worksite health promotion and publishes materials on topics such as small business and health promotion, cost savings from worksite programs, and integration of health promotion with employee benefits. Publications include *Healthy People 2000 at Work: Strategies for Employers, Directory of Worksite Health Promotion Resources*, and *Directory of State Health Promotion Resources for Employers*. Call for a publications order form.

ODPHP National Health Information Center. The ODPHP (Office of Disease Prevention and Health Promotion) National Health Information Center offers information and referral services on all health-related topics. Most inquiries concern the availability of publications and referrals to other organizations. When possible, the center

629

directly answers inquiries from health professionals and the general public. Otherwise, callers are referred to other special Federal information centers and private organizations. The DIRLINE, maintained by the center, is a database of 1,200 health-related organizations with descriptions of their publications and services. The center produces Healthfinders, a series of publications on a variety of topics, including a directory of Federal health information resources, a list of toll-free numbers for health information, and a list of national health observances.

Special Help for Minority Employers and Employees

Office of Minority Health Resource Center, U.S. Department of Health and Human Services. The Federal Government's Office of Minority Health Resource Center responds to requests for information on minority health, locates sources of technical assistance through the Resource Persons Network, and refers requesters to relevant organizations. Activities concentrate on areas with priority for minority health. Bilingual staff members are available to serve Spanish-speaking requesters.

Special Help for Local, State, and Federal Government Employers and Employees

Federal Occupational Health Program, U.S. Public Health Service. The Federal Occupational Health Program offers a variety of occupational health consultation services and technical assistance to all **Federal Government** agencies. The program covers occupational safety and health programs as well as health promotion programs such as fitness and high blood pressure control.

These services help Federal managers to increase productivity, decrease health care liability, enhance employee well-being, and improve work environments. The program has published standards and criteria documents for occupational health, fitness, and employee assistance programs to assist occupational health professionals in developing and evaluating them.

A 30-minute videotape describing a comprehensive management approach to occupational health is available for preview. All services are provided in accordance with the Economy Act via simple, reimbursable interagency agreements.

National Association for Public Employee Wellness (NAPEW). If you are planning a wellness program for **public** employees, you can contact NAPEW for ideas, information, and additional contacts. The NAPEW is a nonprofit group of wellness program directors who work for states, cities, counties, Federal agencies, and state-supported colleges and universities.

The association promotes and strengthens public employee wellness programs through communication and exchange of program leaders' expertise. The NAPEW publishes a quarterly newsletter and a membership roster and sponsors an annual conference in September. Call for resource packets and other information available through the NAPEW clearinghouse.

Office of Personnel Management (OPM), Employee Health Services Branch. OPM can assist **Federal Government** employers by providing policy guidance and technical assistance regarding health promotion programs. Federal Personnel Manual Letter 792-20 issued by OPM permits Federal agencies to use appropriated funds to pay the costs of agency-authorized stop-smoking programs for employees.

NHLBI Primary Cardiovascular Disease Liaisons in State Health Departments

Alabama
Richard G. Adams, M.S.
Director
Hypertension Branch
Alabama Department of Public Health
434 Monroe Street
Montgomery, AL 36130-1701
(205) 242-5128

Alaska
Patty Owen
Health Social Services Planner
Division of Public Health
Alaska Department of Health and Social Services
320 West Willoughby, #101
Juneau, AK 99801-0616
(907) 465-3140

631

Arizona
Carol Vack, C.H.E.S.
Office of Health Promotion and Education
Arizona Department of Health Services
3008 North Third Street
Phoenix, AZ 85012
(602) 230-5803

Arkansas
David Bourne, M.D.
Director
Chronic Disease Program
Section of Health Maintenance
Arkansas Department of Health
Mail Slot 3
4815 West Markham
Little Rock, AR 77205-3867
(501)661-2168

California
Neal D. Kohatsu, M.D., M.P.H.
Chief
Epidemiology and Disease Prevention Section
California Department of Health Services
601 North Seventh Street
P.O. Box 942732
Sacramento, CA 94234-7320
(916) 324-2281

Colorado
Linda Dusenbury, R.N., M.S.
Director Cardiovascular Disease Control Program
Division of Prevention Programs
Colorado Department of Health
4210 East 11th Avenue
Denver, CO 80220
(303) 331-8303

Connecticut
Teri Klein, M.P.H.
Regional Coordinator
Division of Chronic Disease
Connecticut Department of Health Services
150 Washington Street
Hartford, CT 06106
(203) 566-7867

Delaware
Lori Christiansen
Program Director
Cardiovascular Disease Program
Health Monitoring and Program Consultation
Delaware Division of Public Health
Jesse Cooper Building
Federal & Water Streets
P.O. Box 637
Dover, DE 19903
(302) 739-6621

District of Columbia
Marcia Timoll, M.S.
Chief, Health Promotion
D.C. Cardiovascular Disease Control Program
D.C. Commission of Public Health
1660 L Street, NW., Room 809
Washington, DC 20036
(202) 673-6738

Florida
Vickie Pryor, R.N., M.P.H.
Nursing Consultant
Florida Department of Health and Rehabilitative Services
1317 Winewood Boulevard
Tallahassee, FL 32399-0700
(904) 488-2834

Georgia
Jerry P. Brown
Program Manager
Stroke and Heart Attack Prevention Program
Georgia Department of Human Resources
878 Peachtree Street, NE., Room 102
Atlanta, GA 30309
(404) 894-6640

Hawaii
Barbara Yamashita
Acting Chief
Preventive Health Services Branch
Hawaii State Department of Health
P.O. Box 3378
Honolulu, HI 96801
(808) 586-4670

Idaho
Joanne Mitten, M.H.E.
Health Promotion Coordinator
Health Promotion Section
Bureau of Public Health Services
Division of Health
Idaho Department of Health and Welfare
Statehouse Mail
Boise, ID 83720-9990
(208) 334-5927

Illinois
D. Keith Rowley, M.A.
Assistant Chief
Division of Adult and Senior Health
Illinois Department of Public Health
535 West Jefferson Street
Springfield, IL 62761
(217) 782-3300

Indiana
Charles Barrett, M.D., M.S.P.H
Medical Epidemiologist
Epidemiology Resource Center
Indiana State Department of Health
1330 West Michigan Street
P.O. Box 1964
Indianapolis, IN 46206-1964
(317) 633-8421

Iowa
Connie Betterley, M.S., R.D.
Chief, Bureau of Health Promotion
Division of Substance Abuse and Health Promotion
Iowa Department of Public Health
Lucas State Office Building
Third Floor
Des Moines, IA 50319-0075
(515) 281-7097

Kansas
Paula F. Marmet, M.S., R.D.
Director
Office of Chronic Disease and Health Promotion
Division of Health
900 Southwest Jackson, Room 1051
Topeka, KS 66612-1290
(913) 296-1207

Kentucky
Carol Forbes
Administrator
Cardiovascular Disease Program
Division of Epidemiology
275 East Main Street
Frankfort, KY 40621
(502) 564-7996

Louisiana
Shirley Kirkconnell, M.S.W., M.P.H.
Director of Adult Services
Louisiana Department of Health and Hospitals
Office of Public Health
P.O. Box 60630
325 Loyola Avenue, Room 414
New Orleans, LA 70160-0629
(504) 568-7210

Maine
Randy Schwartz, M.S.P.H.
Director
Division of Health Promotion & Education
Maine Department of Human Services
Bureau of Health
State House Station #11
Augusta, ME 04333
(207) 287-5180

Maryland
John Southard, M.D., M.P.H.
Director
Office of Chronic Disease Prevention
Maryland Department of Health and Mental Hygiene
Local and Family Health Administration
P.O. Box 13528
Baltimore, MD 21203
(410) 225-6778

Massachusetts
Lily S. Hsu, M.S., R.D.
Director
Division of Chronic Disease Prevention
Massachusetts Department of Public Health
150 Tremont Street, Seventh Floor
Boston, MA 02111
(617) 727-2662

Michigan
Jean Chabut
Chief
Center for Health Promotion and Chronic Disease Prevention
Michigan Department of Public Health
3423 North Logan St./M.L.K. Jr. Blvd.
Lansing, MI 48909
(517) 335-8368

Minnesota
Richard Welch
Division Director
Health Promotion and Education
Minnesota Department of Health
717 Southeast Delaware Street
P.O. Box 9441
Minneapolis, MN 55440
(612) 623-5699

Mississippi
Wendell Cox
Director
Chronic Illness Program
Division of Health
Mississippi State Department of Health
P.O. Box 1700
Jackson, MS 39215-1700
(601) 960-7857

Missouri
Carol Smith
Assistant Division Director
Division of Chronic Disease Prevention and Health Promotion
Missouri Department of Health
201 Business Loop/70 West
Columbia, MO 65203
(314) 876-3200

Montana
Robert W. Moon, M.P.H.
Health Services Manager
Health Promotion and Chronic Disease
Montana Department of Health and Environmental Services
Cogswell Building
Helena, MT 59620
(406) 444-4488

Nebraska
Jim Dills
Director
Health Promotion and Education
Nebraska Department of Health
301 Centennial Mall South
P O. Box 95007
Lincoln, NE 68509-5007
(402) 471-2101

Nevada
Sandra Fairburn, R.D.
Chief
Community Health Services
Nevada State Division of Health
505 East King Street, Room 300
Carson City, NV 89710
(702) 687-6944

New Hampshire
Elizabeth Donahue-Davis
Health Promotion Advisor
Bureau of Health Promotion
New Hampshire Division of Public Health Services
6 Hazen Drive
Concord, NH 03301-6527
(603) 271-4551

New Jersey
Phyllis Dower, R.N., M.P.H.
Coordinator
Cardiovascular Disease Program
New Jersey State Department of Health
CN #364
Trenton, NJ 08625-0364
(609) 984-6138

New Mexico
Estella Trujillo, B.S.N.
Coordinator
Chronic Disease Prevention and Control Section
New Mexico Department of Health
1190 St. Francis Drive
P.O. Box 26110
Santa Fe, NM 87502-6110
(505) 827-2475

New York
David Momrow, M.P.H.
Acting Director
Bureau of Adult and Gerontological Health
New York State Department of Health
Empire State Plaza
Corning Tower Building, Room 557
Albany, NY 12237
(518) 474-0512

North Carolina
Kathie Paterson, R.N., M.P.H.
Program Coordinator
Division of Adult Health
North Carolina Department of Environment, Health, and Natural Resources
P.O. Box 27687
1330 St. Mary's Street
Raleigh, NC 27611-7687
(919) 733-7081

North Dakota
Sandra Adams, M.S., R.D., C.H.E.S.
Director
Division of Health Promotion and Education
North Dakota State Department of Health & Consolidated Laboratories
Judicial Wing, Second Floor
600 East Boulevard Avenue
Bismarck, ND 58505-0200
(701) 224-2367

Ohio
Kathy Boyle, R.N., M.S.
Nursing Consultant
Bureau of Chronic Diseases
Ohio Department of Health
246 North High Street
Columbus, OH 43266-0588
(614) 466-2144

Oklahoma
Adeline Yerkes, R.N., M.P.H.
Chief
Chronic Disease Service
Oklahoma State Department of Health
1000 Northeast 10th Street
Oklahoma City, OK 73117-1299
(405) 271-4072

Oregon
Donna Clark
Assistant Administrator of Health Services
Oregon Health Division
State of Oregon Department of Human Resources
Suite 850
800 Northeast Oregon Street, #21
Portland, OR 97232
(503) 731-4016

Pennsylvania
Robert McAllister
Director
Cardiovascular Disease Risk Reduction Program
Pennsylvania Department of Health
P.O. Box 90
Harrisburg, PA 17108
(717) 787-2957

Rhode Island
Francis Donahue
Office of Chronic Disease
Rhode Island Department of Health
3 Capitol Hill
Providence, RI 02908-5097
(401) 277-2853

South Carolina
Fran C. Wheeler, Ph.D.
Director
Center for Health Promotion
South Carolina Department of Health and Environmental Control
Robert Mills Complex, Box 101106
Columbia, SC 29211
(803) 737-4121

South Dakota
Norma Schmidt
Division of Health Services
South Dakota Department of Health
118 West Capitol
Pierre, SD 57501-3182
(605) 773-3737

Tennessee
William E. Duncan
Director
Chronic Disease Services
Tennessee Department of Health
Cordell Hull Building, Room 546
Nashville, TN 37247-5201
(615) 741-7366

Texas
Cheryl Cortines Lackey, M.P.H., C.H.E.S.
Director
Division of Public Health Promotion
Texas Department of Health
1100 West 49th Street
Austin, TX 78756-3199
(512) 458-7405

Utah
Joan Ware, R.N., M.S.P.H.
Director
Cardiovascular Disease Program
Bureau of Chronic Disease
Utah Department of Health
P.O. Box 16660
Salt Lake City, UT 84116-0660
(801) 538-6141

Vermont
Marge Hamrell, R.N., M.Ed.
Chief
Health Promotion
Vermont Department of Health
P.O. Box 70
Burlington, VT 05401
(802) 863-7330

Virginia
Ramona Schaeffer, M.S., E.D.
Director
Division of Chronic Disease Control
Virginia Department of Health
Main Street Station
P.O. Box 2448
Richmond, VA 23218
(804) 786-4065

Washington
Karen Krueger, R.N., M.N., M.B.A.
Nurse Consultant
Office of Heart Disease and Cancer Prevention
Department of Health
P.O. Box 47835, LK-13
Airdustrial Park Building #10
Olympia, WA 98504-7835
(206) 586-6082

West Virginia
Sharon Lansdale, R.Ph., M.S.
Director
Division of Health Promotion
West Virginia Bureau of Public Health
1411 Virginia Street East
Charleston, WV 25301-3013
(304) 558-0644

Wisconsin
Patrick L. Remington, M.D., M.P.H.
Chronic Disease Unit
Wisconsin Division of Health
1400 East Washington Avenue
Madison, WI 53703
(608) 267-3835

Wyoming
Jackie Cushing, R.N., M.S.
Consultant
Public Health Nursing
Wyoming Division of Public Health
Hathaway Building, Fourth Floor
Cheyenne, WY 82002
(307) 777-6096

American Samoa
Dr. Edgar Reid
Deputy Director for Preventive Services
L.B.J. Tropical Medical Center
Pago Pago, AS 96799
011 (684) 633-2243

Guam
Angelina G. Mummert, M.P.A.
Health Services Administrator
Bureau of Community Health Services
Department of Public Health and Social Services
P.O. Box 2816
Agana, GU 96910
011 (671) 734-4589, ext.201

Puerto Rico
Raul Castellanos Bran, M.D.
Program de Corazón/HIP
Call Box 70184
San Juan, PR 00936
(809) 763-6240

Virgin Islands
Olaf Hendricks, M.D.
Assistant Commissioner
Division of Prevention, Health Promotion, and Protection
Virgin Islands Department of Health
516 Strand Street
Frederiksted, St. Croix, VI 00840
(809) 772-5895

Resource Organizations, Addresses and Telephone Numbers

A

American Association of Occupational Health Nurses
50 Lenox Pointe
Atlanta, GA 30324
(800) 241-8014

American Cancer Society
National Office
1599 Clifton Road, NE.
Atlanta, GA 30329
(800) ACS-2345
Contact your local American Cancer Society for publications and information.

American College of Occupational and Environmental Medicine
55 West Seegers Road
Arlington Heights, IL 60005
(708) 228-5850

The American Dietetic Association
216 West Jackson Boulevard
Suite 800
Chicago, IL 60606-6995
(312) 899-0040

American Health Consultants
3525 Piedmont Road, Building 6
Suite 400
Atlanta, GA 30305
(800) 688-2421

American Health: Fitness of Body and Mind
P.O. Box 3015
Harlan, IA 51537-3015

American Heart Association
National Center
7320 Greenville Avenue
Dallas, TX 75231
(214) 373-6300
Contact your local American Heart Association for publications and information.

American Hospital Association
Public Relations Division
840 North Lake Shore Drive
Chicago, IL 60611

American Institute for Preventive Medicine
24450 Evergreen Road, Suite 200
Southfield, Ml 48075-5518
(810) 352-7666

American Journal of Health Promotion
1812 South Rochester Road, Suite 200
Rochester Hills, Ml 48307
(810) 650-9600

American Lung Association
1740 Broadway
New York, NY 10019
(212) 315-8700
Contact your local American Lung Association for publications and information.

American Red Cross
18th and D Streets, NW
Washington, DC 20006
Contact your local American Red Cross for publications and information.

Association for Fitness in Business
200 Marott Center
342 Massachusetts Avenue
Indianapolis, IN 46204-2161
(317) 636-6621

B

Baxter Healthcare Corporation
1500 Waukegan Road
McGaw Park, IL 60085-9934
(800) 766-3646

Being Healthy, Inc.
5211 Nebraska Avenue, NW.
Washington, DC 20015
(202) 966-0007

Bloomington Heart and Health Program
1900 West Old Shakopee Road
Bloomington, MN 55431
(612) 887-9603

Bureau of Business Practice
24 Rope Ferry Road
Waterford, CT 06386
(800) 243-0876

Business & Health
Medical Economics Subscriber
Services Dept.
P.O. Box 2082
Marion, OH 43306
(800) 833-0197

C

California Department of Health Services
Health Promotion Section
Health Education-Risk Reduction Program
P.O. Box 942732
Sacramento, CA 94234-7320
(916) 322-6851

Cancer Information Service
Office of Cancer Communications
National Cancer Institute
Building 31, Room 10A24
9000 Rockville Pike
Bethesda, MD 20892
(800) 4-CANCER
(808) 524-1234 (Hawaii—neighbor islands call collect)
(301) 496-8664 (project officer)

Carter Center of Emory University
Health Risk Appraisal Program
One Copenhill
Atlanta, GA 30307
(404) 872-2100

Center for Corporate Health
10467 White Granite Drive
Suite 300
Oakton, VA 22124
(800) 745-1333
(703) 218-8400

Center for Science in the Public Interest
1875 Connecticut Avenue, NW.
Suite 300
Washington, DC 20009-5728
(202) 332-9110

Choose to Lose
P.O. Box 2053
Rockville, MD 20847-2053
(301) 530-5835

Citizens for Public Action on Blood Pressure and Cholesterol, Inc.
7200 Wisconsin Avenue
Suite 1002
Bethesda, MD 20814
(301) 907-7790

Consumer Information Center
Pueblo, CO 81009

Consumer Reports on Health
Box 56356
Boulder, CO 80322-6356

Cooking Light
P.O. Box 830549
Birmingham, AL 35282-981

Cornell University
Resource Center
7 Business and Technology Park
Ithaca, NY 14850
(607) 255-7660

Corporate Health Designs
P.O. Box 55056
Seattle, WA 98155
(206) 364-3448

Creative Walking, Inc.
P.O. Box 50296
Clayton, MO 63105
(314) 721-3600

D

Denice Ferko-Adams & Associates
425 Fairview Street
Coopersburg, PA 18036
(215) 282-2384

Diet Workshop, Inc.
10 Brookline Place West
Suite 107
Brookline, MA 02146
(617) 739-2222

DINE Systems, Inc.
586 North French Road, Suite 2
Amherst, NY 14228
(716) 688-2492

E

Eating Well: The Magazine of Food and Health
Ferry Road
P.O. Box 1001
Charlotte, VT 05445-9977

Emory University School of Medicine
Department of Community and Preventive Medicine
69 Butler Street, SE.
Atlanta, GA 30303-3219
(404) 616-3612

Environmental Improvement Associates
P.O. Box 1
Salem, NJ 08079
(609) 935-4200

Environmental Nutrition
P.O. Box 3000
Dept. BBB
Denville, NJ 07834

F

Federal Occupational Health Program
U.S. Public Health Service
5515 Security Lane, Suite 901
Rockville, MD 20852
(301) 443-2257

Feeling Fine Programs, Inc.
3575 Cahuenga Boulevard West
Suite 440
Los Angeles, CA 90068
(800) 332-3373

Food and Drug Administration
Office of Regulatory Affairs
Consumer Affairs and Information Staff
5600 Fishers Lane (HFC-110)
Rockville, MD 20857
(301) 443-4166

Food and Nutrition Information Center
National Agricultural Library
10301 Baltimore Boulevard
Room 304
Beltsville, MD 20705-2351
(301) 344-3719

H

Hall-Foushee Productions, Inc.
1313 Fifth Street, SE.
Suite 214B
Minneapolis, MN 55414
(612) 379-3829

Harvard Health Letter
P.O. Box 420300
Palm Coast, FL 32142-0300
(800) 828-9045

Health Promotion Services, Inc.
500 Wood Street, Suite 1400
Pittsburgh, PA 15222
(412) 392-3163

Health Prospects
1801 Rockville Pike, Suite 500
Rockville, MD 20852
(301) 770-7519

HealthKit
7021 Barkwater Court
Bethesda, MD 20817
(301) 320-2825

651

Healthtrac
2 North Point, First Floor
San Francisco, CA 94133
(415) 445-5217

Holtyn & Associates
719 Turwill
Kalamazoo, MI 49007
(616) 382-5898

Hope Heart Institute
HOPE Publications/International
Health Awareness Center
350 East Michigan Avenue
Suite 301
Kalamazoo, MI 49007
(800) 334-4094

Human Nutrition Information Service
U.S. Department of Agriculture
6505 Belcrest Road
Hyattsville, MD 20782
(301) 436-8617
(301) 436-5078 (electronic bulletin board)

I

Information Transfer Systems
307 North First
Ann Arbor, Ml 48103
(313) 994-0003

It's YOUR Cholesterol!
2700 Prosperity Avenue
Fairfax, VA 22031
(800) 654-7134
(703) 204-0100

L

Lowfat Lifeline
Dept. 44
626 Benton Street
P.O. Box 1889
Port Townsend, WA 98368
(206) 379-9724

M

Macmillan Publishing Company
866 Third Avenue
New York, NY 10022

Mayo Clinic Health Letter
Subscription Services
P.O. Box 53889
Boulder, CO 80322-3889
(800) 333-9037

Medical Care Affiliates/Health Promotion Affiliates
One Boylston Plaza
Prudential Center
Boston, MA 02199
(800) 922-4749

Minnesota Coalition for a Smoke-Free Society 2000
525 Ford Center
420 North Fifth Street, Suite 525
Minneapolis, MN 55401
(612) 338-8193

N

National Association of Governor's Councils on Physical Fitness and Sports
201 South Capitol Avenue
Suite 440
Indianapolis, IN 46225-1072
(317) 237-5630

National Association for Public Employee Wellness
The Council of State Governments
Iron Works Pike
P.O. 11910
Lexington, KY 40578-1910
(606) 231-1948

National Business Coalition Forum on Health
777 North Capitol Street, NE.
Suite 800
Washington, DC 20002
(202) 408-9320

National Center for Chronic Disease Prevention and Health Promotion
Centers for Disease Control
1600 Clifton Road, NE.
Koger Center
Atlanta, GA 30333
(404) 488-5524

National Center for Health Promotion
3920 Varsity Drive
Ann Arbor, MI 48108
(313) 971-6077
(800) 843-6247

National Kidney Foundation
30 East 33rd Street
New York, NY 10016
(212) 889-2210
(800) 622-9010
Contact your local National Kidney Foundation for publications and information.

National Resource Center on Worksite Health Promotion
Washington Business Group on Health
777 North Capitol Street, NE.
Suite 800
Washington, DC 20002
(202) 408-9320

National Technical Information Service
Department of Commerce
5285 Port Royal Road
Springfield, VA 22161
(703) 487-4650

National Wellness Institute, Inc.
South Hall
1319 Fremont Street
Stevens Point, WI 54481-3899
(715) 346-2172

New Jersey Group Against Smoking Pollution (GASP)
105 Mountain Avenue
Summit, NJ 07901
(908) 273-9368

NHLBI Information Center
National Heart, Lung, and Blood Institute
P.O. Box 30105
Bethesda, MD 20824-0105
(301) 951-3260

O

ODPHP National Health Information Center
P.O. Box 1133
Washington, DC 20013-1133
(800) 336-4797
(301) 565-4167

Office of Disease Prevention and Health Promotion
Switzer Building, Room 2132
330 C Street, SW.
Washington, DC 20201
(202) 472-5307

Office of Minority Health Resource Center
P.O. Box 37337
Washington, DC 20013
(800) 444-6472
(301) 587-1938

Office of Personnel Management
Employee Health Services Branch
Office of Labor Relations and Workforce Performance
U.S. Office of Personnel Management
1900 E Street, NW., Room 7412
Washington, DC 20415
FTS (202) 606-1269

Office on Smoking and Health
Technical Information Center
Centers for Disease Control
Rhodes Building, Mailstop K12
1600 Clifton Road, NE.
Atlanta, GA 30333
(404) 488-5705

P

Pawtucket Heart Health Program
Memorial Hospital of Rhode Island
111 Brewster Street
Pawtucket, RI 02860
(401) 722-6000

Penn State Nutrition Center
Pennsylvania State University
417 East Calder Way
University Park, PA 16801-5663
(814) 865-6323

Performance Resource Press
1863 Technology Drive
Suite 200
Troy, Ml 48083
(810) 588-7733

Physicians Committee for Responsible Medicine
P.O. Box 6322
Washington, DC 20015
(202) 686-2210

President's Council on Physical Fitness and Sports
450 Fifth Street, NW., Suite 7103
Washington, DC 20001
(202) 272-3430

Pyramid Film & Video
Box 1048
Santa Monica, CA 90406-1048
(800) 421-2304
(213) 828-7577

S

Scott Publishing, Inc.
400 Dayton, Suite B
Edmonds, WA 98020
(206) 775-8777
(800) 888-7853

Simon & Schuster
Simon & Schuster Building
Rockefeller Center
1230 Avenue of the Americas
New York, NY 10020

Slack Incorporated
6900 Grove Road
Thorofare, NJ 08086-9447
(800) 257-8290

Smokenders
1430 East Indian School Road
Suite 102
Phoenix, AZ 85014
(800) 828-HELP

Society for Nutrition Education
2001 Killebrew Drive, Suite 340
Minneapolis, MN 55425-1882
(612) 854-0035

Society for Public Health Education
2001 Addison Street, Suite 220
Berkeley, CA 94704
(510) 644-9242

South Carolina Center for Health Promotion
South Carolina Department of Health and Environmental Control
2600 Bull Street
Columbia, SC 29201
(803) 737-4120

Stanford University
Health Promotion Resource Center
1000 Welch Road
Palo Alto, CA 94304-1885
(415) 723-1000

Superintendent of Documents
P.O. Box 371954
Pittsburgh, PA 15250-7954
(202) 783-3238
(202) 512-2250 (FAX)

T

TopHealth: The Health Promotion and Wellness Letter
74 Clinton Place
P.O. Box 203
Newton, MA 02159
(617) 244-6965

Tufts University Diet and Nutrition Letter
P.O. Box 57857
Boulder, CO 80322-7857
(800) 274-7581

U

United Way of America
701 North Fairfax
Alexandria, VA 22314
(703) 683-7852
Contact your local United Way for information.

University of California at Berkeley Wellness Letter
Subscription Department
P.O. Box 420148
Palm Coast, FL 32142

U.S. Pharmacopeial Convention, Inc.
12601 Twinbrook Parkway
Rockville, MD 20852
(301) 881-0666

V

Visiting Nurse Associations of America
3801 East Florida Avenue
Suite 206
Denver, CO 80210
(800) 426-2547
Contact your local Visiting Nurse Association for information.

Vitality Magazine
1 East Wacker, #2430
Chicago, IL 60601
(312) 828-9897

W

Washington Business Group on Health
777 North Capitol Street, NE.
Suite 800
Washington, DC 20002
(202) 408-9320

Weight Watchers International, Inc.
Jericho Atrium
500 North Broadway
Jericho, NY 11753-2196
(516) 949-0476
Contact your local Weight Watchers for information.

Wellness Councils of America (WELCOA)
1823 Harney Street, Suite 201
Omaha, NE 68102
(402) 444-1711

Williams & Wilkins
428 East Preston Street
Baltimore, MD 21202-3993
(800) 638-6423
(800) 638-4007 in Maryland

Worker Health Program
Institute of Labor and Industrial Relations
The University of Michigan
1111 East Catherine
Ann Arbor, Ml 48109-2054
(313) 763-1187

Workplace Health Fund
815 16th Street, NW., Suite 301
Washington, DC 20006
(202) 842-7832

Y

YMCA of the USA
101 North Wacker Drive
Suite 1400
Chicago, IL 60606
(312) 977-0031
Contact your local YMCA for information.

Index

Index

663

calories, continued 456, 458, 459, 464, 522-527, 529-531, 534, 535, 548, 550, 552, 554, 561, 565-574, 583-585, 591, 592, 599
Cancer Information Service 647
canola oil 71, 460
capillaries 5, 305, 307
Capoten 443, 500
Capozide 500
captopril 407, 441-443, 478
carbohydrates 70, 72, 73, 95, 248, 252, 258, 263, 458, 459, 470, 522, 523, 528, 534
carbon dioxide 5, 6, 8
cardiac arrest 40, 52, 54, 333, 334, 337, 340, 350
cardiac catheterization 24, 38, 116, 117, 119-121, 218, 219, 424
Cardiac Pacemakers Inc. 352
cardiac rehabilitation 411, 431
cardiac tamponade 330
cardiologists 25, 217, 219, 223, 224, 230, 319, 330, 348, 403
cardiomyopathy 23-27, 402
cardiomyoplasty 49, 54
cardiopulmonary resuscitation (CPR) 10, 415
Cardiovascular and Renal Drugs Advisory Committee 279
cardiovascular deaths *see* mortality
cardiovascular reactivity 180
cardioversion 39, 338, 350
cardioverter defibrillator 333, 350, 352
carotid arteries 596
carotid atherosclerosis 491
carteolol 440
Carter Center of Emory University 648
cataracts 299
catecholamine 495
catheters 12, 18, 20, 21, 24, 38, 104, 117-119, 218, 219, 278, 317-322, 328, 330, 347-349, 351, 353, 412, 413, 424, 427, 503
causes of death *see* mortality
cell membranes 243
Center for Biologics Evaluation and Research 306
Center for Chronic Disease Prevention and Health Promotion 578, 654
Center for Corporate Health 648

Center for Devices and Radiological Health 104, 314, 328, 335, 348
Center for Exercise Science 616
Center for Science in the Public Interest 648
Centers for Disease Control and Prevention (CDC) 176, 202, 205, 331, 578, 617, 654, 656
cereals 72, 74, 77, 92, 200, 201, 226, 252, 258, 259, 261, 455, 459, 528, 534
cerebral hemorrhage 300, 497, 499
cerebral hypoperfusion 478
cerebrovascular disease 159, 161, 163, 166, 489, 490
cheese 71, 72, 75, 77-79, 87, 95, 201, 255, 256, 258-264, 266, 268, 318, 454, 524, 531-533, 535, 560, 572
chelation therapy 301, 302
chest X-ray 23, 48, 404
childbirth 69, 178, 549
children *see* age groups, children
Children's Liver Foundation 386
Children's Organ Transplant Association 386
Children's Transplant Association 387
chlorthalidone 488
cholesterol 15-17, 19, 20, 45, 46, 53, 63-79, 82, 89, 94, 95, 125, 126, 132, 133, 138-140, 142, 144, 145, 160, 161, 163, 166-168, 170, 176, 179, 190, 192, 195, 198, 199, 201, 211, 212, 241-260, 262-264, 266, 268-270, 285, 286, 288, 321, 328, 421, 451-454, 456-461, 470, 493, 509, 510, 512, 516-518, 520-536, 538, 539, 542, 543, 546-549, 551, 553, 558-560, 565-575, 582, 586, 587, 620, 622, 624, 625, 627, 629, 648, 652
cholesterol measurement 67
cholesterol profile 247, 547
cholesterol testing 547
cholesterol-lowering drugs 20
cholestyramine 20, 456, 458
cholorthalidone 546
Choose to Lose 648
chronic hypertension 485, 486, 497-499
chronic obstructive pulmonary disease 116, 493
chronic renal failure 491
Ciba-Geigy 500
cigarette smoking *see* smoking

circadian rhythm 505
circulation 10-12, 44, 47, 49, 56, 59, 66, 100, 102, 103, 217, 223, 284, 297, 299, 302, 307, 310, 323, 329, 336, 344, 349, 439, 476, 477, 494
circulatory conditions 208
circulatory support system 349
circulatory system 208, 244, 309
Citizens for Public Action on Blood Pressure and Cholesterol, Inc. 648
Cleveland Clinic Foundation 311, 317, 322
click murmur syndrome 59
clonidine 487, 494, 496, 499
coarctation of the aorta 218, 219
cocaine 100, 475, 483, 495
coconut oil 71, 78, 259, 534, 536
cold medicines 33
colestipol 20, 456, 458
collagen 27, 319, 321
collagen-vascular diseases 27
colorectal cancer 299
Combined Health Information Database 629
commissures 342
community resources 622
Compassionate Friends, Inc. 387
complex carbohydrates 70, 72, 73, 258, 459, 522, 528, 534
compliance 174, 184, 349, 373
congenital defects 100
congenital heart defects 116, 215, 393
congestive heart failure 25, 44, 54-57, 209, 219, 292, 293, 313, 471, 489, 490, 549
Consolidated Omnibus Budget Reconciliation Act 376
Consumer Information Center 575, 648
Consumer Nutrition Hotline 457
Consumer Reports on Health 648
contraceptives 85, 102, 122, 544, 550, 551
Cook Inc. 351
cooking classes 195, 624
Cooking Light 649
cooking tips 535, 536
Cornell University 610, 649
coronary angiography 18
coronary arteries 8, 9, 15, 16, 18, 20, 21, 29, 30, 238, 297, 306, 317, 320, 323,

coronary arteries, continued 327, 329, 330, 347, 348, 402, 412, 413, 419, 421, 423, 424, 426, 585
coronary artery bypass graft surgery 20, 31, 57, 204, 324, 327, 330, 413, 428
coronary care unit 11-13
Coronary Club, Inc. 416
coronary heart disease 15, 45, 52, 63, 64, 66, 68, 69, 140, 141, 147, 149, 155, 169, 242, 279, 288, 452, 466, 509, 518, 519, 521, 541-543, 546-550, 553, 558, 562, 564, 575, 581
Corporate Health and Fitness Program 626
corticosteroids 494
costs 7, 139-141, 143, 147, 155, 185, 207, 238, 315, 359, 365, 371, 376, 377, 379, 380, 388, 413, 464, 473, 505, 553, 579, 631
coughing 47, 50, 57, 324, 325, 439
Creative Walking, Inc. 649
cryopreservation 343
Current Population Survey 125, 126, 129, 159, 161, 163, 166
cyanosis 115, 218-222
cyclosporine 367, 379, 395, 475, 496
cystic fibrosis 394

D

Dacron 309, 343
dairy products 71, 72, 74, 75, 95, 252, 253, 255, 460, 528, 531, 546, 561
death rates *see* mortality
deep breathing exercises 324, 325
deep vein thrombosis 99, 105, 106
defibrillation 11, 335, 337, 338, 350
defibrillator 11, 39, 333-335, 337-340, 350-352
dehydration 443
Denice Ferko-Adams & Associates 649
dental care 440, 445, 577
dentist 440, 445, 446
Department of Agriculture 70, 552, 576, 652
depression *see* emotions, depression
desirable weight 72, 74, 86, 252, 511, 523, 528, 549, 583, 585, 587, 589
dextran 106

J

J-curve hypothesis 477
Janssen Pharmaceutica, Inc. 40
Jarvik-7 311
Jefferson Medical College 309
Johnson & Johnson Interventional Systems Co. 104
Journal of the American Medical Association 288, 397
jumping rope 89, 558, 582, 584, 593, 594, 597, 598, 600

K

Kabikinase 277
KabiVitrum AB 278
Kawasaki syndrome 237-240
ketoconazole 40
kidney dialysis 379
kidney disease 81, 85, 300, 363, 383, 384, 544, 545, 549
kidney failure 383, 500
kidney transplants 355, 356, 366, 377, 379, 382
kidneys 50, 72, 73, 75, 77, 81, 83, 85, 99, 180, 181, 187, 254, 258, 300, 307, 329, 355, 356, 361, 363-366, 375, 377, 379, 380, 382-385, 388, 389, 391, 395, 407, 429, 443, 454, 491, 495, 500, 530, 534, 544, 545, 549, 609, 612, 627, 654
Korotkoff 486, 498, 504
Korotkoff sounds 504

L

labetalol 439, 440, 487, 489, 493, 496, 499
Lanoxin 408, 416
laser angioplasty 21
Laser Angiosurgery System 317
laser microsurgery 317
Lasix 407
LDL *see* low density lipoproteins (LDLs)
LeBonheur Children's Medical Center 609
left atrium 5, 26, 60, 61, 223
left ventricle 5, 8, 26, 59, 113, 220, 221, 311, 312, 354, 405

left ventricular assist devices 49
left-ventricular systolic dysfunction 401
leg cramps 407
leg ulcers 99, 103
leg veins 106, 323
licorice-containing substances 475
life expectancy 159, 163, 173
lifestyle modifications 19, 20, 48, 49, 57, 302, 411, 465-467, 470, 471, 476, 479, 481, 482, 484, 485, 489, 492, 493, 553, 581
lipid specialist 457
lipids 319, 460, 461, 493, 587
lipoproteins 67, 178, 243, 285, 287, 288, 460, 547
lisinopril 407, 443
lithotripsy 495
liver 40, 55, 65, 67, 72, 73, 75, 94, 186, 187, 197, 243, 254, 285, 287, 300, 355, 356, 361, 365-367, 369-372, 374, 377-379, 384, 386, 395, 429, 454, 459, 460, 486, 499, 530, 548
liver disease 40, 73, 384, 386
living wills 415
loop diuretics 491, 493
losing weight 19, 48, 68, 69, 86, 87, 89, 96, 244, 302, 560
lovastatin 20, 456, 461
low density lipoproteins (LDLs) 67-69, 133, 190, 192, 243, 247, 248, 285-287, 452, 455, 456, 459-461, 517, 518, 547, 548
low-dose birth control pills 551
low-dose estrogen 285, 287, 288
Lowfat Lifeline 653
lung cancer 543, 544, 554
lymph nodes 237

M

Macmillan Publishing Company 653
magnesium 94, 95, 469, 470, 499
magnesium sulfate 499
magnetic resonance imaging 101, 339
mail-order prescription services 408
malignant hypertension 185, 478, 485
managing heart failure 404, 405, 414
Manoplax 292, 293
mapping the heart 12

Treatment of Mild Hypertension Study 184
Trials of Antihypertensive Intervention and Management 510
Trials of Hypertension Prevention 510, 515
tricuspid valve 6, 221, 222, 341
triglyceride levels 69, 144, 247, 286, 395, 455, 461, 548
triglycerides 67, 69, 144, 192, 199, 247, 285, 286, 395, 455, 460, 461, 493, 518, 548
tropical oils 257, 258
truncus arteriosus 222
Tufts University Diet and Nutrition Letter 658
Tylenol® 426
type A behavior 550

U

U.S. Department of Agriculture 70, 552, 652
U.S. Dietary Guidelines for Americans 552
U.S. Pharmacopeial Convention, Inc. 659
U.S. Preventive Services Task Force 299
U.S. Public Health Service 143, 418, 630, 650
United Auto Workers of America 144
United Network for Organ Sharing 361, 362, 373, 390, 394
United Scleroderma Foundation, Inc. 111
United Way 622, 626, 659
University of Arizona 311
University of California 199, 308, 659
University of California at Berkeley Wellness Letter 659
University of Cincinnati 306
University of Florida 615
University of Tennessee 609
University of Utah 311
unsaturated fats 70-72, 257, 259, 469, 527, 528, 533, 535
unstable angina 298, 419-426, 431-433, 478
Upjohn Co. 279
urinary kallikrein 181
urination 407-409

urine 56, 301, 408, 443, 610
USCI Gruntzig catheter 348
USCI Probe I 348
USDA Cooperative Extension Service 628
uterine cancer 562, 564

V

valvar pulmonary stenosis 218
valve incompetence 342
valve stenosis 342
varicose veins 102
vasculitis 238
Vaseretic 500
vasodilators 25, 57, 109, 119, 293, 472, 477, 490, 494
vasospasm 107, 499
Vasotec 443, 500
vegetable oils 71, 76, 77, 257-259, 454, 460, 533, 535
vegetarianism 252
vein inflammation 105
veins 5, 6, 55, 102, 103, 105, 106, 218, 222, 223, 301, 305, 323, 334, 413
venous lesions 103
venous switch 221
ventricles 3, 5-8, 23, 26, 27, 34-36, 38, 59, 113, 115, 118, 120, 187, 216, 218, 220-223, 230, 311, 312, 333-336, 340, 354, 405
ventricular arrhythmias 35, 39, 291, 292
ventricular assist device 54, 311
ventricular ectopy 469
ventricular fibrillation 11, 36, 333
ventricular septal defect 216, 217, 220-222
ventricular tachycardia 36, 230, 231
venules 5, 6, 305
verapamil 281, 496
vibratory murmur 233
Visiting Nurse Associations of America 627, 659
Vitality Magazine 659
vitamin B1 461
vitamin D 181, 243, 459
vitamins 87, 248, 258, 262, 522, 530, 531, 534
vocational rehabilitation 326

682

W

Y

Z